PSYCHOPHARMACOLOGY OF SEXUAL DISORDERS

This volume is based upon a conference
held in Jerusalem, Israel
Papers originally presented at that meeting
have been updated and others added in
order to provide a broad view of
the subject

PSYCHOPHARMACOLOGY OF SEXUAL DISORDERS

Editor
MARK SEGAL

Biological Psychiatry — New Prospects: 4

John Libbey
LONDON · PARIS

First published 1985 by

John Libbey & Company Limited
80-84 Bondway, London SW8 1SF

British library cataloguing in publication data
Psychopharmacology of sexual disorders
(Biological psychiatry - new prospects;
1. Sexual disorders — Chemotherapy
2. Psychopharmacology
I. Segal, M. II. Series
616.6'9061 RC 556

ISBN 0-86196-022-X

Printed and bound in Great Britain by Whitstable Litho Ltd., Whitstable, Kent.

Contributors

S. AHLENIUS (Sodertalje, Sweden)
T. A. BAN (Tennessee, USA)
B. N. BARWIN ((Ottawa, Ontario, Canada)
O. BENKERT (Mainz, Federal Republic of Germany)
N. J. BOWDEN (Amsterdam, The Netherlands)
F. H. DE JONGE (Amsterdam, The Netherlands)
E. DEL BENE (Firenze, Italy)
S. DICKSTEIN (Jerusalem, Israel)
M. FANCIULLACCI (Firenze, Italy)
W. GUY (Tennessee, USA)
F. HOLSBOER (Mainz, Federal Republic of Germany)
A. J. HUNTER (London, England)
V. A. KRAL (London, Ontario, Canada)
K. LARRSON (Gothenburg, Sweden)
H. E. LEHMANN (Montreal, Canada)
M. R. MURPHY (Texas, USA)
W. M. PETRIE (Tennessee, USA)
M. POGGIONI (Firenze, Italy)
L. PRINCIPE (Firenze, Italy)
J. M. H. REES (Manchester, England)
D. C. RENSHAW (Maywood, Illinois, USA)
H. SCHNIEDEN (Manchester, England)
M. SEGAL (Jerusalem, Israel)
F. SICUTERI (Firenze, Italy)
H. H. SWANSON (Amsterdam, The Netherlands)
N. E. VAN DE POLL (Amsterdam, The Netherlands)
H. G. VAN OYEN (Amsterdam, The Netherlands)
C. A. WILSON (London, England)
W. H. WILSON (Tennessee, USA)

Preface

Sexual desire dawned with the birth of man. It is most probable that sexual disorders were not far behind. However, although sexual desire dawned at this early stage and nurtured for a millenia, it is only recently that modern medicine has begun to recognize abnormalities in sexual desires, drug-physiological- and psychologically-induced sexual disorders and begun to devise methods with which to test them. Only as we become more aware of the mechanisms underlying the normal physiology, pharmocology and biochemistry of the desires themselves will we be in a position to understand the course of their disorders and be able to design optimal therapies.

Despite the vastly expanding literature on this subject, I sincerely feel that this volume makes a significant contribution towards an understanding of mechanisms and current therapies. I, therefore extend my deepest gratitude to all the contributers whose efforts have made this volume possible.

Mark Segal
Editor

To my wife Joyce whose keen
understanding of my drives
nurtured this volume to its
completion

Mark Segal

Contents

Contributors v
Preface vii
Introduction: H. E. Lehmann 1

I: BASIC SCIENCE

1. A role for phenylethylamine in adult male rat mounting behaviour: Mark Segal and Shabtay Dikstein 5
2. Masculine sexual behavior and brain monoamines: Knut Larrson and Sven Ahlenius 15
3. Mechanisms of action of p-chlorophenylalanine (PCPA) and its effects on female sexual behavior in the rat: A.J. Hunter and C.A. Wilson 33
4. Endogenous opiates and the mechanism of male sexual behavior: Michael R. Murphy 51
5. Gonadal hormonal influences upon aggressive behaviors in male and female rats: N.E. van de Poll, N.J. Bowden, H.G. van Oyen, F.H. de Jonge and H.H. Swanson 63

II: CLINICAL SCIENCE

6. The sexual side-effects of drugs: Domeena C. Renshaw 79
7. Pharmacological aspects of sexual dysfunction caused by drugs of abuse: H. Schnieden and J.M.H. Rees 99
8. Neuroleptics and sexual behavior of male schizophrenics: Thomas A. Ban, William Guy and William H. Wilson 115
9 The sexual effects of antipsychotic, antidepressant and psychomotor stimu lant drugs: William M. Petrie 121
10. Sexual dysfunction in male patients — biological indices and classification: O. Benkert and F. Holsboer 133
11. Apomorphine and other dopamine modifiers on human sexual and nocicep tive tonus: E. Del Bene, M. Faniullaci, M. Poggioni, L. Principe and F. Sicuteri 145
12 Psychopharmacology of sexual disorders of old age: V.A. Kral 155
13. Prolactin and sexuality: B. Norman Barwin 161

Author Index 167
Subject Index 169

Introduction

H. E. LEHMANN

Division of Psychopharmacology, McGill University, 1033 Pine Avenue West, Montreal, Quebec H3A 1A1, CANADA

The four most powerful physiological forces that periodically influence the behavior of all mammals are thirst, sleep, hunger and sexual drive, in this order of biological urgency. There is good evidence that all are regulated by subcortical brain mechanisms which are controlled and mediated by neurotransmitters, polypeptides and hormones. In addition, all have compelling cortical representations in the form of a subjective need-awareness. Three of these forces are excitatory appetitive drives while the fourth, sleep, is a state of global inhibition. While thirst, hunger and sleep are essential functions for individual survival in all mammals, sexual activity is a necessary condition for the survival of the species.

Other features that uniquely characterize sexual drive and function are the need for a partner and the absence of a direct and immediate biological goal — as, for instance, water is to thirst, food is to hunger and the state of sleep is to fatigue — since the biological result of sexual activity, ie the offspring, is far removed in time from its cause, although the relief from sexual tension is immediate. The fact that normal satisfaction of the sexual drive requires the need for a partner, leads, in many species, to intersubjective relationships and the formation of social groups that last long beyond the immediate relief of sexual tension and even the successful rearing of offspring. The need to secure sexual partners frequently involves competition and thus aggression, and so does the maintenance of the partnership role in the social group, on a scale from dominance to submission. It is, therefore, not surprising that the same hormones and transmitters that play significant roles in the regulation of sexual activity, eg testosterone and catecholamines, also determine agonistic behavior, ie competitive aggression and dominance.

During his evolutional ascendence, *Homo sapiens* has acquired the capacity to supplement, enhance, inhibit or completely override his physiological controls of sexual drive and function. He has achieved this through cultural and cognitive measures (such as moral principles, religious roles, cultural values, customs, traditions and taboos) as well as by means of scientific artifacts (such as inhibitory and excitatory drugs).

For humans today, sexuality has become not only one of the most powerful, but also one of the most complex forces that motivates our social existence. Because our biological, reproductive maturity does not, as a rule, coincide with maturity of the psychological aspects of our sexuality, this maturity-gap of sexual libido often has destructive effects on the development of personality and frequently causes dangerous problems and the development of tensions in the social adaptation of whole generations.

Many centuries ago, Helen's beauty and erotic appeal, 'the face that launched a thousand ships', started the Trojan war, and throughout history Eros, or sexual love, has probably been responsible for as many battles, duels, human sacrifices and murderous crimes as have the strivings for power and wealth. Sexual images and symbols are dominant motivational forces in the commercial markets of industrialized countries, and sexual permissiveness and freedom, or sexual restriction and suppression, have significantly shaped whole cultures. It was the libido's awesome potential for good and evil that revealed to Freud the secrets of the unconscious and became the cornerstone of the first theoretical structure that sought to probe the innermost depths of human existence.

This book takes a deliberate, measured step towards the clarification, if not as yet the full understanding, of one fundamental aspect of sexuality: the biological roots of its representation in the central nervous system. In doing this, the book perhaps comes closer than most other reported research in this field to the possibilities of opening pragmatic doors, or at least methodological avenues, for the pharmacological control of sexual awareness and functioning in man, as far as these phenomena are mediated by the brain.

Larssen & Ahlenius describe the interdependence of gonadal hormones and the biosynthesis and transport of essential brain amines in the regulation of male sexual behavior. The rostral part of the cerebral cortex, the medial preoptic-anterior part of the hypothalamus and the amygdaloid nuclei are important structures involved in sexual arousal, and all receive projections from dopamine and noradrenaline pathways with terminals in the nucleus accumbens and the tuberculum olfactorium.

Hunter & Wilson, in discussing the action of p-chlorophenylalanine (PCPA) on female sexual behavior in the rat, come to the surprising conclusion that, contrary to the traditional view, serotonin does not play an inhibitory role in the control of female sexual behavior, but has, in fact, a stimulatory effect on female sexual behavior and that the stimulatory action of the serotonin synthesis inhibitor PCPA may be explained by its effects on progesterone production or by its stimulation of serotonin release.

The role of endorphins in human sexual behavior is discussed by Murphy, who, on the basis of his experiments, proposes that endogenous opiates may influence the regulation of testosterone levels and thus modulate the activity of certain neurotransmitters that mediate sexual motivation in the brain. He suggests that opiate antagonists may prove useful in the treatment of sexual dysfunction.

Abnormal reactivity of migraine sufferers who respond with attack symptoms and sexual excitement to small doses of dopaminergic substances, such as apomorphine and bromocriptine, has been observed by Del Bene and his colleagues and is explained by them on the basis of the many similarities existing between the biochemical and pharmacological characteristics of the nociceptive and sexual apparatus as they relate to dopamine and endorphins.

Writing mainly as a clinician, Barwin reports the good news that sexual dysfunction from hyperprolactinemia, if correctly diagnosed, is one form of sexual disorder that can today be treated simply and successfully with the dopaminergic compound bromocriptine which normalizes prolactin levels and thus eliminates dysfunctional symptoms, such as loss of libido and problems of erectile response.

The complex interdependence of aggressive behavior, sex, testosterone level and assimilated experience is analyzed by van de Poll and his coworkers. Their experiments seem to show that male rats are both the more fearful and the more aggressive sex. If male rats have been defeated in a fight, they become more submissive than females who are less interested in their status. However, if aversive experiences are minimized, testosterone stimulates attack behavior equally in male and female rats. In a study on humans, other investigators have shown that aggressive responsiveness of professional hockey players to threatening behavior correlated significantly with their testosterone plasma levels.

Segal & Dickstein propose the interesting hypothesis that phenylethylamine (PEA), or PEA receptor, may be a common unifying mechanism between the clinical antidepressant effectiveness of different compounds in humans and their experimentally observed enhancing action on sexual mounting behavior in the male rat. The authors' bold approach tries to link the confusing variety of action mechanisms that have been postulated for different antidepressants with those of the many different substances that, dependent upon dosage, either inhibit or enhance sexual behavior in rat models.

The relative experimental and methodological security of animal models is lost when one enters the clinical field and deals with human subjects. Although, in animal experiments, too, many complexities may arise and not all variables can always be controlled; but rats, at least, do not seem to be plagued by distressing guilt feelings, nor are they likely to repress sexual stirrings or disguise them in symbolic form. Human beings, however, are subject to such contingencies and the clinicians who study human subjects have to rely on observations rather than on experiments.

In his chapter on the effects of psychopharmacological treatment of sexual disorders of the elderly, Kral points to the role of minor tranquilizers and antidepressants as useful adjuvants to psychotherapy which is indicated as the principal management of many of the sexual problems in the elderly. Neuroleptic drugs, antidepressants and lithium are, as in younger patients, prescribed for sexual dysfunction associated with psychotic or affective disorders. Pharmacotherapy for the processes involved in dementia, however, is unspecific and can only be symptomatic given our present state of knowledge.

With the introduction of the third edition of the Diagnostic Statistical Manual (DSM III) of the American Psychiatric Association, a need for reconsidering the diagnosis of sexual dysfunction has arisen. Benkert & Holsboer propose a new classification that adds six different new axes to the existing diagnostic system of sexual disorders. These authors point out that it is now generally accepted that 30 per cent of cases with sexual dysfunction are not psychogenic in origin, instead of the 10 per cent as was thought not very long ago; in addition, they review the role of various hormones in the treatment of sexual disorders.

In four different chapters, Petrie, Ban & coworkers, Renshaw and Schnieden & Rees review the effects of prescribed drugs and substances of abuse on sexual function. Antipsychotic drugs, probably through some inhibitory action on the pituitary-gonadal axis as well as through blocking dopaminergic neurons, and antidepressants, through antiparasympathetic and antisympathetic effects, reduce sexual libido and often interfere with erection and ejaculation in the male and with orgasmic potency in both sexes. Stimulants of the amphetamine type and cocaine, by releasing dopamine centrally, may increase sexual activity but frequently also cause delayed ejaculation and orgasm. Alcohol, sedatives, and minor tranquilizers may sometimes improve sexual performance by removing excessive inhibitions. The reports on the sexual effects of marijuana, LSD, amyl nitrite and other abuse substances are anecdotal and inconclusive. Opiates, however, are clearly responsible for decreased sexual libido, activity and performance in all those addicted to them.

Finally, most antihypertensive drugs tend to interfere with normal sexual function and this may frequently be the reason for the non-compliance with treatment that is so commonly observed among hypertensives.

In summary, many drugs are known to impair sexual functioning in man but very few, if any, are known to improve it. There is, thus, a clear challenge to further research for which this volume provides a sound and stimulating basis.

1

A role for phenylethylamine in adult male rat mounting behaviour

Mark SEGAL[1] and Shabtay DIKSTEIN*

*Psychopharmacology Research Laboratory, Hadassah University Hospital, Jerusalem; and *Unit of Cell Pharmacology, School of Pharmacy, The Hebrew University of Jerusalem, Jerusalem, ISRAEL*

Introduction

Antidepressants: clinical effectiveness and potential mechanisms

Antidepressant drugs consist of a variety of groups of chemically different entities claimed to reverse the clinical state of depression in humans, their onset of action varying from several days onwards (Laakmann, 1982). Not all antidepressants are equivalently effective in all patients. The reasons for this are numerous — for example, misdiagnosis (Maj, 1981), hormonal imbalances (Langer *et al.*, 1982), neurotransmitter imbalances (Mass, 1979; Waldmeier, 1981) etc.

Pharmacologically, the different classes of antidepressants have been claimed to exert their effect(s) through one or more of a variety of mechanisms. These include: imipramine through its inhibition of the re-uptake of both 5-hydroxytryptamine (5-HT) and norepinephrine (NE) (Maitre *et al.*, 1980); clorgyline through monoamine oxidase-Type A inhibition (MAOI-Type A) (Thornton *et al.*, 1980); deprenyl through its monoamine oxidase-Type B (MAOI-Type B) inhibition (Thornton *et al.*, 1980); mianserin by an action on adrenergic alpha receptors (Hughes, 1978); nomifensine through a dopaminergic agonist-type reaction (Le Fur & Uzan, 1980) through metabolic reactions to potentially active metabolites and/or by a metabolic time-lag to reach an active steady state plasma level (Leakmann, 1982), and so on. However, despite their varied pharmacological mechanisms in animal experimental models, all have proven clinically effective (Laakmann, 1982). This means that whether their clinical effectiveness is due to a direct effect of the drug itself upon one or more specific receptors, through the inhibition of the enzyme monoamine oxidase (Type A and/or B), through the inhibition of the re-uptake or of the release of one or more neurotransmitters, neuromodulators or through some other, as yet unknown, entity, remains to be resolved.

Depression and biological rhythms: towards a possible basic understanding of mechanisms

It has recently been reported that patients suffering from mental depression demonstrate a phase-advancement in one or more of their biological circadian rhythms (Wehr & Goodwin, 1981). This, together with the effectiveness of sleep deprivation therapy (Schilgen & Tolle, 1980) and the effectiveness of alterations in the time

[1]Present address: Sci Con, 611/16 Adam St, Maalot Moriah, Jerusalem, Israel.

sequence of rapid-eye-movement (REM) dream sleep (Wehr & Goodwin, 1978), has led to postulating a theory of altered biological rhythms accounting for certain, 'if not all', clinical states of depression (Goodwin *et al.*, 1982). Even more recently, several clinically effective antidepressants (eg imipiramine, clorgyline) have been reported to phase-delay biological circadian rhythms in normal experimental models (using the rat as a model, Wirz-Justice & Campbell, 1982). These data open further experimental avenues in research on common or related and/or interrelated mechanism(s) which may account for the clinical effectiveness of antidepressant drugs.

Antidepressant drugs and induced sexual disorders

Despite all the recent advances and the remaining controversies relating to how antidepressants exert their clinical effect, one clear fact remains. This is that, after initial reversal of the decreased libido in the depressed patient, in one way or another, through a centrally- or peripherally-mediated antiadrenergic or anticholinergic effect (Barnes *et al.*, 1979; Le Fur & Uzan, 1980; Petrie, 1980), antidepressants interfere with human sexual response on chronic administration. Whether this is by inducing impotency in the male, an altered time sequence of orgasm in the male and/or female or in some other manner, the end result is a reduction in libido (see the chapter by Kral).

Antidepressants: sexually-induced side effects and new avenues for exploration

The observations outlined above suggest a number of areas which could be explored: for example, the mechanisms by which antidepressants adversely affect sexual function could be studied; pharmacological agents could be sought which would specifically reverse the antidepressant-induced reduction in sexual function (ie agents identified which could be administered concurrently with the antidepressant); an antidepressant could be developed which, during chronic administration, would not reduce sexual function or which might even directly enhance it, and its potential mehcnaism(s) of action studied. Our own decision was to pursue the last option.

Recent advances into mechanisms accounting for sexually-enhanced and/or induced behaviour(s)

In our laboratory, we initiated a study of the mechanism(s) by which pharmacological agents inhibit, enhance and/or induce sexual behaviour(s) (Segal *et al.*, 1977, 1978; Segal & Dikstein, 1981*a*, 1981*b*) and we also undertook a search for a compound which would induce sexual behaviour(s) on chronic administration (Segal & Dikstein, 1981*b*).

Antidepressants and sexual behaviour

A recent finding was that there are three antidepressants, amitriptyline, nomifensine and mianserin, with different basic pharmacological mechanisms of action in animal models (Laakmann, 1982) which both inhibit (at a dose of 10 mg/kg sc) and slightly enhance (at a dose of 0.003 mg/kg sc) mounting (sexual) behaviour in the naive male rat (strain of the Hebrew University; Segal & Schnieden, unpublished observations).

This led us to ask the question of whether an antidepressant's initial reversal of decreased libido in depressed patients resulted from its antidepressant effect or whether, conversely, there was direct stimulation by an as yet unknown central mechanism or some combination of these. We also asked whether proglonged antidepressant administration interferes with sexual function through peripheral antiadrenergic or anticholinergic side-effects or through some, again as yet unknown, direct central mechanism.

Sexual activity and para-chlorophenylalanine (PCPA)

Numerous reports have appeared claiming that the tyrosine hydroxylase inhibitor PCPA enhances and/or induces sexual behaviour(s) in experimental animals (Sheard, 1969; Shilito, 1969; Tagliamonte *et al.*, 1969; Wilson *et al.*, 1982) which do not demonstrate such behaviour(s) when untreated (Sheard, 1969; Shilito, 1969; Tagliamonte *et al.*, 1969). One report also claims that PCPA is effective in man (Benkert, 1973), but this result could not be replicated (Benkert, 1977). PCPA is also a toxic material (Gay *et al.*, 1975) whose effectiveness in either male or female experimental animals is dependent on their basic level of sexual activity: sexually sluggish animals are affected, while more sexually vigorous animals remain unaffected (Hyyppa *et al.*, 1971; Da Prada *et al.*, 1972; Benkert *et al.*, 1973; Dewesbury, 1975). The scientific literature is also already saturated with controversial data relating to PCPA's potential mechanism(s) of action which have been well-reviewed by many investigators (eg Gessa & Tagliamonte, 1975; Karczmar, 1975; Shilito, 1975; Vogt, 1975; Wilson *et al.*, 1982, etc).

PCPA: potential mechanism(s) of action — present evidence

In this volume alone, excellent data are presented, and claims made, that PCPA's mechanism of action in the male rat is due to a lack of 5-HT at central receptor sites (see the chapter by Larsson & Ahlenius), to an abundance of 5-HT at specific central receptor sites in the female rat (see the material presented by Wilson & Hunter), or that endogenous peptides are also involved in the complex mechanism of action underlying alterations in sexual behaviour (see Murphy's chapter).

Recent evidence relating to sexual behaviour(s) in male rats

Preliminary evidence from our own laboratory allows us to postulate that some mechanism(s) other than those implicated in the 5-HT-dopamine balance hypothesis (Gessa & Tagliamonte, 1975) account(s) for PCPA's influence on sexual behaviour(s) (Segal *et al.*, 1977; Segal & Dikstein, 1981*b*). This arises from an extensive structure-activity relationship investigation of a series of phenylethylamine (PEA) derivatives on both male and female rat sexual behaviours. In this study, one derivative in particular, ortho-methoxyphenylethylamine (OMPEA), was observed as the most potent in the series (Segal & Dikstein, 1981*b*). This was of great interest because Hwang & van Woert (1980) have reported that in a series of PEA derivatives studied for their effectiveness on serotonergic mechanisms (uptake, re-uptake, block, release, binding, etc) OMPEA was, for all practical purposes, ineffective.

This, therefore, directed us to explore other avenues for potential mechanisms because, as with the story relating to antidepressants (ie antidepressants with a variety of mechanisms of action all being clinically effective), we had already observed that, dependent on the dose administered, several different classes of pharmacological agents effectively inhibited, enhanced and/or induced sexual behaviour(s) in rats. These agents include, for example, the alpha-adrenergic agonist clonidine; a series of beta-adrenergic blocking agents of the mixed $beta_1$-$beta_2$ variety (d,l-propranolol and l-propranolol: d-propranolol being ineffective), of the pure $beta_1$ variety (metoprolol) and of the pure $beta_2$ variety (butoxamine); the 5-HT antagonist cyprohepotidine; microgram quantities of 5-hydroxytryptophan (which in higher doses has been reported to reverse the sexual activity induced by lowering central levels of 5-HT (Biggio *et al.*, 1974); the three different antidepressants, amitriptyline, nomifensine and mianserin (Segal & Schnieden, unpublished observations) as outlined earlier; rats on a 48-hour starvation schedule; corn-fed rats and, so forth (Segal & Dikstein, 1981*b*). This means that, as with antidepressants, some common underlying basic mechanism or mechanisms must account for the fact that such a variety of pharmacological agents can behave so similarly in terms of affecting sexual behaviour.

Methodology

Details of the development of our basic methodology for the assessment of sexual behaviour(s) and their potential mechanism(s) are given in the Appendix to this chapter.

New evidence relating directly to a role for phenylethylamine (PEA) in male rat mounting behaviour and discussion

Within the last few years, Knoll and his group in Hungary have reported that the MAOI-Type B deprenyl increased sexual activity in sluggish male rats to a degree 10 times greater than the MAOI-Type A clorgyline (Knoll, 1981). Since deprenyl has also been reported to possess antidepressant activity (Vargas & Tinger, 1967) and its major substrate is PEA (Knoll, 1976), this led us to consider that PEA, or a PEA-type receptor (Hauger *et al.*, 1982), might be a possible linking mechanism accounting for the effectiveness of a compound as an antidepressant and its effectiveness as an enhancer of mounting behaviour in the male rat.

In an earlier report, Segal and Dikstein (1981*b*) suggested that chronic administration of d-phenylalanine (in doses of 0.001 to 10 mg/kg po), a direct precursor of PEA (Heller *et al.*, 1976), induced male rat mounting. On the other hand, d-tyrosine, an amino acid with reported pharmacological activity on the cardiovascular system (Shalita & Dikstein, 1979), was totally ineffective in inducing male rat mounting behaviour when administered for a prolonged period over the same dose range as that used with d-phenylalanine (Segal & Dikstein, 1981*b*). Even more recently (Segal & Dikstein, unpublished observations), we have observed that the chronic administration of l-phenylalanine, also pharmacologically active in several behavioural models (Barrett *et al.*, 1976; Blum *et al.*, 1978; Gibson *et al.*, 1982) and a precursor in the synthesis of catecholamines (Blashko, 1939), was also totally ineffective in inducing male rat mounting behaviour.

In another series of experiments, PEA itself was chronically administered in a dose range of 0.01 to 1.0 mg/kg po and found to be effective at inducing male rat mounting behaviour (Segal *et al.*, 1984 and Segal & Dikstein, unpublished observations). Although it could possibly be assumed that this was due to some peripheral mechanism of action of PEA, we have also observed, in collaboration with D.M. Jacobowitz of the NIMH, and using the brain microdissection technique of Palkovitz (1973), that doses of PEA which induced male rat mounting behaviour also significantly increased the levels of NE in the nucleus pre-opticus medialis (POM, determinations were carried out by high performance liquid chromatography; Shohami *et al.*, 1983). This effect appeared to be specific to the POM since neither NE nor dopamine levels were found to be altered in the nucleus interstitialis stria terminalis, the anterior hypothalamic nucleus, the median eminence, the arcuate nucleus, the habenula and the amygdaloid nucleus (Segal, Shohami & Jacobowitz, 1984, in press).

Several studies have implicated the POM in sexual activity in both animals (Bermond, 1982) and humans (Lisk, 1967). It has also been shown that NE levels in the POM are significantly decreased in sexually sluggish male rats (Moyer *et al.*, 1974). In addition, it is known that the antideprerssant imipramine can raise the central levels of PEA (Sabelli *et al.*, 1978; Reynolds, 1979).

Hypothesis relating a role for PEA in male rat mounting behaviour

Although considerable research is still warranted, and notwithstanding the complex pharmacological and behavioural activities of the materials used in our experimental studies, in addition to the existing postulated theories involving 5-HT, dopamine and endogenous peptides, we would like to propose that phenylethylamine (PEA) may serve as a possible common mechanism linking the similar sexual effectiveness of so many different types of pharmacological agents or, at least, play a role of some importance in their basic mechanism(s).

Even though it has been shown that prolonged administration of PEA to intact female rats does not interfere with their normal oestrus (Hartzshtark & Dikstein, personal communication), it is still possible that PEA's mechanism of action in both female and male rats may be through modulating or regulating mechanisms at the level of a central oestrogen or other hormonal receptor (Nock & Feder, 1981).

Directions for future research

Further research should be directed towards elucidating the role played by phenylethylamine in the induction of male rat mounting behaviour, as well as in other sexual behaviour(s) and functions, and to determine its interrelationships with other central amines, hormones and peptides.

APPENDIX

Development of basic methodology for assessing sexual behaviour(s) and their potential mechanism(s)

In excellent reviews, Dewesbury (1975) and Whalen *et al.* (1975) have already outlined the complexity of studying sexual function and behaviour(s) and have discussed the various methods available. It is not, therefore, necessary to proceed in that direction.

Carefully evaluating the total picture in terms of methodological complexity, time involved and cost accounting, we decided to study whether various pharmacological compounds could inhibit and/or enhance male rat mounting behaviour. The second step was to follow active compounds and determine whether they inhibited or enhanced female lordotic behaviour. The third and final step was to determine whether the most active compound in any series could actually induce mounting behaviour (male rats) and/or lordotic behaviour (female rats) when administered either acutely or chronically in a dose related manner. In summary, this was carried out as described below.

Inhibition of male rat mounting behaviour (Segal et al., 1977)

A standard dose of PCPA (defined as an effective dose, totalling 500 mg/kg ip; 300 mg/kg ip on the first day of the experimental period, followed 24 h later by a dose of 200 mg/kg ip) is administered to groups of 4 male rats (weighing 180–220 g), housed in individual cages until the time of testing: twenty-four hours after the last dose of PCPA (ie on the third day of the experiment). With several years experience, with no pre-selection of animals according to their base-line sexual activity and with an 'n' in the hundreds, we found that this dose of PCPA induces 20.4 ± 3.9 mounts (Segal, Schnieden & Dikstein, unpublished observation) over a 15-min period per group of 4 rats placed together in a single open-topped plastic chamber measuring 44 × 57 × 23 cm; the bottom of the chamber was covered with wood shavings.

Any pharmacological agent which, when administered simultaneously along with PCPA (using the 2-day administration schedule as outlined above), significantly reduced the control values of 20.4 ± 3.9 mounts during a 15-min observation period was considered to be an inhibitor of male rat mounting behaviour. In this model, all animals were maintained on a regular 12 h-12 h light-dark cycle.

Enhancement of male rat mounting behaviour (Segal et al., 1977)

In this case, a standard dose of PCPA (defined as a subliminal dose, totalling 150 mg/kg ip 75 mg/kg ip on the first day of the experiment, followed 24 h later by a dose of 75 mg/kg ip) is administered to groups of 4 male rats in the same manner as outlined in the previous section. The animals were tested (over a 15-min observation period in groups of 4, also as outlined above) on the third day, 24 h following the last administration of PCPA. Again, with no pre-selection of the animal's base-line sexual activity and an 'n' in the hundreds, this dose of PCPA was found to induce 2.5 ± 0.6 male mounts in groups of 4 over the 15-min observation period. Any pharmacological agent which significantly increased this value was considered an enhancer of male rat mounting behaviour. As in the model outlined above, the experimental animals were also maintained in a regular 12 h-12 h light-dark cycle.

The most active compound in any pharmacological series assessed was then studied to see whether it influenced female lordotic behaviour. This was carried out as follows.

Inhibition of female lordotic behaviour (Segal et al., 1978)

A set dose of oestrogen (10 μg/rat im) was administered to a group of unselected normal intact female rats. Twenty-four hours later, a second dose of oestrogen (10 μg/rat im) was administered, and on the third day, 5 to 7 hours prior to testing, a dose of 500 μg/rat im of progesterone was given. Each female was maintained in a single holding cage. To ensure an active male partner, all males, again with no pre-selection as to base-line sexual activity, were treated with the effective dose of PCPA (see above) and when presented to a hormone-treated intact female rat produced a 1:1 lordosis:mount ratio resulting in a lordosis quotient (ie lordoses/mounts) equal to one (15-min observation period). Any pharmacological agent which significantly reduced this value was considered as an inhibitor of female lordotic behaviour. All animals in this model were maintained on a regular 12 h-12 h light-dark cycle. However, as opposed to the observations of male-to-male rat mounts which were generally carried out between 08:00 to 13:00 hours, male-female sexual responses were tested 5 to 7 hours into the female's dark cycle; the rats being observed in a dark room with only the aid of a 40 watt red bulb for illumination.

Enhancement of female lordotic behaviour (Segal et al., 1978)

Normal, intact, female rats, unselected as to base-line sexual activity, were titrated with oestrogen-progesterone until a dose regimen of oestrogen alone (2 doses of 0.05 μg/rat im at 24 h intervals) was found which induced a lordosis quotient equivalent to that observed for a completely normal, hormonally-untreated, female rat (0.1 ± 0.1, over the 15-min observation period in the female's dark cycle on the third day). Again, active male partners were ensured by treating them with an effective dose of PCPA. Any pharmacological agent which, when administered concurrently with the oestrogen regimen, significantly increased this value (during the 15-min test period of the third day) was considered to be an enhancer of female lordotic behaviour.

However, because of the complexity of trying to understand and/or unravel the basic mechanisms accounting for the effectiveness of compounds in a model involving the co-administration of an active test compound with PCPA (male rat, Segal *et al.*, 1977) or with oestrogen (female rat, Segal *et al.*, 1978), we began to determine whether the most active compounds in any series could effectively induce such behaviours (male mounts or female lordoses) when administered alone, acutely or chronically. This was carried out as follows.

Induction of male rat mounting behaviour (Segal & Dikstein, 1981b)

Compounds previously found active in the PCPA male rat model were administered (po, in a dose-response manner) daily for one, 2, 3 and 14 days respectively to individually housed rats. Testing (the observation of a group of 4 rats over a 15-min period) was carried out 24 hours after the last administration of the compound, ie on the 15th day. We found that potentially active compounds required more than 7 days of chronic administration for activity to be induced (Segal & Dikstein, unpublished observation). Therefore, to ensure reproducibility of activity data, we carried out all further testing by arbitrarily selecting the 14-day chronic administration schedule. Untreated or vehicle administered animals do not mount when observed in groups of 4 for 15-min on the 15th day; 24 h after the last administration of vehicle or at any time in the 15th day for untreated animals (Segal & Dikstein, unpublished observations). Any compound found to induce activity after 14 days of chronic administration was considered an inducer of male rat mounting behaviour.

Induction of female lordotic behaviour (Segal et al., 1978)

Unselected, normal, intact females were administered the potentially active compounds for 14 days (arbitrary selection) and confronted with an active male partner (PCPA-treated) 24 hours after the final administration of the drug (15-min observation period on the 15th day). Any compound found to significantly induce a lordosis quotient greater than that observed in normal, untreated, intact females (control value of 0.1 ± 0.1) was considered to be an active inducer of female lordotic behaviour.

Again, the authors wish to stress their careful consideration of the complexities involved in assessing rat sexual behaviour in relation to male and female mounting, female, and even male, lordotic behaviour, female soliciting behaviour, male intromissions, ejaculations and so on.

Methodological selection for our mechanism studies

In order to achieve a possible understanding of some of the underlying mechanisms in the complexities of rat sexual behaviour(s), the mechanisms studies discussed in the text of this article were based on the study of male-to-male rat mounting behaviour chronically-induced by microgram quantities of active agents (Segal & Dikstein, 1981*b*). At present, we have not extrapolated beyond this point. Inhibitory studies, generally requiring large doses, are even more complicated to interpret and, therefore, were not discussed in this chapter.

Acknowledgements—The authors acknowledge the invaluable collaboration of Dr D.M. Jacobowitz, Chief, Histopharmacology Section, NIMH, Bethesda, Maryland, without whose expertise in the technique of brain microdissection the data relating to the effects of phenylethylamine on central levels of norepinephrine could not have been obtained.

The authors also gratefully acknowledge the financial assistance of Biotechnology General (Israel) Limited.

References

Barrett, E.S., Adams, P.M., Poffenberger, P.L., Fritz, R.R. & Abell, C.W. (1976): Effects of rapid depletion of phenylalanine and tyrosine in sleep and behaviour. *Pharmacol. Biochem. Behav.* **5,** 47-53.

Barnes, T.R.E., Bamber, R.W.K. & Watson, J.P. (1979): Psychotropic drugs and sexual behaviour. *Brit. J. Hosp. Med.* **211,** 594-600.

Beckmann, H., Strauss, M.A. & Ludolph, E. (1974): D,L-Phenylalanine in depressed patients: an open study. *Jour. Neural. Trans.* **41,** 123-134.

Benkert, O. (1973): In *Psychopharmacology of sexual disorders and drug abuse.* Amsterdam: North Holland Publishing Co. Pp. 489-496.

Benkert, O. (1977): *Sexuelle Impotenz. Neuroendocrinologische und Pharmakotherapeutische Untersuchungen.* Berlin: Springer-Verlag.

Benkert, O., Renz, A. & Matussek, N. (1973): Dopamine, noradrenaline and 5-hydroxytryptamine in relation to motor activity, fighting and mounting behavior. *Neuropharmacol.* **12,** 187-193.

Bermond, B. (1982): Effects of medial preoptic hypothamaic anterior lesions on three kinds of behavior in the rat: inter-male aggression, male sexual and mouse-killing behavior. *Aggressive Behavior* **8,** 335-354.

Biggio, G., Fadda, P., Fanni, P., Tagliamonte, A. & Gessa, G.L. (1974): Rapid depletion of serum tryptophan, brain tryptophan, serotonin and 5-hydroxyindoleacetic acid by a tryptophan-free diet. *Life Sci.* **14,** 1321-1329.

Blum, B., Segal, B., Shtachem, G. & Shohatz, B. (1979): Spacticity phenomenon caused by N-substituted phenylalanines. *Pharmacol. Biochem. Behav.* **8,** 19-23.

Da Prada, N., Carruba, N., O'brion, R.A., Sener, A. & Pletscher, A. (1972): The effect of 5,6-dihydroxytryptamine on sexual behavior of male rats. *Europ. J. Pharmac.* **19,** 288-290.

Dewesbury, D.A. (1975): The normal heterosexual pattern of copulatory behavior in male rats: effects of drugs that alter brain monoamine levels. In *Sexual behavior: pharmacology and biochemistry,* eds Sandler, M. & Gessa, G.L. New York: Raven Press. Pp. 169-179.

Gay, R., Newmeyer, J.A., Elion, R.A. & Weider, S. (1975): *Drug-sex practice in the Haight-Ashbury or "The Sensuous Hippie".* In *Sexual behavior: pharmacology and biochemistry,* eds Sandler, M. & Gessa, G.L. New York: Raven Press. Pp. 63-84.

Gessa, G.L. & Tagliamonte, A. (1975): Role of brain serotonin and dopamine in male sexual behavior. In *Sexual behavior: pharmacology and biochemistry,* eds Sandler, M. & Gessa, G.L. New York: Raven Press. Pp. 117-128.

Gibson, C.J., Deikel, S.M., Young, S.M. & Binik, Y. (1982): Behavioral and biochemical effects of tryptophan, tyrosine and phenylalanine in mice. *Psychopharmacol.* **76,** 118-121.

Goodwin, F.K., Wirz-Justice, A. & Wehr, T.A. (1982): Evidence that the pathophysiology of depression and the mechanism of action of antidepressant drugs both involve alterations in circadian rhythms. In *Typical and atypical antidepressants: clinical practice,* Vol. 32. eds Costa, E. & Racagni, G. New York: Raven Press. Pp. 1-11.

Hauger, R.L., Skolnick, P. & Paul, S.M. (1982): Specific [^{3}H] beta-phenylethylamine binding sites in rat brain. *Europ. J. Pharmac.* **83,** 147-148.

Heller, B., Fischer, E. & Martin, R. (1976): Therapeutic action of D-phenylalanine in Parkinson's Disease. *Arzneim. Forsch.* **26,** 577-579.

Hughes, I.E. (1978): The effect of amitriptyline in presynaptic mechanisms in noradrenergic nerves. *Brit. J. Pharmac.* **63,** 315-321.

Hwang, E.C. & van Woert, M.H. (1980): Comparative effects of substituted phenylethylamines on brain serotonergic mechanisms. *Jour. Pharmac. Exp. Therap.* **213,** 254-260.

Hyyppa, M.T., Lahtinen, P. & Rinne, U.K. (1971): Effect of L-DOPA on the hypothalamic, pineal and striatal monoamines on sexual behavior in the rat. *Brain Res.* **30,** 265-272.
Karczmar, A.G. (1980): Drugs, transmitters and hormones, and mating behavior. *Mod. Probl. Pharmacopsychiat.* **15,** 1-76.
Knoll, J. (1976): Analysis of the pharmacological effect of selective monoamine oxidase inhibitors. In *Monoamine oxidase and its inhibition,* Ciba Foundation Symposium 39. Amsterdam: Exerpta Medica. Pp. 135-161.
Knoll, J. (1981): The pharmacology of selective MAO inhibitors. In *Monoamine oxidase inhibitors: the state of the art,* eds Youdim, M.B.H. & Paykel, E. New York: John Wiley & Sons Ltd. Pp. 45-61.
Kral, V.A. (1985): Psychopharmacology of sexual disorders in the elderly. In *Psychopharmacology of sexual disorders,* ed Segal, M. London: John Libbey & Co. Pp. 155-159.
Laakmann, G. (1982): Antidepressants. In *Psychopharmacology 1, Part 2, clinical psychopharmacology,* eds Hippius, H. & Winokur, G. Amsterdam: Exerpta Medica. Pp. 86-96.
Larsson, K. & Ahlenius, S. (1985): Masculine sexual behaviour and brain monoamines. In *Psychopharmacology of sexual disorders,* ed Segal, M. London: John Libbey & Co. Pp. 15-32.
Langer, G., Schönbeck, G., Konig, G. & Aschauer, H. (1982): Neuroendocrine mechanisms in the therapeutic effects of antidepressant drugs: the "thyroid-axis" hypothesis. In *Typical and atypical antidepressants: clinical practice,* Vol. 32, eds Costa, E. & Racagni, G. New York: Raven Press. Pp. 297-302.
Le Fur, G. & Uzan, A. (1977): Effects of 4-(3-indolyl-alkyl) piperidine derivatives on uptake and release of noradrenaline, dopamine and 5-hydroxytryptamine in rat brain synaptosomes, rat heart and human blood platelets. *Biochem. Pharmac.* **26,** 497-503.
Lisk, R.D. (1967): Sexual behavior: normal control. *Neuroendocrinol.* **2,** 197-239.
Maitre, L., Mosser, L., Baumann, P.A. & Waldmeier, P.C. (1980): Amine uptake inhibitors: criterion of selectivity. *Acta Psychiat. Scand.* 61, suppl. 280, 97-110.
Maj, J. (1981): Antidepressant drugs: will new findings change the present theories of their action. *Trends Pharmac. Sci.* **2,** 80-83.
Mann, J. & Gershon, S. (1980): L-deprenyl, a selective monoamine oxidase type B inhibitor in endogenous depression. *Life Sci.* **26,** 877-882.
Mass, J.W. (1979): Neurotransmitters and depression: too much, too little, or too unstable. *Trends Neurol. Sci.* 1-3.
Moyer, J.A., Herrenkohl, L.R. & Jacobowitz, D.M. (1974): Stress during pregnancy: effect of catecholamines in discrete regions of offsprings as adults. *Brain Res.* **144,** 173-178.
Murphy, M.R. (1985): Endogenous opiates and the mechanism of male sexual behavior. In *Psychopharmacology of sexual disorders,* ed Segal, M. London: John Libbey & Co. Pp. 51-62.
Nock, B. & Feder, H. (1981): Neurotransmitter modulation of steroid action in target cells that mediate reproduction and reproductive behavior. *Neurosci. Biobehav. Revs.* **5,** 437-447.
Palkovitz, M. (1973): Isolated removal of hypothalamic and other brain nuclei in the rat brain. *Brain Res.* **59,** 449-450.
Petrie, W.M. (1980): Sexual effects of antidepressants and psychomotor stimulant drugs. *Mod. Probl. Pharmacopsychiat.* **15,** 77-90.
Reynolds, G.P. (1979): Phenylethylamine — a role in mental illness. *Trends Neurosci.* 1-3.
Sabelli, H.C., Borison, R.L., Diamond, B.I., Havdala, H.S. & Narasimhachari, N. (1978): Phenylethamine and brain function. *Biochem. Pharmac.* **27,** 1729-1730.
Schilgen, B. & Toffe, R. (1980): Partial sleep deprivation as therapy for depression. *Archs Gen. Psychiat.* **37,** 267-271.
Segal, M. & Dikstein, S. (1981*a*): Recent advances in the mechanisms of action of pharmacological agents influencing sexual function. 5th World Congress of Sexology, Haifa, Israel.
Segal, M. & Dikstein, S. (1981*b*): Structure activity relationship (SAR) and mechanism studies of phenylethylamine (PEA) derivatives partially effective in influencing male rat mounting behaviour. In *Sexology,* International Congress Series No. 566, eds Hoch, Z. & Lief, H.I. Amsterdam: Exerpta Medica. Pp. 103-109.
Segal, M., Edelstein, E. & Dikstein, S. (1977): Effect of paramethoxyphenylethylamine and its derivatives on rat male-to-male mounting behaviour. *Res. Comm. Psychol. Psychiat. Behav.* **2,** 161-177.

Segal, M., Edelstein, E.L., Dikstein, S. & Hartzshtark, A. (1978): A method for quantifying lordosis behaviour in the normal female rat: effect of para-methoxyphenylethylamine. *Res. Comm. Psychol. Psychiat. Behav.* **3,** 359-367.
Segal, M., Shohami, E. & Jacobowitz, D.M. (1984): Phenylethylamine, norepinephrine and mounting behaviour in the male rat. *Pharmacol. Biochem. Behav.* **20**, 133-135.
Shalita, B. & Dikstein, S. (1979): D-tyrosine prevents hypertension in DOCA-saline treated uninephrectomized rats. *Pflügers Arch. Physiol.* **379,** 245-250.
Sheard, M.H. (1969): The effect of p-chlorophenylalanine on behavior in rats: relation to brain serotonin and 5-hydroxy-indoleacetic acid. *Brain Res.* **15,** 524-528.
Shilito, E.E. (1969): The effect of para-chlorophenylalanine on normal and pinealectomized rats. *Br. J. Pharmac.* **38,** 305-315.
Shilito, E.E. (1975): Comparison of the effects of behavior of methiothepin and parachlorophenylalanine I. Behavior studies. In *Sexual behavior: pharmacology and biochemistry,* eds Sandler, M. & Gessa, G.L. New York: Raven Press. Pp. 129-132.
Shohami, E., Segal, M. & Jacobowitz, D.M. (1983): Application of high-performance liquid chromatography with electro chemical detection to the determination of catecholamines in microdissected regions of the rat brain. *J. Neurosci. Methods* **8**, 275-281.
Tagliamonte, A., Tagliamonte, P., Gessa, G.L. & Brodie, B.B. (1969): Compulsive sexual activity induced by p-chlorophenylalanine in normal and pinealectomized rats. *Science* **166,** 1433-1435.
Thornton, C., Dore, C.J., Elsworth, J.D., Herbert, M. & Stern, G.M. (1980): The effect of deprenyl, a selective monoamine oxidase inhibitor, on sleep and mood in man. *Psychopharmacology* **70,** 163-166.
Vargas, E. & Tringer, I. (1967): Clinical trial of a new type of promptly acting psycoenergetic agent (phenyl-isopropyl-methyl-propinyl-amine-HCl. E-250). *Acta Med. Acad. Sci. Hung.* **23,** 289-295.
Vogt, M. (1975): Comparison of the effects of behavior of methiothepin and parachlorophenlethylamine. II. Relation of metabolism of 5-HT: chemical findings. *Sexual behavior: pharmacology and biochemistry,* eds Sandler, M. & Gessa, G.L. New York: Raven Press. Pp. 133-136.
Waldmeier, P.C. (1981): Noradrenergic transmission in depression: under- or over-function. *Pharmacopsychiat.* **14,** 3-9.
Wehr, T.A. & Goodwin, F.K. (1979): Rapid cycling in manicdepressives induced by tricyclic antidepressants. *Archs Gen. Psychiat.* **36,** 555-559.
Wehr, T.A. & Goodwin, F.K. (1981): Biological rhythms and psychiatry. In *American handbook of psychiatry,* Vol. 7, eds Arieti, S., Kieth, H. & Brodie, H. Pp. 46-74.
Whalen, R.E., Gorzalka, B.B. & De Bold, J. (1975): Methodologic considerations in the study of animal sexual behaviors. In *Sexual behavior: pharmacology and biochemistry,* eds Sandler, M. & Gessa, G.L. New York: Raven Press. Pp. 33-43.
Wilson, C.A. & Hunter, A.J. (1985): Mechanisms of action of p-chlorophenylalanine (PCPA) and its effects on female sexual behaviour in the rat. In *Psychopharmacology of sexual disorders,* ed Segal, M. London: John Libbey & Co. Pp. 33-49.
Wilson, C.A., Bonney, R.C., Everard, D.M., Parrott, R.F. & Wise, J. (1982): Mechanisms of action of p-chlorophenylalanine in stimulating sexual receptivity in the female rat. *Pharmacol. Biochem. Behav.* **16,** 777-784.
Wirz-Justice, A. & Campbell, I.C. (1982): Antidepressant drugs can slow or dissociate circadian rhythms. *Experientia* **38,** 1301-1309.

2

Masculine sexual behavior and brain monoamines

Knut LARSSON and Sven AHLENIUS

University of Göteborg, Department of Psychology, Unit of Psychobiology, Box 14158, S-400 20 Göteborg, SWEDEN; Astra Läkemedel AB, Research and Development Laboratories, Pharmacology, S-151 85 Södertälje, SWEDEN

Introduction

Experimental evidence is reviewed showing that both catecholamines (CA) and 5-hydroxytryptamine (5-HT) are involved as neurotransmitters in the neural circuits mediating masculine sexual behavior in the rat, CA exerting a stimulatory and 5-HT an inhibitory influence on the behavior. Drastic changes in sexual behavior are produced by the administration of ergot drugs like lisuride and pergolide or by a group of new aminotetralin compounds. Possible monoaminergic mechanisms mediating these effects are discussed.

Drugs have long been used to study the chemistry of sexuality. In 1938, on the basis of studies performed by themselves and others, Semans & Langworthy suggested that penile erection and emission of semen from the meatus of the urethra are reflexes mediated by the parasympathetic system and that penile detumescence and emission of semen into the urethra are mediated by the sympathetic system. During the 1950s, the Soulairacs' pioneered studies on drugs and mating behavior of male rats (Soulairac, 1952, 1961). A leading investigator on drugs and sexuality during the 1960s was Meyerson, who studied female rat sexual behavior (Meyerson, 1964*a,b*). Since then, a wealth of studies on the pharmacology of sexual behavior has appeared. We have ourselves maintained a modest program of research on brain monoamines (MA) and masculine sexual behavior. These studies have lately been focussed on aminotetralins, some of which drastically change the mating pattern of rats, presumably due to interference with brain MA metabolism. In this communication, we report on this work, beginning by reviewing the literature on the role of brain MA in masculine sexual behavior. Almost all experimental evidence available, including our own, has been obtained on rats and we, therefore, focus on this species.

The copulatory behavior of the male rat consists of several stereotyped patterns: mount, intromission and ejaculation. Mounts are recognized by an approach to the rear of the stimulus animal, forepaw palpitations of the flanks of the stimulus animal, and shallow, repetitive, pelvic thrusting by the mounting animal. Intromission consists of mount terminated by a quick pelvic thrust. Ejaculation is characterized by mounts terminated by a deep pelvic thrust which is maintained for several seconds while repeated flexures of the hindquarters occur. During intromission and ejaculation, intravaginal insertion of the penis is usually achieved. However, male rats sometimes display these behavior patterns without vaginal insertion and female rats may exhibit intromissive and ejaculatory patterns although lacking the phalic development necessary to achieve insertion. The terms intromission and ejaculation refer only to the display of the respective motor components. Ejaculation does not imply emission of fluid from the penis.

When presented with a receptive female, the experienced male mounts her immediately and after repeated mounts and intromissions, spaced in time by some tenths of second intervals, ejaculates. The latency of the initial mount and intromission, the time from the first intromission to ejaculation (the ejaculatory latency), the number of mounts and intromissions preceding ejaculation, and the period of sexual inactivity following ejaculation (postejaculatory interval) represent the main parameters used to quantify the sexual performance of the rat (Dewsbury, 1979).

Although the main features of the mating behavior are species-typical, much variation occurs in timing and frequency of the various response patterns. Strain, age, experience, and other factors contribute to this variation. For instance, young rats just having reached puberty, use more mounts and intromissions to ejaculation than older rats (Larsson, 1956). Inexperienced rats usually are more variable in their behavior than experienced ones. A source of variability is the female estrous condition. Failing consideration of these sources of variability may partly explain the inconsistency in the results reported and many apparent contradictions that characterize this area of research (Whalen *et al.*, 1975).

The successive intromissions are supposed to generate a central state of sexual arousal culminating in ejaculation (Carlsson & Larsson, 1974). A decrease in the number of intromissions to ejaculation produced by a drug treatment may be thought of as a stimulatory action of the drug. Conversely, an increase in the intromission frequency, or an increase in the number of mounts without vaginal penetration, represent signs of a depressive action of the drug.

Effects of drugs interfering with catecholamine (CA) neurotransmission

A nonspecific increase of brain MA in intact animals produced by treatment with monoamine oxidase inhibitors, such as iproniazid (25 mg/kg × 3), nialamide (50–100 mg/kg) or pargyline (25–50 mg/kg), results in some prolongation of the ejaculatory latency and the postejaculatory interval, and an increase in the number of mounts and intromissions preceding ejaculation (Dewsbury *et al.*, 1972). The effects, however, are weak and not always observed (Butcher *et al.*, 1969).

Administration of pargyline (40 mg/kg) or nialamide (250 mg/kg) (Malmnäs, 1973) decreased the sexual activity of castrated male rats maintained at subthreshold doses of testosterone. A nonspecific decrease of brain MA caused by administration of small doses of reserpine (0.25 mg/kg) was reported by Soulairac & Soulairac (1961) to result in a decrease in the number of intromissions preceding ejaculation and a shortening of the ejaculatory latency. This observation was confirmed by Dewsbury & Davis (1970) and was extended to include another antipsychotic agent, tetrabenazine (1.5–5.0 mg/kg) (Dewsbury, 1972). The facilitatory effect, found after treatment with reserpine or tetrabenazine, is probably due to the decrease in central 5-HT produced by these drugs (Carlsson, 1966).

Administration of L-Dopa (100 mg/kg) combined with benserazide (50 mg/kg), an inhibitor of aromatic amino acid decarboxylase (Bartholini *et al.*, 1969), had no effects upon sexual behavior (Hyyppä *et al.*, 1971). When L-Dopa is administered to animals showing a low base level of sexual activity, a clear stimulatory effect can be observed. Tagliamonte *et al.* (1974) administered L-Dopa (150 mg/kg) combined with benserazide to a group of sexually sluggish rats. As a result of this treatment, the proportion of mounting and intromitting animals increased, the ejaculatory latency and the postejaculatory interval shortened and the number of mounts and intromissions before ejaculation decreased. The same effect was observed by these authors after treatment with apomorphine (0.5 mg/kg), a selective dopamine (DA) receptor agonist, suggesting a role of DA rather than noradrenaline (NA) in this effect. The stimulatory effect of both drugs was blocked by the administration of the DA receptor blocking agent haloperidol (1.0 mg/kg) (Andén *et al.*, 1970*a*).

Evidence for a role of CA, especially DA, in mediating sexual activity is provided by experiments involving administration of apomorphine or amphetamine to animals pretreated with tetrabenazine, which activates DA receptors directly and indirectly respectively (Andén, 1970; Carlsson, 1970). Amphetamine (0.8 mg/kg) and apomor phine (0.8 mg/kg) counteracted the sedating effect of tetrabenazine (5 mg/kg) (Butcher *et al.*, 1969). Bignami (1966) reported an increased number of intromissions per min in normal rats treated with 0.5 mg/kg amphetamine. Apomorphine has repeatedly been found to have a biphasic effect upon sexual behavior. In doses not exceeding 0.4–0.8 mg/kg, apomorphine shortens the ejaculatory latency and reduces the number of mounts and intromissions before ejaculation while in higher doses, it abolishes sexual activity (Butcher *et al.*, 1969; Tagliamonte *et al.*, 1974; Gessa & Tagliamonte, 1975). Finally, the work of Malmnäs (1973) on castrated rats maintained on subthreshold testosterone levels may be mentioned. He found that apomorphine (0.03–0.30 mg/kg) significantly increased the proportion of sexually active animals while no such increase was seen after the administration of clonidine (0.003–0.03 mg/kg), an NA receptor agonist (Andén *et al.*, 1970*b*). Further, he found L-Dopa (1–10 mg/kg) to be ineffective while α-methyl-p-tyrosine (75 mg/kg), a tyrosine hydroxylase inhibitor (see Uden friend, 1966), lowered the proportion of copulating animals. The decrease in intromission frequency and the shortening of the ejaculatory latency seen after the administration of apomorphine may either be interpreted as due to an increased sensory feedback from the intromissions or an increased tonus in central mechanisms. Under either condition, central DA stimulation appears to stimulate sexual activity.

Effects of drugs interfering with 5-hydroxytryptamine (5-HT) neurotransmission

The administration of 5-hydroxytryptophan (5-HTP) (50 mg/kg), combined with benserazide (25 mg/kg), to intact male rats prolonged the ejaculatory latency and increased the number of intromissions to ejaculation (Ahlenius *et al.*, 1979, 1980*a*). These effects were effectively counteracted by the administration of metergoline (1 mg/kg) (Ahlenius *et al.*, 1980*a*), a 5-HT receptor blocking agent (Fuxe *et al.*, 1978). These observations support the contention that central 5-HT plays an inhibitory role in male rat sexual behavior.

A decrease in brain 5-HT levels may be accomplished by the administration of the inhibitor of 5-HT synthesis, parachlorophenylalanine (PCPA). Both CA and 5-HT synthesis are initially inhibited by this drug. However, while the CA levels recover relatively rapidly, the 5-HT level remains lowered for a longer period (Koe & Weissmann, 1966).

Several independent groups have reported that grouped male or female rats show a striking increase in the number of male-to-male and female-to-female mounting responses after the administration of PCPA (Sheard, 1969; Tagliamonte *et al.*, 1969; Shillito, 1970; Mitler *et al.*, 1972). Also, a facilitation of heterosexual behavior of male rats has been shown following treatment with PCPA (Ahlenius *et al.*, 1971; Salis & Dewsbury, 1971; Mitler *et al.*, 1972). This facilitatory effect of PCPA was particularly marked in rats showing a low base-line level of sexual activity (Ginton, 1976; Dalló, 1977) and in castrated rats maintained on subthreshold doses of testosterone (Malmnäs, 1973). Södersten *et al.* (1976*a*) injected male rats daily with testosterone-propionate in doses insufficient to cause any sexual activity. After treatment with PCPA, the majority of the testosterone propionate-injected rats started to copulate, displaying full mating behavior. Treatment with 5-HTP but not L-dopa counteracted the stimulatory effect of PCPA, suggesting that the stimulatory effect of PCPA was related to the decrease in 5-HT synthesis rather than the CA synthesis. The effect of PCPA on masculine copulatory behavior was also demonstrated in castrated animals not given testosterone (Södersten *et al.*, 1976*a*). Again, the facilitatory action of PCPA on the expression of sexual behavior was counteracted by the administration of 5-HTP, but not L-Dopa.

The marked stimulatory effects of PCPA observed by us in castrated rats was surprising in view of previous negative findings and prompted us (Emery & Larsson, 1979) to explore factors that might influence the responsiveness of the animals to this drug. We found that one of the factors was the strain of animals used. Wistar rats, which were employed by us were significantly more responsive to PCPA than Sprague-Dawley rats, a species used by most other authors. For example, at Day 21 post-castration, the administration of PCPA (100 mg/kg × 4) caused intromission and ejaculation behavior in 85 per cent of the Wistar rats, while none of the Sprague-Dawley rats tested showed any intromission behavior. Another important factor was the time of castration. While 85 per cent of the tested animals ejaculated on Day 21 post-castration, only 20 per cent ejaculated 90 days after castration. Although both Wistar and Sprague-Dawley strains displayed a decline in their behavioral responsiveness to PCPA, the Wistar rats showed a slower rate of decline.

As was demonstrated by Södersten *et al.* (1976*b*), treatment with PCPA may facilitate the display of male sexual behavior not only in the male but also in the female. Following the administration of PCPA, a significantly higher number of ovariectomized females displayed a mount and intromission pattern in response to a receptive female as compared to saline treated controls and 6 out of 21 females showed an ejaculatory pattern. The female mating pattern, including the ejaculatory behavior, had all the characteristics of the behavior normally seen in the male, except for the postejaculatory refractory period which was considerably shorter. The occurrence of ejaculatory behavior in the female is particularly remarkable since display of this behavior by normal female rats has previously been described in one report only (Emery & Sachs, 1976).

The technique of histofluorescence reveals serotonergic pathways rising from cell bodies in the nucleus raphe in the mesencephalon and entering the forebrain (Dahlström & Fuxe, 1964). Relatively selective disruption of the ascending serotonin pathways can be accomplished by localized injection of the neurotoxin, 5,7-dihydroxytryptamine (5,7-DHT) (Baumgarten *et al.*, 1978). We injected 5,7-DHT into the dorsal medial mesencephalic tegmentum, thereby destroying the medial component of the 5-HT pathways (Larsson *et al.*, 1978). The rats used were inexperienced and postpuberally castrated. The animals were tested for sexual behavior before and after treatment with testosterone propionate (150 μg/kg daily for 30 days). Prior to the hormone treatment, the rats displayed only occasional mounts and intromissions. Following the treatment, the drug-injected animals began to copulate sooner and at a higher frequency than the sham-operated controls. At the end of the testing period, 12 out of 19 rats in the experimental group displayed the ejaculatory pattern as compared to 2 out of 9 sham-operated rats. Statistical analysis revealed a significant correlation between the facilitation of sexual behavior caused by the lesion and the reduction of (^{3}H)-5-NA uptake in the hypothalamus. Also, although NA uptake was reduced, this reduction did not reach statistical significance.

Similar results were reported by Södersten *et al.* (1978) after treatment with either 5,7-DHT or *p*-chloroamphetamine, another neurotoxin that selectively destroys 5-HT neurons (see Fuller, 1978). The effect was reversed by pretreatment with the 5-HT uptake inhibitor zimelidine (Ross *et al.*, 1976). They also found that treatment with 5,7-DHT had a clear stimulatory effect on the mounting behavior of ovariectomized, hormonally untreated, female rats.

Summary of findings

— An increase in central CA neurotransmission produces a facilitation of male rat sexual behavior as evidenced by a moderate decrease in the number of intromissions preceding ejaculation and a shortening of the ejaculatory latency.

— An inhibition of central CA neurotransmission impairs the capacity to display sexual behavior.

— An increase in central 5-HT neurotransmission depresses the sexual activity of male rats, as evidenced by a prolonged ejaculatory latency and postejaculatory intervals, an increased number of mounts and intromissions preceding ejaculation, and an increase in the number of animals that fail to start to copulate.

— A decrease in central 5-HT neurotransmission facilitates the expression of sexual activity. The ejaculatory latency shortens, fewer mounts and intromissions precede ejaculation and the number of copulating animals increases. This facilitatory effect is particularly marked in castrated animals, which may show full mating behavior by the administration of drugs which block 5-HT neurotransmission.

— Surgical interference with 5-HT neurotransmission by brain lesions or local application of neurotoxins which selectively destroy 5-HT neurons in the central nervous system produce a facilitation of sexual behavior similar to systemic drug injections, thus demonstrating that the behavioral effects are related to interference with specific neuronal systems in the brain.

The above evidence supports the conclusion reached by others (Gessa & Tagliamonte, 1974) that male rat sexual behavior is under the neural control of CA which exerts a stimulatory influence and 5-HT which exerts an inhibitory influence. These neuronal systems may not necessarily be specific to masculine sexual behavior, but could be systems that are of global importance in the control of motor and arousal mechanisms.

Effects of ergot drugs and aminotetralins

Our analysis of the role of monoamines as neurotransmitters in the neural regulation of sexual behavior has, so far, been based on treatment with drugs having relatively well established mechanisms of action. We will now turn to a group of compounds, ergots and ergot congeners, which interact with monoaminergic receptors in the central nervous system in a complex way which is not well understood (Fuxe *et al.*, 1979). Ergot drugs derive their interest in this context from their effects on masculine sexual behavior which, in some cases (to be discussed below) far exceed those produced by any other experimental treatments.

The ergot first discovered to produce abnormal changes in the mating behavior of rats was lisuride. From observations on grouped male and female rats treated with lisuride, Da Prada *et al.* (1977) reported increased male-to-male and female-to-female mounting behavior, an effect resembling that produced by the administration of PCPA. This observation stimulated us to investigate the action of lisuride on heterosexual

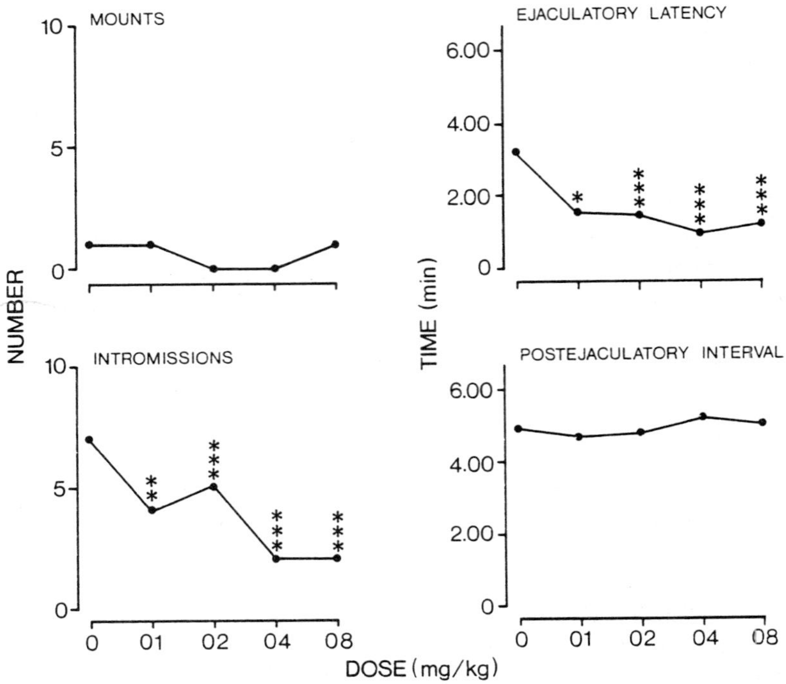

Fig. 1. *Effects of lisuride (−15 min) on male rat copulatory behavior.* The animals were injected ip every second day in a balanced order 0.1, 0.2, 0.4 and 0.8 mg/kg lisuride hydrogen maleate. The figure shows median values based on the performance of 16 animals: ejaculation latency (χ^2 =22.24, n = 16, $P <$ 0.001, Friedman two-way analysis of variance by ranks); intromissions before ejaculation (χ^2 =18.82, n = 16, $P < 0.001$); mounts before ejaculation (χ^2 = 2.02, n = 16, N.S.); and postejaculatory interval (χ^2 = 4.10, n = 16, N.S.); $^*P < 0.05$; $^{**}P < 0.02$; $^{***}P < 0.01$. Wilcoxon matched-pairs signed rank test was used for comparison with control (From: Ahlenius *et al.,* 1980*b*).

behavior (Ahlenius *et al.,* 1980*b*). Following the administration of lisuride, we found a dose-dependent decrease in the number of intromissions preceding ejaculation and a shortening of the ejaculatory latency (Fig. 1). No changes were seen in other components of the mating pattern including mount latency, intromission latency and postejaculatory interval. When administered to rats rendered sexually inactive by castration, lisuride induced copulatory behavior in a dose-dependent manner (Fig. 2). Some males displayed full mating behavior, while others showed intromissions or mounts only. In castrated animals, the effect had a gradual onset and repeated injections were necessary in order to cause ejaculatory behavior.

We have tested two other ergot drugs, pergolide and bromocriptine. The administration of pergolide (1.6–3.2 mg/kg), but not bromocriptine (5–20 mg/kg), caused changes in the mating pattern similar to those obtained with lisuride (Ahlenius *et al.,* 1982).

Lisuride is structurally similar to LSD-25 (Zikán & Semonský, 1960). Biochemical experiments have shown that lisuride, like many other chemically related ergot alkaloids, reduces turnover and synthesis of 5-HT and DA in the brain and, at higher doses, increases brain NA turnover (Kehr, 1977). Animal behavior experiments have shown that lisuride produces effects resembling those of amphetamine and apomorphine. Lisuride also induces hind limb abduction similar to that seen after treatment with 5-HTP, indicating central CA and 5-HT receptor activation respectively (Horowski & Wachtel, 1976, 1979; Kehr, 1977). These biochemical and behavioral

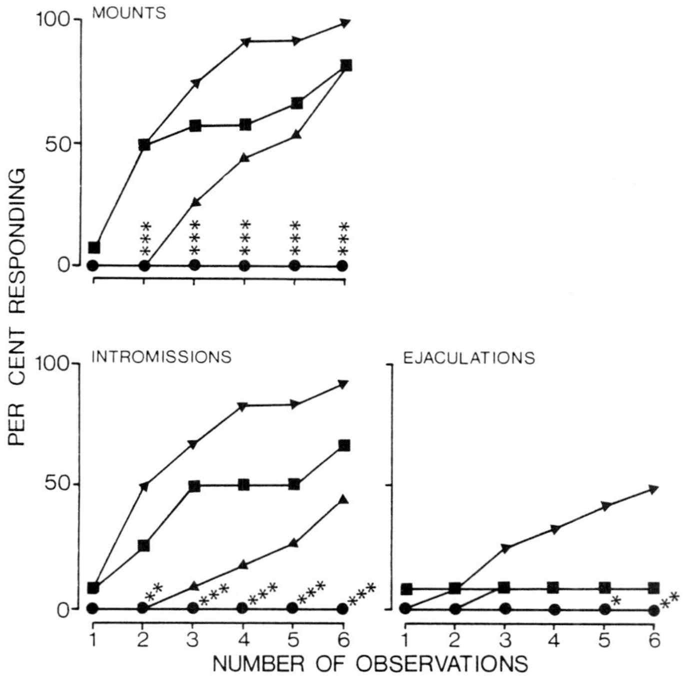

Fig. 2. *Effects of lisuride (−15 min) on copulatory behavior in castrated male rats.* The drug tests began 31 days after castration and were continued every second day for 12 days. The figures show the cumulative percentage of rats displaying various components of the mating pattern. Number of animals in the various groups was: saline (n = 18); 0.1 mg/kg (n = 12); 0.2 mg/kg (n = 12) and 0.4 mg/kg (n = 12). Differences between the various treatments at each observation were calculated by means of a χ^2-test. $^*P < 0.05$; $^{**}P < 0.01$; $^{***}P < 0.001$. 0.0 ●——●; 0.1 ▲——▲; 0.2 ■——■; 0.4 ▼——▼. (From Ahlenius *et al.,* 1980*b*).

observations have led to the conclusion that lisuride is a potent 5-HT and DA receptor agonist. In addition, biochemical experiments indicate that lisuride is a weak NA receptor blocking agent.

Like apomorphine and amphetamine, lisuride causes a shortening of the ejaculatory latency and a decrease in the intromission frequency and these effects may be interpreted as being due to DA stimulation. However, directly or indirectly acting DA receptor agonists such as apomorphine or amphetamine have much weaker effects on sexual behavior and an action of lisuride on classic DA receptors is, therefore, not probable. Further, treatment with lisuride but not amphetamine (Ahlenius & Larsson, unpublished observations) induced sexual behavior in castrated rats. The alterations in sexual behavior following treatment with lisuride resemble those produced by the administration of PCPA. It is particularly noted that lisuride, like PCPA, induces full mating behavior in castrated rats. Since lisuride blocks firing in dorsal raphe 5-HT neurons, presumably by acting upon presynaptic receptors (Rogawski & Aghajanian, 1978), the changes produced by lisuride might, like those of PCPA, be due to impairment of brain 5-HT neurotransmission. The ergot drugs and PCPA may thus affect central 5-HT neurotransmission similarly. It should be observed, however, that lisuride also elicits symptoms of post-synaptic 5-HT receptor activation as indicated above.

Changes in sexual behavior, even more pronounced than those occurring after treatment with lisuride, have recently been observed in our laboratories following the administration of two new compounds, 8-OMe-2-(di-n-propylamino)tetralin (8-OMe-

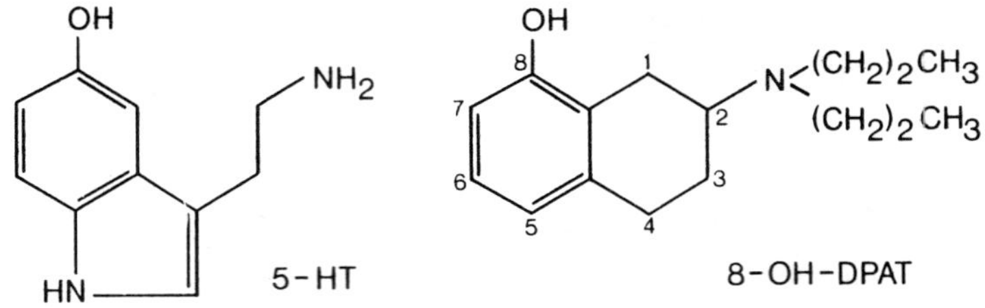

Fig. 3. *Structural formula of 8-OH-2-(di-n-propylamino) tetralin (8-OH-DPAT). The structural formula of 5-hydroxy-tryptamine (5-HT) has been included for comparison.*

DPAT) and 8-OH-2-(di-n-propylamino)tetralin (8-OH-DPAT) (Fig. 3). Treatment with 8-OMe-DPAT caused a dose-dependent decrease in the number of mounts and intromissions and a shortening of the ejaculatory latency as demonstrated in Fig. 4. At higher dose levels, several of the males ejaculated at the very first intromission. Two isomers of this drug were tested and both produced the same drastic changes in the coital pattern. Treatment with the closely related compound, 8-OH-DPAT, produced similar effects but the drug was about 10-fold as potent as 8-OMe-DPAT. A dose-dependent reduction was found in the number of intromissions preceding ejaculation and in the ejaculatory latency. Again, several of the males ejaculated at the very first intromission, particularly at the higher doses.

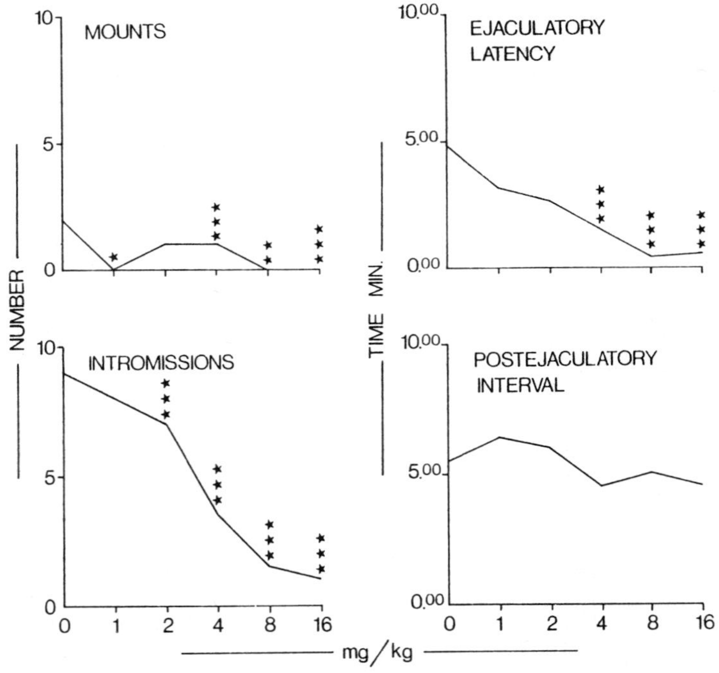

Fig. 4. *Effects of 8-OMe-DPAT on male rat sexual behavior.* The figure shows the results of two separate experiments: 1 and 2 mg/kg (n = 12) and 4, 8 and 16 mg/kg (n = 14). The drug or saline vehicle was given 15 min before presenting the male with a female. Using a balanced design the animals served as their own controls in the two experiments respectively. Shown are the medians and the two control groups are represented by the grand median. Statistical comparisons with the respective control group were made by means of Wilcoxon matched-pairs signed-ranks test. *$P < 0.05$; **$P < 0.02$; ***$P < 0.01$. (From Ahlenius *et al.,* 1981).

Treatment with either 8-OMe-DPAT or 8-OH-DPAT also induced sexual activity in castrated animals. Four weeks after castration, when the animals did not show any sexual activity, the rats were injected repeatedly with either compound. Injection of 8-OMe-DPAT every second day for 12 days produced a dose-dependent increase in the number of mounts and intromissions. 8-OH-DPAT was given to three groups of castrated rats in the doses of 0.25 and 0.50 mg/kg every second-third day for 9 days. There was a significant increase in the number of mounts and intromissions in the drug-treated groups. Two of the nine animals given 0.25 mg/kg and four of the nine animals given 0.50 mg/kg of 8-OH-DPAT ejaculated. In a final test, the rats were observed for sexual behavior without any drug treatment. Except for one animal which showed some mounts, none of the animals showed any sexual activity in this test (Ahlenius *et al.*, 1981).

We have also investigated the effects of the two ergot drugs methysergide (5–20 mg/kg) (Kehr, 1977) and LSD-25 (0.125–0.50 mg/kg) on sexual behavior. The administration of methysergide shortened the ejaculatory latency and reduced the number of

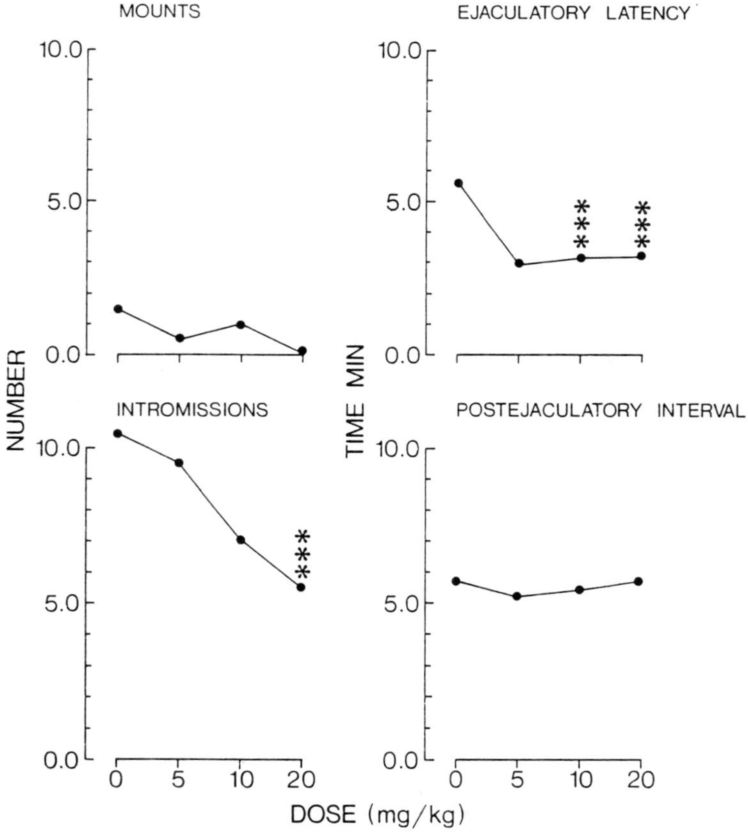

Fig. 5. *Effects of methysergide on male rat sexual behavior.* Methysergide, 0–20 mg/kg i.p. was administered 15 min before the observations started. The animals served as their own controls using a balanced design. Shown are the medians based on the performance of 16 animals. Statistical analysis was performed by means of Friedman two-way ANOVA followed by Wilcoxon matched-pairs signed-ranks test (Siegel, 1956). Comparisons are made with controls or as indicated by brackets. Mounts: χ^2 (3) = 3.13, N.S. ($P > 0.05$); Intromissions: χ^2 (3) = 11.47, $P < 0.01$; Ejaculatory latency: χ^2 (3) = 11.32, $P < 0.02$; Postejaculatory latency: χ^2 (3) = 2.04, N.S. *$P < 0.05$; **$P < 0.01$; ***$P < 0.001$; N.S. $P > 0.05$.

intromissions to ejaculation but the effects obtained were less marked than those seen after treatment with 8-OMe-DPAT or 8-OH-DPAT (Fig. 5). Administration of LSD-25 did not produce any alterations in sexual behavior (Ahlenius *et al.*, 1981).

Biochemical data indicate that the investigated aminotetralins are potent postsynaptic 5-HT receptor agonists (Hjorth *et al.*, 1982; Arvidsson *et al.*, 1981). With regard to central 5-HT neurotransmission, the effects of 8-OH-DPAT increased 5-HT levels and decreased 5-HIAA levels, 5-HT-synthesis rate and 5-HT utilization; results which are virtually identical to those reported with the administration of lisuride or LSD. In contrast to lisuride and LSD, however, which are potent DA agonists (Pieri *et al.*, 1977), 8-OH-DPAT appears to lack appreciable effects on central CA receptors, at least in the doses investigated. Animals treated with lisuride or the aminotetralins show a behavioral syndrome inclusive of a flat body posture, forepaw extension and treading, abducted hindlimbs, tremor in the forelimbs and Straub tail. This syndrome can also be induced by the administration of 5-HTP, thus suggesting increased postsynaptic 5-HT stimulation.

There is evidence that 8-OH-DPAT, like lisuride, inhibits firing in 5-HT neurons of

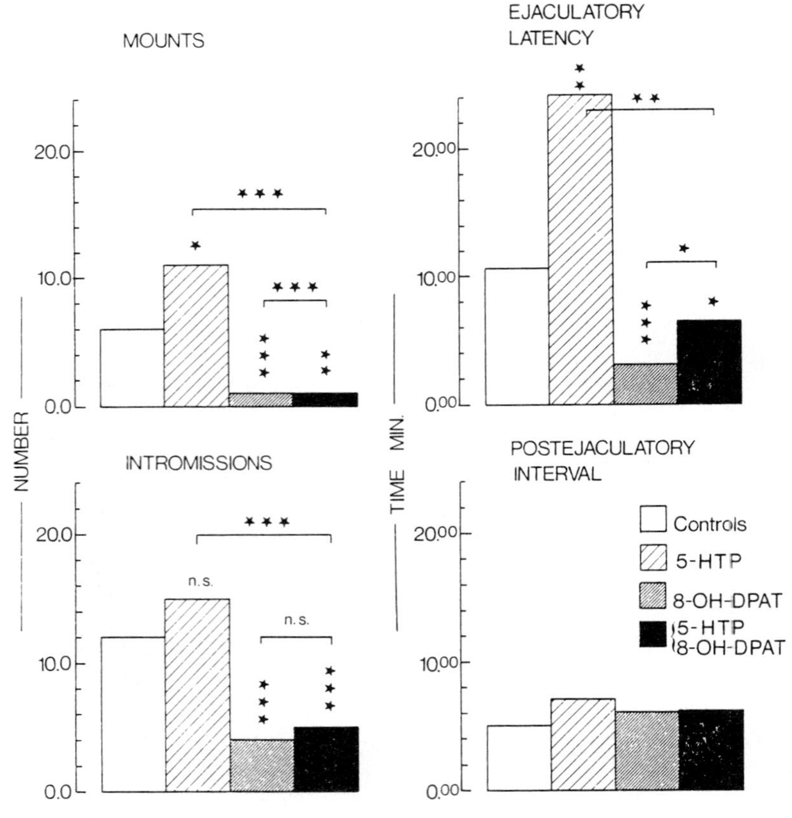

Fig. 6. *Effects of 5-HTP on 8-OH-DPAT-induced facilitation of male rat sexual behavior.* 5-HTP, was given in a dose of 25 mg/kg i.p. (−60 min) and 8-OH-DPAT in a dose of 0.25 mg/kg i.p. (−15 min). Peripheral decarboxylation of 5-HTP was prevented by the administration of benserazide 25 mg/kg i.p. (−90 min). The animals served as their own controls using a balanced design. Shown are the medians based on the performance of 17 animals. Statistical analysis as described in the legend to Fig. 5. Mounts: χ^2 (3) = 20.36, $P < 0.001$; Intromissions: χ^2 (3) = 21.24, $P < 0.001$; Ejaculatory latency: χ^2 (3) = 28.50, $P < 0.001$; Postejaculatory latency: χ^2 (3) = 7.25, N.S. ($P > 0.05$).

the dorsal raphe (T.H. Svensson, personal communication). One possible explanation is that activation of 5-HT autoreceptors is the predominant effect of both these drugs on the serotonergic system involved in the mediation of sexual behavior of the rat. However, as a result of treatment with 5-HTP, we found an increase in the ejaculatory latency whereas administration of 8-OH-DPAT, alone and in combination with 5-HTP, caused a decrease of the ejaculatory latency to 30 and 60 per cent of controls respectively (Fig. 6). The results obtained do not indicate any antagonizing effect of 5-HTP on the effects of the aminotetralins and do not support an action of 8-OH-DPAT at 5-HT autoreceptors.

Further attempts to antagonize the action of the aminotetralins have involved treatment with drugs which are believed to block DA and 5-HT receptors postsynaptically. To the former category belongs haloperidol and to the latter metergoline and methiothepin (Lloyd & Bartolini, 1974). None of these drugs, however, were able to antagonize 8-OH-DPAT-induced changes in sexual behavior (Figs 7–8 and unpublished observations).

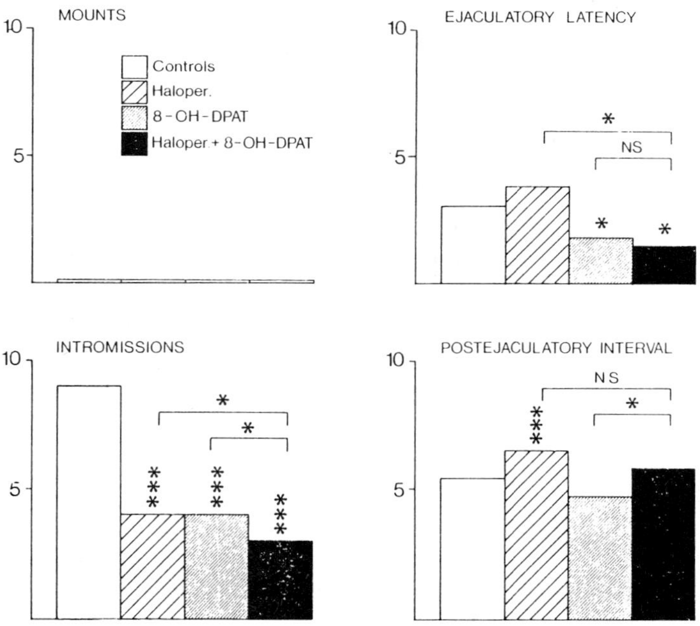

Fig. 7. *Effects of haloperidol on 8-OH-DPAT-induced facilitation of male rat sexual behavior.* Haloperi-dol was given in a dose of 0.16 mg/kg i.p. (−20 min) and 8-OH-DPAT in a dose of 0.25 mg/kg (−15 min). The animals served as their own controls using a balanced design. Shown are the medians based on the performance of 17 animals. Statistical analysis as in legend to Fig. 5. Mounts: χ^2 (3) = 1.07, N.S. ($P >$ 0.05); Intromissions: χ^2 (3) = 23.2, $P < 0.001$; Ejaculatory latency: χ^2 (3) = 17.17, $P < 0.001$; Postejaculatory latency: χ^2 (3) = 13.88, $P < 0.01$.

It has been suggested that the effects of lisuride on rat sexual behavior may be due to a combined impairment of 5-HT neurotransmission and activation of central CA neurotransmission (Da Prada *et al.*, 1977). We tried to mimick the action of 8-OH-

DPAT by treating the animals with PCPA in combination with another aminotetralin compound, 5-OH-2-(di-n-propylamino)tetralin (5-OH-DPAT), which is a potent DA receptor agonist (McDermed *et al.*, 1978; Hacksell *et al.*, 1979). Figure 9 shows the results of this experiment. The administration of PCPA and 5-OH-DPAT decreased

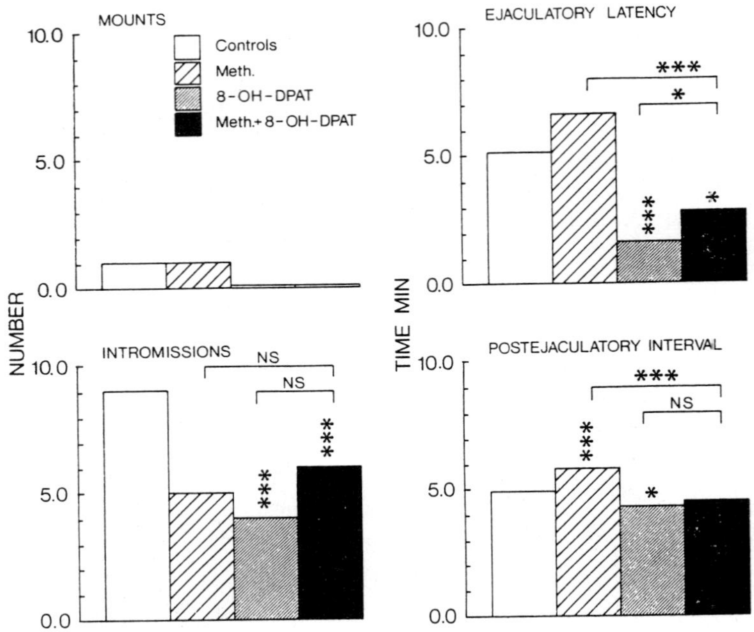

Fig. 8. ***Effects of methiothepin on 8-OH-DPAT-induced facilitation of male rat sexual behavior.*** Methiothepin was given in a dose of 0.2 mg/kg i.p. (−30 min) and 8-OH-DPAT in a dose of 0.2 mg/kg i.p. (−15 min). The animals served as their own controls using a balanced design. Shown are the medians based on the performance of 13 animals. Statistical analysis as in legend to Fig. 5. Mounts: χ^2 (3) = 5.35, N.S. ($P > 0.05$); Intromissions χ^2 (3) = 13.45, $P < 0.01$; Ejaculatory latency: χ^2 (3) = 20.53, $P < 0.001$; Postejaculatory latency: χ^2 (3) = 21.55, $P < 0.001$.

the ejaculatory latency to 67 and 49 per cent of the controls respectively. When combined, the two drugs decreased the ejaculatory latency to 29 per cent of the control values. However, the strong effects induced by 8-OMe-DPAT or 8-OH-DPAT could not be reproduced.

In conclusion, several biochemically related compounds with 5-HT receptor stimulating properties, lisuride, 8-OMe-DPAT and 8-OH-DPAT, have been found to produce a highly dramatic reduction in ejaculatory latency and in the number of intromissions to ejaculation in the male rat. Current pharmacological means of activating central 5-HT receptors produce the opposite effects, whereas a reduction in central 5-HT receptor activation is associated with effects in the same direction as those produced by the above-mentioned drugs. On the assumption that they act at central 5-HT receptors, we suggest that the drugs act preferentially as agonists at 5-HT autoreceptors or, alternatively, as selective 5-HT receptor antagonists. Available biochemical and behavioral evidence does not, however, allow a precise conclusion of the mechanisms of action of these drugs to be made at present and a role of DA activation in these effects should not be excluded.

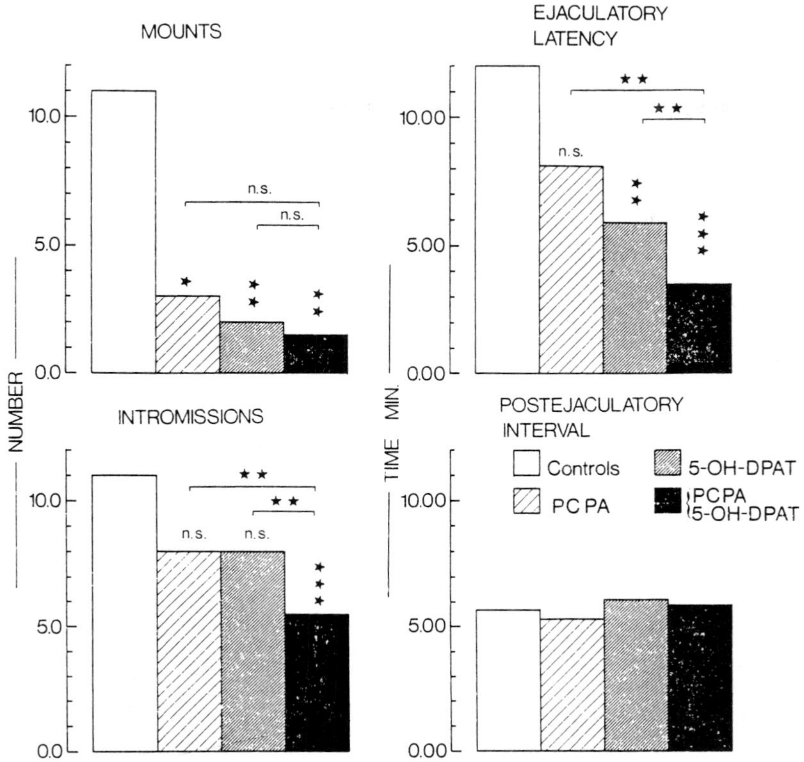

Fig. 9. *Effects of PCPA and 5-OH-DPAT combined on male rat sexual behavior.* PCPA was administered, 100 mg/kg i.p. × 4, in daily doses (−24 h) and 5-OH-DPAT 0.1 mg/kg i.p. (−15 min). Shown are the medians based on the performance of 9-10 animals/group. Statistical analysis was performed by means of Kruskal-Wallis one-way ANOVA followed by Mann-Whitney U-test for individual comparisons (Siegel, 1956). Mounts χ^2 (3) = 11.43, $P < 0.01$; Intromissions: χ^2 (3) = 14.28, $P < 0.01$; Ejaculatory latency: χ^2 (3) = 18.62, $P < 0.001$; Postejaculatory latency: χ^2 (3) = 3.99, N.S. ($P > 0.05$).

Discussion

Mating is a final outcome of physiological activities on several different levels of the neuraxis. It is dependent on sensory receptors of the genitals which are stimulated during coitus and on postganglionic efferent nerves. The basic components of the mating pattern, including penile erection, pelvic thrusting, emission of semen into the urethra and ejaculation of semen are controlled by neural centra in the lower spinal cord which, in turn, are under an inhibitory and excitatory influence of descending spinal nerves. The brain includes a multitude of neuronal systems activated during sexual arousal. Systemic administration of drugs may produce alterations in physiological processes at all these levels. An obvious task for future research is to delimit the action of drugs including those which interfere with MA neurotransmission to specific areas within the central nervous system.

A characteristic of sexual behavior is its dependence on gonadal hormones. These hormones may influence the various steps in the biosynthesis of DA, NA and 5-HT. They may influence the transport of the transmitter to the synaptic membrane; influence its release into the synaptic space and its reuptake; interact with the enzymes within and outside the terminal that degrade the transmitter substance; interact with the receptors at the postsynaptic membrane and influence the processes occurring in the postsynaptic axons. Apart from the fact that castration and subsequent treatment with gonadal steroids may alter the synthesis rate of DA, NA and 5-HT in brain nuclei believed to be involved in mediating sexual behavior (Engel *et al.*, 1979), little is known about the interaction between sex steroids and brain MA.

Beach (1967) proposed that dual neural mechanisms are involved in sexual behavior, one determining sexual arousal and another determining the execution of the copulatory acts; the activity of the latter being partially under the control of the former. Beyer (1976) suggested a third modulatory mechanism that exerts an inhibitory influence on the other mechanisms. We thus may ask to what extent the drug treatments discussed may influence these three hypothetical mechanisms.

Conditions facilitating sexual arousal include the presence of a mating partner and other stimuli associated with mating, such as genital and perhaps proprioceptive stimuli produced during execution of the copulatory performance and any environmental stimuli increasing the level of responsiveness of the male to the mating partner. Finally, there are the gonadal hormones. Various experimental approaches, such as brain lesion and electrical stimulation experiments, hormone implantation and autoradiographic techniques, have provided evidence indicating the importance for sexual arousal of an area encompassing the rostral part of the cerebral cortex, the medial preoptic-anterior part of the hypothalamus and the corticomedial amygdaloid nuclei. A characteristic feature of the parts of the brain that have been implicated in the sexual arousal mechanism is that they all receive projections from ascending DA and NA pathways and probably various structures in the ventral forebrain closely connected with the olfactory lobe. Thus, the mesolimbic DA system has its terminals i.a. in the bed nucleus of stria terminalis, nucleus accumbens and tuberculum olfactorium. Noradrenergic pathways terminate i.a. in the preoptic area, hypothalalmus, bed nucleus of stria terminalis, amygdala and hippocampus (Ungerstedt, 1971). The partial coincidence of the projection areas of the ascending CA pathways and the area containing hormone-concentrating neurons gives some support to the idea that CA are involved as neurotransmitters in the copulatory arousal mechanism. Important observations pertaining to this question were recently reported by Hansen *et al.* (1982*a*). They found that the administration of lisuride to animals that were made sexually inactive by lesions in the medial preoptic area temporarily restored full mating behavior. Thus following medial preoptic area injury, the remains of a neural circuitry underlying the male mating pattern can be made functional again by altering the activity of central MA systems.

The copulatory mechanism includes neural circuits mediating basic genital reflexes. Aside from the fact that genital reflexes can be elicited at the level of the spinal cord, virtually nothing is known of the neural substrate of the copulatory mechanism.

Several lines of research point to the existence of a modulatory mechanism of sexual behavior. This mechanism comprises neurons having neural connections capable of deactivating sexual behavior and sensory pathways transmitting information to these neurons. Evidence for the existence of brain regions exerting inhibitory effects on sexual behavior comes mainly from lesion studies. Thus, lesions in the neocortex and parts of the limbic system may result in increased sexual activity in males of several species (Larsson, 1979). Besides a tonic inhibitory effect, there also appear to be brain structures exerting a phasic inhibitory effect on sexual behavior. The postejaculatory refractory period is probably determined by an active physiological process since lesions in the mesodiencephalic area may shorten markedly the postejaculatory refractory period in male rats (Heimer & Larsson, 1964; Barfield *et al.*, 1975; Clark *et al.*, 1975; Hansen *et al.*, 1982*b*).

Monoaminergic neurons and pathways are probably part of the neural substrate for modulating sexual behavior in rats. The 5-HT cell bodies in the medulla-oblongata-pons generally give rise to descending bulbospinal pathways whereas the ascending 5-HT pathways generally originate from the caudal raphe nuclei in the mesencephalon (Dahlström & Fuxe, 1964). Some ascending axons terminate in the rostral end of the hypothalamus and the preoptic area. Other axons, located medial and dorsal to those terminating in the hypothalamus, enter the diagonal band of Broca and, passing rostral to the septum, terminate in the cingulum. Some axons may continue caudally, terminating in the amygdala. All these various projection areas of 5-HT axons encompass structures probably involved in the mediation of masculine sexual behavior in rats (Larsson, 1979).

Acknowledgements—This work was supported by the Swedish Humanities and Social Research Council.

We thank Mrs Elisabeth Wallin for expert technical assistance and Mrs Claery Persson for typing the manuscript. The figures were prepared at 'Läromedelscentralen' at the University of Göteborg. Drugs were generously donated by Hoffman-La Roche, Basel, Switzerland (methiothepin), Leo AB, Helsingborg, Sweden (haloperidol) and Swedish Sandoz AB, Stockholm, Sweden (methysergide).

References

Ahlenius, S., Eriksson, H., Larsson, K., Modigh, K. & Södersten, P. (1971): Mating behavior in the male rat treated with p-chlorophenylalanine methyl ester alone and in combination with pargyline. *Psychopharmacol.* **20,** 383-388.

Ahlenius, S., Heimann, M. & Larsson, K. (1979): Prolongation of the ejaculation latency in the male rat by thioridazine and chlorimipramine. *Psychopharmacol.* **65,** 137-140.

Ahlenius, S., Larsson, K. & Svensson, L. (1980*a*): Further evidence for an inhibitory role of central 5-HT in male rat sexual behavior. *Psychopharmacol.* **68,** 217-220.

Ahlenius, S., Larsson, K. & Svensson, L. (1980*b*): Stimulating effects of lisuride on masculine sexual behavior of rats. *Eur. J. Pharmacol.* **64,** 47-51.

Ahlenius, S., Larsson, K., Svensson, L., Hjorth, S., Carlsson, A., Lindberg, P., Wikström, H., Sanchez, D., Arvidsson, L.-E., Hacksell, U. & Nilsson, J.L.G. (1981): Effects of a new type of 5-HT receptor agonist on male rat sexual behavior. *Pharmacol. Biochem. Behav.* **15,** 785-792.

Ahlenius, S., Engel, J., Larsson, K. & Svensson, L. (1982): Effects of pergolide and bromocriptine on male rat sexual behavior. *J. Neural Transmission* **54,** 165-170.

Andén, N.-E. (1970): Effects of amphetamine and some other drugs on central catecholamine mechanisms. In *Amphetamines and related compounds,* eds E. Costa & S. Garattini. New York: Raven Press. Pp 447-462.

Andén, N.-E., Butcher, S.G., Corrodi, H., Fuxe, K. & Ungerstedt, U. (1970*a*): Receptor activity and turnover of dopamine and noradrenaline after neuroleptics. *Eur. J. Pharmacol.* **11,** 303-314.

Andén, N.-E., Corrodi, H., Fuxe, K., Hökfelt, B., Hökfelt, T., Rydin, L. & Svensson, T. (1970*b*): Evidence for a central noradrenaline receptor stimulation by clonidine. *Life Sci.* **9,** 513-523.

Arvidsson, L.-E., Hacksell, U., Nilsson, J.L.G., Hjorth, S., Carlsson, A., Lindberg, P., Sanchez, D. & Wikström, H. (1981): 8-Hydroxy-2-(di-n-propylamino)-tetralin, a new centrally acting 5-HT receptor agonist. *J. Med. Chem.* **24,** 921-923.

Barfield, R.J., Wilson, C. & McDonald, P.G. (1975): Sexual behavior: extreme reduction of postejaculatory refractory period by midbrain lesions in male rats. *Science* **189,** 147-149.

Bartholini, G., Blum, J.E. & Pletscher, A. (1969): Dopa-induced locomotor stimulation after inhibition of extracerebral decarboxylase. *J. Pharm. Pharmacol.* **21,** 297-301.

Baumgarten, H.G., Klemm, H.P., Lachenmayer, L., Björklund, A., Lovenberg, W. & Schlossberger, H.G. (1978): Mode and mechanism of action of neurotoxic indoleamines: a review and a progress report. *Annals of the New York Academy of Sciences* **305,** 3-24.

Beach, F.A. (1967): Cerebral and hormonal control of reflexive mechanisms involved in copulatory behavior. *Physiol. Rev.* **47,** 289-316.

Beyer, C. (1976): Neuroendocrine mechanisms in sexual behavior. In *Subcellular mechanisms in reproductive neuroendocrinology,* eds F. Naftolin, K.J.. Ryan & J. Davies. Amsterdam: Elsevier. Pp 471-484.
Bignami, G. (1966): Pharmacological influences on mating behavior in the male rat. *Psychopharmacologia (Berl.)* **10,** 44-58.
Butcher, L.L., Butcher, S.G. & Larsson, K. (1969): Effects of apomorphine, (+)-amphetamine, and nialamide on tetrabenazine-induced suppression of sexual behavior in the male rat. *Eur. J. Pharmacol.* **1,** 283-288.
Carlsson, A. (1966): Drugs which block the storage of 5-hydroxytryptamine and related amines. In *Handbook of experimental pharmacology,* eds O. Eishler & A. Farah, Vol. 19. Berlin-Heidelberg-New York: Springer. Pp 529-592.
Carlsson, A. (1970): Amphetamine and brain catecholamines. In *Amphetamines and related compounds,* eds E. Costa & S. Garattini. New York: Raven Press. Pp 289-300.
Carlsson, S.G. & Larsson, K. (1974): Comments on the rat-sex model. In *Motivation control systems analysis,* ed D.J. McFarland. New York: Academic Press. Pp 504-507.
Clark, T.K., Caggiula, A.R., McConnell, R.A. & Antelman, S.M. (1975): Sexual inhibition is reduced by rostral midbrain lesions in the male rat. *Science* **190,** 169-171.
Dahlström, A. & Fuxe, K. (1964): Evidence for the existence of monoamine containing neurons in the central nervous system. *Acta Physiol. Scand.* **62** (Suppl.), 1-55.
Dalló, J. (1977): Effect of two brain serotonin depletors on the sexual behavior of male rats. *Po. J. Pharmacol. Pharm.* **29,** 247-251.
Da Prada, M., Bonetti, E.P. & Keller, H.H. (1977): Induction of mounting behavior in female and male rats by lisuride. *Neurosci. Lett.* **6,** 349-353.
Dewsbury, D.A. & Davis, H.N. (1970): Effects of reserpine on the copulatory behavior of male rats. *Physiol. Behav.* **5,** 1331-1333.
Dewsbury, D.A. (1972): Effects of tetrabenazine on the copulatory behavior of male rats. *Eur. J. Pharmacol.* **17,** 221-226.
Dewsbury, D.A. (1979): Description of sexual behavior in research on hormone-behavior interactions. In *Endocrine control of sexual behavior,* ed C. Beyer. New York: Raven Press. Pp 3-32.
Dewsbury, D.A., Davis, Jr. H.N. & Jansen, P.E. (1972): Effects of monoamine oxidase inhibitors on the copulatory behavior of male rats. *Psychopharmacologia (Berl.)* **24,** 209-217.
Emery, D.E. & Larsson, K. (1979): Rat strain differences in copulatory behavior after *para*-chlorophenylalanine and hormone treatment. *J. Comp. Physiol. Psychol.* **93,** 1067-1084.
Emery, D.E. & Sachs, B.D. (1976): Hormonal and monoaminergic influences on masculine copulatory behavior in the female rat. *Horm. Behav.* **7,** 341-352.
Engel, J., Ahlenius, S., Almgren, O., Carlsson, A., Larsson, K. & Södersten, P. (1979): Effects of gonadectomy and hormone replacement on brain monoamine synthesis in male rats. *Pharmacol. Biochem. Behav.* **10,** 149-154.
Fuller, F.W. (1978): Structure-activity relationships among the halogenated amphetamines. *Annals of the New York Academy of Sciences* **305,** 147-159.
Fuxe, B.B., Fredholm, L., Agnati, F., Ögren, S.-O., Everitt, B.J., Jonsson, G. & Gustafsson, J.-A. (1978): Interaction of ergot drugs with central monoamine systems. *Pharmacology* **16** (Suppl. 1), 99-314.
Fuxe, K., Schwarz, R., Agnati, L., Fredholm, B., Ögren, S.-O., Köhler, Ch. & Gustafsson, J.-A. (1979): Actions of ergot derivatives at dopamine synapses. In *Dopaminergic ergot derivatives and motor function,* eds K. Fuxe & D.B. Calne. London: Pergamon Press. Pp 141-157.
Gessa, G.L. & Tagliamonte, A. (1974): Role of brain monoamines in male sexual behavior. *Life Sci.* **14,** 425-436.
Gessa. G.L. & Tagliamonte, A. (1975): Role of brain serotonin and dopamine in male sexual behavior. In *Sexual behavior: pharmacology and biochemistry,* eds M. Sandler & G.L. Gessa. New York: Raven Press. Pp 117-118.
Ginton, A. (1976): Copulation in noncopulators: effect of PCPA in male rats. *Pharmacol. Biochem. Behav.* **4,** 357-359.
Hacksell, U., Svensson, U., Nilsson, J.L.G., Hjorth, S., Carlsson, A., Wikström, H., Lindberg, P. & Sanchez, D. (1979): N-Alkylated 2-aminotetralins: central dopamine receptor stimulating activity. *J. Med. Chem.* **22,** 1469-1475.

Hansen, S., Köhler, C. & Ross, S.B. (1982*a*): On the role of the dorsal mesencephalic tegmentum in the control of masculine sexual behavior in the rat: effects of electrolytic lesions, ibotenic acid and DSP4. *Brain Res.* **240,** 311-320.

Hansen, S., Köhler, Ch., Goldstein, M. & Steinbusch, H.V.M. (1982*b*): Effects of ibotenic-induced neuronal degeneration in the medial preoptic area and the lateral hypothalamic area on sexual behavior in the male rat. *Brain Res.* **239,** 213-232.

Heimer, L. & Larsson, K. (1964): Drastic changes in the mating behavior of male rats following lesions in the junction of diencephalon and mesencephalon. *Experientia* **20,** 460.

Hjorth, S., Carlsson, A., Lindberg, P., Sanchez, D., Wikström, H., Arvidsson, L.-E., Hacksell, U. & Nilsson, J.L.G. (1982): 8-Hydroxy-2-(di-n-propylamino)-tetralin, 8-OH-DPAT, a potent and selective simplified ergot congener with central 5-HT-receptor stimulating activity. *J. Neural Transmission,* **55,** 169-188.

Horowski, R. & Wachtel, H. (1976): Direct dopaminergic action of lisuride hydrogen maleate, an ergot derivative, in mice. *Eur. J. Pharmacol.* **36,** 373-383.

Horowski, R. & Wachtel, H. (1979): Pharmacological effects of lisuride in rodent mediated by dopaminergic receptors: mechanism of action and influence of chronic treatment with lisuride. In *Dopaminergic ergot derivatives and motor functions,* eds K. Fuxe & D.B. Calne. Oxford: Pergamon Press. Pp 237-251.

Hyyppä, M.T., Lehtinen, P. & Rinne, U.K. (1971): Effect of L-DOPA on the hypothalamic, pineal and striatal monoamines and on the sexual behavior of the rat. *Brain Res.* **30,** 265-272.

Kehr, W. (1977): Effect of lisuride and other ergot derivatives on monoaminergic mechanisms in rat brain. *Eur. J. Pharmacol.* **41,** 262-273.

Koe, B.K. & Weissman, K. (1966): *p*-Chlorophenylalanine: a specific depletor of brain serotonin. *J. Pharmacol. Exp. Ther.* **154,** 499-516.

Larsson, K. (1956): Conditioning and sexual behavior in the male albino rat. *Acta Psychologica Gothoburgensia* 1-269.

Larsson, K., Fuxe, K., Everitt, B.J., Holmgren, M. & Södersten, P. (1978): Sexual behavior in male rats after intracerebral injection of 5,7-dihydroxytryptamine. *Brain Res.* **141,** 293-303.

Larsson, K. (1979): Features of the neuroendocrine regulation of masculine sexual behavior. In *Endocrine control of sexual behavior,* ed C. Beyer. New York: Raven Press. Pp 77-163.

Lloyd, K.G. & Bartholini, G. (1974): The effect of methiothepin on cerebral monoamine neurons. In *Advances in biochemical psychopharmacology,* Vol. 10. New York: Raven Press. Pp 305-309.

Malmnäs, C.O. (1973): Monoaminergic influence of testosterone-activated copulatory behavior in the castrated male rat. *Acta Physiol. Scand.* (Suppl.) **395,** 1-128.

McDermed, J.D., McKenzie, G.M. & Freeman, H.S. (1978): Synthesis and dopaminergic activity of (±), (+)-, and (−)-2-dipropylamine-5-hydroxy-1,2,3,4-tetrahydronapthalene. *J. Med. Chem.* **19,** 547-549.

Meyerson, B.J. (1964*a*): Central nervous monoamines and hormone-induced estrous behavior in the spayed rat. *Acta Physiol. Scand.* (Suppl. 241) **63,** 1-32.

Meyerson, B.J. (1964*b*): Estrus behavior in spayed rats after estrogen or progesterone treatment in combination with reserpine or tetrabenazine. *Psychopharmacologia (Berl.)* **6,** 210-218.

Mitler, M.M., Morden, B., Levine, S. & Dement, W. (1972): The effects of parachlorophenylalanine on the mating behavior of male rats. *Physiol. Behav.* **8,** 1147-1150.

Pieri, M., Schaffer, R. & Haefely, W. (1977): Central dopamine receptor stimulation by LSD and lisuride. *Experientia* **33,** 806.

Rogawski, M.A. & Aghajanian, G.K. (1978): Response of central monoaminergic neurons to lisuride: comparison with LSD. *Life Sci.* **24,** 1289-1298.

Ross, S.B., Ögren, S.-O. & Renyi, A.L. (1976): (2)-Dimethyl-amino-1-(4-bromophenyl)-1-(3-pyridyl) propene (H 102/09), a new selective inhibitor of the neuronal 5-hydroxytryptamine uptake. *Acta Pharmacol. Toxicol. (Kbh)* **39,** 152-166.

Salis, P.J. & Dewsbury, D.A. (1979): *p*-Chlorophenylalanine facilitates copulatory behavior in male rats. *Nature* (Lond.) **232,** 400-401.

Semans, J.H. & Langworthy, O.R. (1938): Observations on the neurophysiology of sexual function in the male rat. *J. Urol.* **40,** 836-846.

Sheard, M.H. (1969): The effect of p-chlorophenylalanine on behavior in rats: relation to brain serotonin and 5-hydroxy-indoleacetic acid. *Brain Res.* **15,** 524-528.
Shillito, E.E. (1970): The effect of *para*-chlorophenylalanine on social interaction of male rats. *Br. J. Pharmac.* **38,** 305-313.
Siegel, S. (1956): *Nonparametric statistics for the behavioral sciences.* New York: McGraw-Hill.
Södersten, P., Larsson, K., Ahlenius, S. & Engel, J. (1976*a*): Sexual behavior in castrated male rats treated with monoamine synthesis inhibitors and testosterone. *Pharmac. Biochem. Behav.* **5,** 319-327.
Södersten, P., Larsson, K., Ahlenius, S. & Engel, J. (1976*b*): Stimulation of mounting behavior but not lordosis behavior in ovariectomized female rats by *p*-chlorophenylalanine. *Pharmacol. Biochem. Behav.* **5,** 329-333.
Södersten, P., Berge, O.G. & Hole, K. (1978): Effects of *p*-chloroamphetamine and 5,7-dihydroxytryptamine on the sexual behavior of gonadectomized male and female rats. *Pharmacol. Biochem. Behav.* **9,** 499-508.
Soulairac, A. (1952): La signification de la période réfractaire dans le comportement sexuel du rat male. *J. Physiol.* (Paris) **44,** 99-113.
Soulairac, A. & Soulairac, M.L. (1961): Action de la réserpine sur le comportement sexuel du rat-male. *C.R. Soc. Biol.* (Paris) **155,** 1010-1013.
Tagliamonte, A., Tagliamonte, P., Gessa, G.L. & Brodie, B.B. (1969): Compulsive sexual activity induced by *p*-chlorophenylalanine in normal and pinealetomized male rats. *Science* **166,** 1433-1435.
Tagliamonte, A., Fratta, W., Del Fiacco, M. & Gessa, G.L. (1974): Possible stimulatory role of brain dopamine in the copulatory behavior of male rats. *Pharmacol. Biochem. Behav.* **2,** 257-260.
Udenfriend, S. (1966): Biosynthesis of the sympathetic neurotransmitter, norepinephrine. In *The Harvey lectures,* Series 60. New York: Academic Press. Pp 57-83.
Ungerstedt, U. (1971): Stereotaxic mapping of the monoamine pathways in the brain. *Acta Physiol. Scand.* (Suppl.) **367,** 1-48.
Whalen, R.E., Gorzalka, B.B. & de Bold, J. (1975): Methodological considerations in the study of animal behavior. In *Sexual behavior: pharmacology and biochemistry,* eds M. Sandler & G.L. Gessa. New York: Raven Press. Pp 33-44.
Zikán, V. & Semonský, M. (1960): Mutterkornalkaloide XVI. Einige N-/D-6-Methyl-isoergolenyl-8/-,N-/D-6-Methylergolenyl-8-/- und N-/D-6-Methylergolin/I/-yl-8/-N'-substituierte Harnstoffe, Kursiv Coll. *Czech. Chem. Commun.* **25,** 1922-1928.

3

Effects and mechanisms of action of p-chlorophenylalanine (PCPA) on sexual behaviour in the female rat

C. A. WILSON and A. J. HUNTER

Department of Obstetrics & Gynaecology, St. George's Hospital Medical School, London SW17 ORE, UNITED KINGDOM

Introduction

The role of central serotonergic systems in various behaviours has been extensively studied, usually by depleting endogenous brain 5-HT and noting the effects of this biochemical manipulation. Methods of depletion include lesions of the midbrain raphe nucleus (the main site of 5-HT cell bodies) or administration of neurotoxic agents such as p-chloroamphetamine (PCA) and 5,7-dihydroxytryptamine (5,7-DHT) or of inhibitors of 5-HT synthesis, such as p-chlorophenylalanine (PCPA).

PCPA reduces the 5-HT concentration in all forebrain areas innervated by the ascending 5-HT pathway originating from the dorsal and median raphe and also areas in the spinal cord innervated by the descending system from the raphe (Ogren *et al.*, 1981). Thus, the administration of PCPA has been shown to increase daytime motor activity (Marsden & Curzon, 1976; Steigrad *et al.*, 1978), increase aggression in rats (Matte & Tornow, 1978; Valzelli *et al.*, 1981), induce hyperphagia (Breisch *et al.*, 1976), reduce REM sleep and increase SW sleep (Borbely *et al.*, 1981). In particular, PCPA has been used to elucidate the role of 5-HT on sexual behaviour and in this chapter we will concentrate on this aspect.

The effect of PCPA on male sexual behaviour

Nearly all the reports in the literature agree that the administration of PCPA stimulates male sexual behaviour in a variety of species, ie in rats, rabbits and cats (Sheard, 1969; Ferguson *et al.*, 1970; Perez-Gruent *et al.*, 1971). This was first shown in 'sluggish' or 'non-copulatory' intact male rats (Tagliomente *et al.*, 1969; Ahlenius *et al.*, 1971; Bertolini, 1971; Salis & Dewsbury, 1971; Mitler *et al.*, 1972; Ginton, 1976), and then in castrated males treated with submaximal doses of testosterone (Malmas & Meyerson, 1971), after bilateral pudentectomy (Dahlof & Larsson, 1979), and after neonatal castration in rats in which the development of the external genitalia was maintained by treatment with dihydrotestosterone (Booth *et al.*, 1979). All these models show a low level of sexual activity. PCPA has no effect in rats or cats that show vigorous sexual behaviour before treatment (Whalen & Luttge, 1970; Zitrin *et al.*, 1970), presumably because activity is already at a maximum. At first, it was thought that the presence of testosterone was required before PCPA could exert its 'aphrodisiac' effect (Gessa *et al.*, 1970), but later experiments showed that PCPA was active in untreated castrated males (Malmas & Meyerson, 1971; Sodersten *et al.*, 1976*a*) and in castrated males treated with oestradiol (Luttge, 1975). Most interestingly, PCPA has been shown to stimulate male sexual behaviour in female ovariectomised rats (in the presence or absence of oestradiol or testosterone) (Singer, 1972; Rodriguez-Sierra *et al.*, 1976; Sodersten *et al.*, 1976*b*; Van de Poll *et al.*, 1977), thus indicating that the neuronal requirements for the male ejaculatory pattern of behaviour is present in both sexes.

The effects summarized above occur whether PCPA is administered as a single injection, chronically over 3-4 days, or, in the case of females, is given over a period of four to 19 days. The onset and duration of these effects correlate with the rate of depletion of brain 5-HT (Sodersten *et al.*, 1976*a*). This has led to the widely held view that 5-HT exerts an inhibitory effect on male sexual behaviour and that PCPA stimulates such behaviour by inhibiting 5-HT synthesis. Supporting this, 5-HTP (the immediate precursor to 5-HT) can reverse the stimulatory effect of PCPA (Tagliomonte *et al.*, 1969; Malmas & Meyerson, 1971; Sodersten *et al.*, 1976*a*), or can inhibit male sexual behaviour in otherwise untreated male rats (Ahlenius *et al.*, 1979, 1980) as can several 5-HT uptake inhibitors that increase the availability of 5-HT in the synapse, such as zimelidine, alaproclate and femoxitine (Hamberger-Bar *et al.*, 1978; Ahlenius *et al.*, 1979, 1980). In addition, serotonin neurotoxic agents (5,7-DHT) and other depletors (PCA) and antagonists of 5-HT (methysergide) stimulate male sexual behaviour (Benkert & Eversmann, 1972; Da Prada *et al.*, 1972; Humphries *et al.*, 1980; Larsson *et al.*, 1978; Sodersten *et al.*, 1978).

The effect of PCPA on female sexual behaviour

In ovariectomised oestrogen-primed females, a single injection of PCPA has stimulated receptive behaviour 4-8 hours after administration in all experiments reported (Meyerson, 1964; Meyerson & Lewander, 1970; Ahlenius *et al.*, 1972; Everitt *et al.*, 1974, 1975*a*; Eliasson & Meyerson, 1977). When rats are primed with higher doses or with multiple daily doses of oestradiol, the effect can also be seen 24 and 48 hours after PCPA administration (Zemplan *et al.*, 1973; Everitt *et al.*, 1975*c*; Davis & Kohl, 1978). Other pharmacological agents that reduce brain 5-HT can also stimulate female sexual behaviour including PCA and 5,7-DHT (Everitt *et al.*, 1975*b*; Zemplan *et al.*, 1977) as well as various 5-HT receptor blockers like methysergide and cinanserin (Zemplan *et al.*, 1973; Ward *et al.*, 1975; Davis & Kohl, 1978; Foreman & Moss, 1978*a*; Franck & Ward, 1981). Based on these reports, it has been concluded that 5-HT exerts an inhibitory control of female sexual behaviour, just as it does on male sexual behaviour. Supporting this, administration of 5-HT itself into specific hypothalamic sites inhibits female receptivity (Foreman & Moss, 1978*a*).

However, unlike the work carried out on the male, there are a number of reports that do not support this hypothesis, and most of these are experiments which involve the use of PCPA. Thus, although a single injection of PCPA can stimulate female sexual behaviour, daily administration over 3 or 4 days reduces the lordosis quotient in animals made receptive with oestrogen plus progesterone priming (Segal & Whalen, 1970; Singer, 1972; Gorzalka & Whalen, 1975) and chronic PCPA treatment is without stimulatory effect in non-receptive animals (Singer, 1972; Sodersten *et al.*, 1976*b*; Eliasson & Meyerson, 1977). A single injection of PCPA administered 24 hours before the expected receptive period can even inhibit sexual behaviour in intact females (Al Satli *et al.*, 1981). In addition, various drugs known to increase 5-HT activity such as the 5-HT uptake inhibitors and quizapine (a 5-HT angonist) can stimulate female receptivity, suggesting that 5-HT has perhaps a positive modulatory effect on female behaviour (Hamberger-Bar *et al.*, 1978; Kow *et al.*, 1979).

The pharmacological actions of PCPA

In order to clarify the role of 5-HT in the control of female sexual behaviour, it is important to understand the mechanism of action of the pharmacological tools used to manipulate this amine in the brain, since conflicting results may be due to any one of a variety of actions possessed by these drugs. Because most of the experiments on sexual behaviour have involved PCPA, we have concentrated on investigating the possible mechanisms of action of this compound on female sexual behaviour.

PCPA is best known as an inhibitor of 5-HT synthesis since it is a potent inhibitor of tryptophan hydroxylase (Koe & Weissman, 1966) and it has been used extensively in behavioural studies to deplete 5-HT under the assumption that this is its predominant activity. However, several reports show that in spite of a significant correlation between 5-HT depletion and behavioural effects, the two may not be causally related. For instance, the hyperphagic action of PCPA may well be due to its structural similarity to its parent amino-acid; administration of the latter having a hyperphagic effect with a similar dose-response curve to PCPA (Coscina *et al.*, 1978).

Depletion of brain indoleamines by inhibiting indoleamine synthesis

PCPA is a potent inhibitor of tryptophan hydroxylase in the brain and liver (Koe & Weissman, 1966) but not in the pineal gland (Deguchi & Barchas, 1972). Its onset of action occurs within two hours, since depletion of the main indoleamine metabolite, 5-hydroxyindoleacetic acid (5-HIAA) appears in this time, and its maximum effect is observed within 24 hours (Wilson *et al.*, 1977). A single injection significantly depletes 5-HT in the hypothalamus for 8 days and elsewhere in the brain for 12 days (Miller *et al.*, 1970).

The effect of PCPA on 5-HT receptors and metabolism

Since PCPA reduces presynaptic serotonergic activity, it also alters postsynaptic function. In the first 24 hours after administration, there is an increase in postsynaptic receptor affinity for exogenous 5-HT. It has been suggested that this is due to a reduction in competition from the lowered levels of endogenous 5-HT. Eight to ten days after PCPA treatment, there is an increase in receptor numbers (B max) indicating super-sensitivity due to reduced presynaptic 5-HT activity. At this time, receptor affinity (K_D) is normal (Steigrad *et al.*, 1978).

Peculiarly, PCPA increases the conversion of 5-HTP to 5-HT and then slows down the disappearance of 5-HT. Although the mechanism of action remains unknown, it does not act by altering 5-hydroxydecarboxylase activity, release of 5-HT or uptake or 5-HTP (McBride *et al.*, 1976). For experimental purposes, one can assume that a PCPA-treated animal is more sensitive to the action of exogenous 5-HTP.

Depletion of brain catecholamines

Many reports have shown that PCPA treatment depletes brain noradrenaline (NA) and, more recently, adrenaline (A) was also found to be affected while dopamine (DA) levels remains unchanged (Miller *et al.*, 1970; Ahlenius *et al.*, 1972; Sloviter *et al.*, 1978; Reader, 1982). In some experiments, the depletion of NA was only transient, levels returning to normal within 24 hours (Ahlenius *et al.*, 1972), whereas in others the depletion lasted for 3 days in the hypothalamus and for 5 days in other brain areas (Miller *et al.*, 1970). PCPA is a weak inhibitor of tyrosine hydroxylase (the rate-limiting enzyme in the catecholamine synthetic pathway), having approximately 1/40th of the activity of α-methyltyrosine. Chronic injections of PCPA over 3 days do not appear to effect tyrosine hydroxylase activity (Koe & Weissman, 1966). A possible explanation of this paradox is that the inhibitory effect on tyrosine hydroxylase is due to the transient release of 5-HT after acute PCPA administration (see later) and this amine is known to inhibit the enzyme (Pujol *et al.*, 1978).

In addition, PCPA can induce a transient release of NA from nerve terminals, thus lowering brain concentrations for a short time; this action is probably via its metabolite p-chlorophenylethylamine (Sloviter *et al.*, 1978). This metabolite also inhibits the enzyme PNMT which converts NA to A (see below).

The actions of p-chlorophenylethylamine (PCPEA) – a metabolite of PCPA

PCPEA is formed from PCPA by decarboxylation and is detroyed by monoamine oxidases. It has a short half-life and after an intra-peritoneal (ip) injection of PCPA, maximum concentrations are present in the brain in 6–8 min, falling to zero by 16 min (Koe & Weissman, 1966). However, it is continuously formed while PCPA is in the circulation (ie for approximately 6 hours, after a single ip injection) (Edwards & Blau, 1972).

PCPEA has a variety of actions, including release of 5-HT and NA from nerve terminals. This may be due to its structural similarity to the two amines and it may thus compete for uptake and/or storage sites. This effect can be seen particularly in the presence of an MAO inhibitor (MAOI) administered together with either PCPA or PCPEA. A decade ago, it was suggested that the behavioural effects of PCPA, in the first 6 hours after administration, could be due to PCPEA (Edwards & Blau, 1972) and, more recently, clear evidence was given that the 'serotonin-behaviour syndrome' seen after PCPA plus an MAOI was due to PCPEA-induced release of 5-HT (Sloviter *et al.*, 1978).

PCPEA has been tested as well as other chlorinated phenylethylamines for inhibition of PNMT. The molar concentration required for 50 per cent inhibition is 3.5×10^4 and although PCPEA is the least potent of the chlorinated analogues it still has significant activity (Fuller *et al.*, 1975) and it significantly reduces brain adrenaline (A) levels (Reader, 1982). It is possible that the reduction in A concentration may account for some of the effects of PCPA. In particular, it is suggested that the PCPA-induced depletion of A correlates better than induced depletion of 5-HT, with its inhibition of gonadotrophin release (Cone, personal communication).

Action of PCPA on steroid metabolism

PCPA increases the activity of the hypothalamic aromatizing enzyme which converts testosterone to oestradiol. Since oestrogens stimulate sexual behaviour in both sexes, an increased production of the latter hormone might explain the stimulatory effect of PCPA (Farabollini & di Prisco, 1981). The mechanism by which PCPA acts on the aromatizing enzyme is unknown.

The effect of PCPA on the adrenal

Many experiments have been carried out to determine whether PCPA acts on adrenal steroidogenesis and hence affects behaviour via this mechanism. In males, adrenalectomy does not alter the stimulatory action of PCPA (Malmas & Meyerson, 1971). In females, the data are conflicting. In two papers, adrenalectomy did not alter the action of PCPA on lordosis (Zemplan *et al.*, 1973; Everitt *et al.*, 1975*c*) and in adrenal-intact ovariectomised guinea pigs, PCPA did not alter progesterone levels (Carter *et al.*, 1978). However, in two other reports, PCPA was inactive in adrenalectomised-ovariectomised-oestrogen-primed animals (Eriksson & Sodersten, 1973; Gorzalka & Whalen, 1975). Both reports state that the animals were in good health, but we and others (Hamberger-Bar *et al.*, 1978; Wilson *et al.*, 1982) have found that PCPA is toxic in adrenalectomised rats. When progesterone plasma concentration was measured in our ovariectomised-oestrogen primed rats, PCPA caused a slight but significant rise 4 hours after administration (Wilson *et al.*, 1982). Farabollini & di Prisco (1981) found that oestrogen and testosterone plasma levels in ovariectomised rats and rabbits were reduced by PCPA. Perhaps PCPA inhibits the conversion of progesterone to other steroids further along the synthetic pathway.

Investigations of the mechanism of action of PCPA on female sexual behaviour

The results in Tables 1–4 have been published previously (Wilson *et al.*, 1982).

Correlation of the stimulatory effect of PCPA on female sexual behaviour and hypothalamic indoleamine depletion

Table 1 shows that in ovariectomised rats primed with 2 μg oestradiol benzoate (OB), a

Table 1. *Effect of PCPA, given 4 hours before, on lordosis and hypothalamine amine concentration*

Treatment[c] *mg/kg IP*	*Number receptive rats*	*Mean LQ% (with range)*		*5-HT*	*Hypothalamic concentration 5-HIAA*	*NA*	*DA*
					(ng/100 mg ± SE)[a]		
Saline	1/23	7.2	(0–65)	163 ± 19	122 ± 29	233 ± 12	320 ± 38
100	9/24*††	39.6**†††	(0–100)	180 ± 29	107 ± 14	300 ± 31*	568 ± 43
150	19/22***	71.6***	(0–100)	157 ± 14	42 ± 9**	197 ± 10[b]	323 ± 35
200	12/15***	42.8***†	(0–95)	—	—	—	
300	13/20***	54.7***†	(0–90)	175 ± 10	37 ± 5**	188 ± 8	365 ± 83

Significance between saline group and treated groups: $*P < 0.05$; $**P < 0.01$; $***P < 0.001$. Significance between group given 150 mg/kg PCPA and other PCPA treated groups: $†P < 0.05$; $††P < 0.01$; $†††P < 0.002$, by the Mann-Whitney U test.
[a]Amine estimations carried out on 7 rats/group.
[b]Significantly different from saline group at $P < 0.05$ according to Student's *t*-test.
[c]All rats primed with 2μg OB 52 hours before testing.

single injection of PCPA, 48 hours later and 4 hours before testing for receptivity (percentage of no. of lordoses to 20 mounts: Lordosis Quotient (LQ)). The maximum effect occurred after 150 mg/kg, while higher doses were less effective. Graded doses of PCPA were, however, increasingly effective in reducing 5-HIAA and NA hypothalamine concentrations. Thus, the dose-respone curves for the two effects of PCPA were not parallel, and this lack of correlation was confirmed completely in two other experiments. The first (see Table 2) showed that administration of 5-HTP together with 150 mg/kg PCPA did not reverse the stimulatory effect of PCPA on sexual behaviour, although hypothalamic indoleamine levels reverted to normal. In the second experiment, when PCPA was given 24 hours after oestrogen-priming and 24 hours before testing, both 5-HT and 5-HIAA levels were significantly depleted

Table 2. *Reversal of the effects of PCPA, given 4 hours before, on lordosis and amine depletion*

Treatment[c]	*Dose mg/kg IP*	*LQ%*	*(range)*	*5-HT*	*5-HIAA*	*NA*	*DA*
				Hypothalamic concentration ng/100 mg ± SE[a]			
Saline (18)	—	23	(0–65)	156 ± 15	190 ± 11***	269 ± 21	219 ± 14
PCPA + (30) Saline	150	76.5***	(0–100)	99 ± 8*	82 ± 14***	187 ± 18	181 ± 7
PCPA + (20) 5-HTP	150 20	80.7***	(5–100)	215 ± 23*†	139 ± 23	194 ± 14	197 ± 34
PCPA + (11) DOPA	150 200	73.0***	(20–100)	80 ± 9**	121 ± 20*	171 ± 25	255 ± 20
PCPA + (4)[d] DOPS	150 250	74.1***	(70–100)	98 ± 5*	87 ± 17***	149 ± 11	217 ± 39
PCPA + (14) Clonidine	150 1.0	2.0†††	(0–65)				
PCPA + (8) Noradrenaline	150 0.3[b]	54.0**†	(24–100)				
Progesterone (7)	2.0[c]	84.4***	(65–100)				
Progesterone + Noradrenaline (7)	2.0[c] 0.3[b]	55.4**†	(0–100)				

All drugs were given intraperitoneally concomitantly with the PCPA except; [b]0.3 mg/kg noradrenaline given intraventricularly 15 minutes before testing. [c]progesterone given SC. () Number of rats per group for behavioural test.
[a]Amine estimations carried out on 8 rats/group, except [d]the group treated with PCPA plus DOPS (n = 4) which was not included in the tests for significance.
Significance between saline group and other treated groups: $*P < 0.05$; $**P < 0.01$; $***P < 0.001$
Significance between group given PCPA alone and other treated groups: $\dagger P < 0.05$; $\dagger\dagger\dagger P < 0.001$ by the Mann-Whitney U test.
Significance between progesterone alone and progesterone plus noradrenaline: $\dagger P < 0.05$.
[c]All rats primed with 2µg OB 52 hours before testing.

although NA levels were unaffected (this is in agreement with the findings of Ahlenius *et al.*, 1972). Despite this, stimulation of sexual receptivity did not occur. Chronic administration of 150 mg/kg PCPA daily for 3 days, which is extremely effective in depleting indoleamine hypothalamic levels, also had no effect on female sexual behaviour (see Table 3).

Table 3. *Effect of PCPA, given 24 hours before, on lordosis and hypothalamic amine concentrations*

Treatment[c] *mg/kg IP*	*Number receptive rats*	*Mean LQ% with range*	*5-HT*	*5-HIAA*	*NA*
			Hypothalamic concentration (ng/100 mg ± SE)[a]		
Saline	0/7	0	195 ± 10	115 ± 10	209 ± 13
100	1/8	12.9 (0–90)	108 ± 8**	74 ± 30***	189 ± 14
150	0/6	0	51 ± 6***	14 ± 3***	193 ± 12
300	1/6 (2 sick)	9.0 (0–55)	59 ± 8***	not detectable	234 ± 34
150 × 3[b]	0/13	5.2 (0–40)	54 ± 4***	not detectable	191 ± 10

Significance between saline group and treated groups: $**P < 0.01$; $***P < 0.001$. by the Mann-Whitney U test.
[a]Amine estimations carried out on 6 rats/group. [b]150 × 3; PCPA given at 150 mg/kg 4, 24 and 48 hours before testing. [c]All rats primed with 2µg OB 52 hours before testing.

Correlation of the stimulatory effect of PCPA on female sexual behaviour and hypothalamic catecholamine depletion

As mentioned earlier, PCPA can cause a transient reduction in NA and A levels, the NA reduction lasting 24 hours in some rats and as long as 3–5 days in others. In our experiments, a single injection of PCPA (150 mg/kg) induced a significant decrease in hypothalamic NA concentrations 4 hours later, a time when sexual behaviour was stimulated (see Tables 1 and 2). Attempts to raise NA levels to normal using DOPA or DOPS were unsuccessful. The ineffectiveness of DOPA was not surprising since its administration rarely affects brain NA, being converted mainly to DA (Hyyppa *et al.*, 1971), but the lack of effect of DOPS was surprising. However, since neither reversed the biochemical effects of PCPA, one would not expect them to reverse the behavioural effect either. Another attempt at reversing NA levels was made using clonidine (an α-adrenergic agonist) in a dose thought to act on postsynaptic receptors (Gold *et al.*, 1978). This, however, was toxic in PCPA-treated animals. Finally, NA itself was administered intraventricularly to rats bearing permanent cannulae in the third ventricle. Administration of this amine at 100 μg/rat caused sedation for approximately 10 minutes but normal motor activity was restored by 15 minutes. Rats, primed 48 hours before with 2 μg OB, were treated with either PCPA or 2 mg progesterone and tested 4 hours later. Then NA or saline was injected intraventricularly and the animals were retested 15 minutes later. NA inhibited the stimulatory effects of both PCPA and progesterone (see Table 2). This inhibitory effect is contrary to some of the data in the literature which show that adrenergic agents stimulate female sexual behaviour in rats and guinea pigs (Everitt *et al.*, 1975*c*; Nock & Feder, 1979; Irving *et al.*, 1981), and that inhibition of presynaptic noradrenergic release and lesions of the noradrenergic ventral bundle reduce receptivity (Davis & Kohl, 1977; Hansen *et al.*, 1980). Foreman & Moss (1978*b*), however, present pharmacological evidence that α-adrenergic activity is inhibitory, although ß-adrenergic activity is stimulatory to female sexual behaviour.

Stimulation of female sexual behaviour and the physicochemical properties of PCPA

Coscina *et al.* (1978) have indicated that the physicochemical properties of PCPA may be responsible for its hyperphagic action and it is possible that the effect of PCPA on female sexual behaviour is also due to these properties. Dalhouse (1976) reports that the parent amino-acid, phenylalanine, had no effect on male sexual behaviour and we found that 150 mg/kg phenylalanine had no effect 4 hours after administration on female lordosis in ovariectomised rats primed with 2 μg OB (controls LQ=3.6%, n=11; phenylalanine LQ=0%, n=6).

Stimulation of female sexual behaviour by the action of PCPA on the adrenal

The conflicting results of the effect of PCPA on adrenalectomised female rats has already been summarised. We found that PCPA administration raised progesterone plasma levels from 2.2 ± 0.18 ng/ml (n=6) to 3.1 ± 0.25 ng/ml (n=5) 4 hours after administration and, although this increase was slight, it was statistically significnt ($P < 0.01$). Thus, it is possible that PCPA stimulates progesterone secretion from the adrenal, perhaps at the expense of testosterone and oestrogen production.

Stimulation of female sexual behaviour by a metabolite of PCPA, ie PCPEA

It has been suggested that the effects of PCPA observed in the first 6 hours after administration may be due to its metabolite PCPEA and Sloviter *et al.* (1978) have gone further, suggesting that the early effects of PCPA are due to a release of 5-HT induced by PCPEA.

We have investigated the possibility that the stimulatory effect of PCPA on female sexual behaviour occurs only after its conversion to PCPEA. Table 4 shows that administration of 20 mg/kg PCPEA, one hour before testing significantly stimulated lordosis. It was not as marked as the effect seen after PCPA, presumably because it is not circulating for a long enough period when administered as an exogenous bolus. In fact, PCPEA appeared to exert an 'all or none' effect, either being completely ineffective or inducing a high lordosis quotient (5/15 showing LQ of 0%; 10/15 showing a mean LQ of 66%).

Most importantly, when PCPA was administered to animals pretreated with an inhibitor of amino-acid decarboxylase (benserazide), thus blocking its conversion to PCPEA, there was a marked reduction in its stimulatory effect. Benserazide did not inhibit the action of PCPEA itself or progesterone.

If PCPEA is the active principle of PCPA, as far as stimulating female sexual behaviour is concerned, what is its mechanism of action? It does not inhibit 5-HT synthesis (Sloviter *et al.*, 1978), but it does stimulate the release of 5-HT and NA.

NA release. Looking at the stimulatory effect of PCPA, it was assumed that the reduction in NA concentration after PCPA was due to a decrease in synthesis rate and this reduced NA activity correlated with increased sexual behaviour. However, it is also possible that the fall in hypothalamic NA concentration was actually due to its enhanced release and thus an increase in NA activity may be what correlates with the behavioural effect. The latter interpretation is supported by the work of others (eg Everitt *et al.*, 1975*c*). It should be noted that the effect of PCPA on NA levels occurs early and is transitory, thus indicating that this effect is due to PCPEA and strongly supporting the observation that the depletion of NA after PCPA is prevented by benserazide (see Table 4).

5-HT release. We have also considered the possibility that PCPEA acts by stimulating a release of 5-HT which then exerts a positive effect on female sexual behaviour. We have confirmed the observation that PCPEA does, indeed, induce 5-HT release biochemically, since it increased 5-HIAA levels at the cost of slightly lowering 5-HT (see Table 4).

Table 5 outlines the effects of two serotonin agonists, 5-HTP and quizapine, and two antagonists, cinanserin and metergoline, on female sexual behaviour in both 'receptive' and 'non-receptive' animals. 5-HTP and quizapine stimulated receptivity in 'non-receptive' rats primed 48 hours before with 10 μg OB. Animals made very receptive with 200 μg OB were not affected by 5-HTP while quizapine increased their lordosis quotient to even higher levels. Conversely, the two 5-HT antagonists slightly reduced receptivity in the animals primed with the high dose of 200 μg and did not significantly affect the less receptive rats primed with 10 μg OB.

These results conflict with most reports in the literature which suggest that both systemic and central administration of 5-HT agonists and antagonists have inhibited and stimulated female sexual behaviour respectively (eg Zemplan *et al.*, 1973; Ward *et al.*, 1975; Foreman & Moss, 1978*a*). Further investigations are being carried out to confirm and explain our results. Meanwhile, two other findings also support the possibility that 5-HT has a stimulatory effect on female sexual behaviour.

We have shown that the administration of 0.5 mg progesterone to ovariectomised rats primed with 2 μg OB increases receptivity 4 hours later and, at the same time, increases 5-HT release and possibly turnover, as indicated by the stable levels of 5-HIAA in the face of a reduction in 5-HT (Table 6). We have also shown that 10 and 100 μg/rat of 5-HT injected into the lateral ventricle significantly stimulated receptive

Table 4. *The role of PCPEA in the stimulatory effect of PCPA on female sexual behaviour*

Treatment[c]	*Dose (mg/kg)*	*Time of administration (hours before testing)*	*Mean LQ% (range)*		*Hypothalamic concentration* *5-HT*	*5-HIAA*	*NA*	*DA*
					ng/100 mg/SE[a]			
Saline (11)	—	4	3.6	(0–20)	144 ± 5	100 ± 9	197 ± 6	246 ± 27
PCPA(11)	150	4	73.0***	(20–100)	134 ± 6	56 ± 5*	165 ± 6[b]	315 ± 16
PCPA +	150	4	16.0†	(0–100)	173 ± 24	71 ± 12*	202 ± 18	279 ± 26
Benserazide (7)	250	4.25						
PCPEA (20)	20	1	44.0*	(0–100)	116 ± 11*	119 ± 16	143 ± 6**	188 ± 12
PCPEA +	250	1.25	33.0*	(0–100)				
Benseradize (5) (3/8 died)								
Progesterone (5)	2	4	83.7***	(60–100)				
Progesterone +	2	4						
Benserazide (5)	250	4.25	92.0***	(80–100)				

() Number of rats per group.
[a]Seven rats/group for amine assays. [b]Significantly different from saline group at $P < 0.02$ according to Student's *t-test.*
Significance between saline group and treated groups: *$P < 0.05$;**$P < 0.02$;***$P < 0.001$.
Significance between PCPA group and PCPA plus Benserazide: †$P < 0.02$ by the Mann-Whitney U test

Table 5. *Effect of 5-HT agonists and antagonists on sexual behaviour in 'receptive' and 'non-receptive' female rats*

Drug[b] Treatment	*Dose mg/kg*	*No. of animals*	*Mean LQ range* 200µg OB 'Receptive gp'		*No. of animals*	10µg OB 'Non-receptive gp'	
			Saline	*Drug*		*Saline*	*Drug*
5-HTP	20	9	78.9 (5–100)	83.9 (40–100)	11	8.0 (0–55)	37.5* (0–90)
Quipazine	5	11	90 (50–100)	99.5*** (95–100)	29	45.0 (0–100)	81.8*** (45–100)
Cinanserin	10	26	94.4 (60–100)	83.2** (25–100)	14	33.2 (0–100)	31.7 (0–90)
Metergoline[a]	5	12	91.6 (65–199)	68.7* (25–100)	14	61.0 (0–100)	55.0 (0–95)

Significance between saline and drug treatments: $*P < 0.02$; $**P < 0.01$; $***P < 0.005$ by the Wilcoxon Matched-pair Test.
[a]1% ascorbic acid in saline used as the control vehicle.
[b]All drugs given 2 hours before test, except 5-HTP which was given 1 hour before test.

behaviour in suitably primed ovariectomised rats. Interestingly, injections of 5-HT into the 3rd ventricle were ineffective (Table 7). Foreman & Moss (1978*a*) report that administering 5-HT into the preoptic area or arcuate nucleus of the hypothalamus inhibited lordosis. Perhaps our injections into the third ventricle lead the amine to an inhibitory site (probably in the hypothalamus), while administration into the lateral ventricle brings the 5-HT to a stimulatory site.

Table 6. *The effect of progesterone on female sexual behaviour and hypothalamic indole compounds*

Treatment of ovariectomised rats primed with 2µg OB	*Dose/rat*	*No. of animals*	*Mean LQ (range)*	*Hypothalamic ng/100 mg* 5-HT ± SE	5-HIAA ± SE
Oil	0.2 ml	10	0%	220 ± 9	114 ± 5
Progesterone[a]	0.5 mg	10	66%*** (20 – 100)	196 ± 6*	126 ± 4

[a]Progesterone given 48 hours after OB and 4 hours before testing for receptivity.
Significance between oil treated and progesterone groups. $*P < 0.05$ compared by Student's *t-test:* $***P < 0.005$ compared by Mann Whitney U test.

Others have also obtained evidence that 5-HT is stimulatory to female sexual behaviour. Thus, selective 5-HT uptake inhibitors stimulated receptivity in ovariectomised-adrenalectomised female rats while inhibiting sexual behaviour in the male rat (Hamberger-Bar *et al.*, 1978). Quizapine has been reported to stimulate lordotic activity in transected spinalised rats but, in this case, it is probably acting on the descending serotonergic pathways (Kow *et al.*, 1979). Lesions of the midbrain raphe which destroy the ascending serotonergic pathway reduce female receptivity (Herndon, 1976).

Table 7. *Effect of intracerebrally administered 5-HT on female sexual behaviour*[a]

Treatment	*Site*	*No. of animals*	*Mean LQ (range)*	
			Pre-injection	*1 hour post-injection*
10μl saline	3rd ventricle	6	24.3% (0–60)	25.7% (0–70)
10μg 5-HT	3rd ventricle	7	20.0% (0–90)	35.7% (0–70)
100μg 5-HT	3rd ventricle	4	12.5% (0–50)	20.0% (0–40)
10μl saline	lateral ventricle	5	30.0% (0–70)	32.0% (0–70)
10μg 5-HT	lateral ventricle	7	20.0% (0–70)	46.2%* (0–100)
100μg 5-HT	lateral ventricle	4	30.0% (0–50)	70.0% (60–80)

[a]Rats primed with 0.25μg OB daily for 3 days followed by 0.2 mg progesterone on 4th day and 4 hours before testing.
Significance between pre and post-injection values: $*P < 0.02$ by the Wilcoxon Matched-pair Test.

Correlation of the inhibitory effect of PCPA on female sexual behaviour and hypothalamic indoleamine depletion

If 5-HT is stimulatory to female sexual behaviour, its depletion in the CNS should be

Table 8. *Investigation of the inhibitory effect of PCPA on female sexual behaviour*

Priming Treatment	*Drug Treatment*	*Dose mg/kg*	*No. of animals*	*Mean LQ% (range)*	*Hypothalamic ng/100 mg*	
					5-HT ± SE	*5/HIAA ± SE*
200μg OB 52 h before testing	—	—	23	77% (0–100)	—	—
,,	PCPA 24 h before testing	150	18	58.3% (15–90)	—	—
,,	PCPA 24 h & 48 h before testing	150 × 2	11	85.4% (45–100)	—	—
2μg OB 52 h before and 0.5 mg P 4 h before testing	—	—	16	74.7% (10–100)	179.5 ± 13.5	132 ± 6.5
,,	PCPA 24 h before testing	150	19	29.5** (0–70)	92.5*** ± 8.5	39*** ± 4
,,	PCPA 24 h before and 5-HTP 4 h before testing	150 20	19	54.5*†† (0–85)	103.5*** ± 11	65***† ± 10

Significance between control group and PCPA treated groups: $*P < 0.02$; $**P < 0.02$; $***P < 0.001$.
Significance between PCPA group and PCPA plus 5-HTP group. $†P < 0.05$; $††P < 0.02$.
Behaviour analysed by Mann-Whitney U test and indole compounds by Scheffés test after analysis of variance.

inhibitory. We have examined this possibility by administering PCPA 24 hours before testing for behaviour. At this time, inhibition of 5-HT synthesis is at its maximum and levels of both 5-HT and 5-HIAA are low. In addition, circulating PCPA has disappered and so no PCPEA is being produced.

Ovariectomised rats were made receptive by either priming with a single injection of 200 μg OB 52 hours before testing or with 2 μg OB followed 48 hours later by 0.5 mg progesterone. When PCPA (150 mg/kg) was administered 24 hours before testing, it had no effect on behaviour in the rats primed with oestrogen alone, but it inhibited receptivity in the group primed with oestrogen plus progesterone (see Table 8). Thus, it appears that 5-HT is not involved at all in the action of oestrogen in inducing receptivity, but that its presence is required for the receptive-inducing action of progesterone. The latter has been suggested before, based on results of two reports from Whalen's group who also showed that PCPA reduced the receptivity normally seen after oestrogen plus progesterone (Segal & Whalen, 1970; Gorzalka & Whalen, 1975). Sodersten *et al.* (1976*b*) report that PCPA did not reduce receptivity after oestrogen plus progesterone, but they used higher multiple priming doses of oestrogen than did Segal & Whalen (1970). The hypothesis was tested by attempting to reverse the inhibitory effect of PCPA by a concomitant injection of 20 mg/kg 5-HTP. Table 8 shows that this reversal did occur and that it correlated with an increase in brain 5-HIAA.

Interrelationship of progesterone and 5-HT on female sexual behaviour

The possible interrelationship between progesterone and 5-HT has been noted. Assuming that 5-HT is inhibitory to female sexual behaviour, Kow *et al.* (1974) have suggested that progesterone disinhibits inhibitory serotonergic neurones and more recently Sietnieks & Meyerson (1980, 1982) have shown that the inhibitory effect of 5-HT agonists on female receptivity increases with increasing concentrations of progesterone. They suggest that progesterone normally acts presynaptically to inhibit 5-HT neuronal release and that this induces a sensitization of the postsynaptic receptors.

We have also presented evidence showing that progesterone and 5-HT are interrelated in their effect on female sexual behaviour, but since we suggest that 5-HT activity is stimulatory to female sexual receptivity our interpretation is different. Because it is known that progesterone can stimulate 5-HT turnover (Ladisch, 1974; Cone *et al.*, 1981; see Table 7) and possibly synthesis rate (Crowley *et al.*, 1979), we suggest that in this manner it then stimulates female sexual behaviour. We further hypothesize that continuously raised 5-HT activity induces desensitization and this might explain the sequential inhibitory effect of progesterone in which refractoriness to a second injection of progesterone occurs (Morin, 1977). This refractoriness can be prevented by a protein synthesis inhibitor (Parsons & McEwen, 1981), possibly by inhibiting 5-HT synthesis enzyme production. It might also explain why 5-HTP and quipazine are inhibitory in rats primed with oestrogen and progesterone (Seitneiks & Meyerson, 1982; Rodriguez-Sierra & Davis, 1979); their administration tending to accelerate the desensitization of the postsynaptic 5-HT receptors and thus terminating the effect of progesterone.

Summary and conclusions

We have shown that the stimulatory effect of PCPA on female sexual behaviour is not due to depletion of brain indoleamines and, therefore, our data do not support the hypothesis that 5-HT plays an inhibitory role in the control of female receptivity in the rodent. We have investigated other possible mechanisms by which PCPA might exert its stimulatory effect and these are: (1) by stimulating production of adrenal progesterone, although this effect is slight; and (2) by acting via its metabolite PCPEA and, in turn, altering NA activity or stimulating the release of 5-HT.

We have presented some preliminary evidence that 5-HT has a stimulatory effect on female sexual behaviour and more clear-cut evidence that depletion of 5-HT is inhibitory to this behaviour. Finally, we have suggested that progesterone exerts its behavioural effects via stimulation of 5-HT turnover.

However, the many results of experiments described in the literature in which administration of 5-HT agonists and antagonists inhibit and stimulate receptivity, respectively, and which thus support the traditional view of the inhibitory role of 5-HT, must be explained. Just as we have shown that the actions of PCPA are multiple and that the interpretation of some of the experiments in which it has been used are open to question, it is possible that experiments using other compounds can be re-interpreted according to the variety of activities these compounds are known to possess. For instance, cinanserin has a direct neuronal depressant action (Segal, 1976), methysergide is a potent DA antagonist (MacLeod & Login, 1977) and both of these compounds are partial 5-HT agonists (Colpaert *et al.*, 1979). Most seriously of all, doubts have been shed on whether the 5-HT receptor blockers actually bind at all to 5-HT receptors within the CNS (Haigler & Aghajanian, 1974; Jacoby *et al.*, 1978). Another example is the drug LSD which has been considered as a 5-HT agonist in behavioural experiments (Everitt & Fuxe, 1977; Sietnieks & Meyerson, 1980) but is also a DA agonist (Creese *et al.*, 1975). Green *et al.* (1981) have stated that behavioural data obtained by using 5-HT agonists and antagonists should be interpreted with 'extreme care'. Our work confirms this statement, and extends it to the serotonin synthesis inhibitor PCPA.

Acknowledgements—We gratefully thank the relevant firms for their gifts of quipazine (Miles Laboratories Ltd), metergoline (Montedison Pharmaceutical Ltd), cinanserin (Squibb & Son Ltd) and benserazide (Hoffman, La Roche & Co). Some of this work was generously supported by the Wellcome Foundation.

References

Ahlenius, S., Eriksson, H., Larsson, K., Modigh, K. & Sodersten, P. (1971): Mating behaviour in the male rat treated with p-chlorophenylalanine methyl ester alone and in combination with pargyline. *Psychopharmalogia* **20,** 383-388.

Ahlenius, S., Engel, J., Eriksson, H., Modigh, K. & Sodersten, P. (1972): Importance of central catecholamines in the mediation of lordosis behaviour in ovariectomised rats treated with oestrogen and inhibitors of monoamine synthesis. *J. Neural. Transm.* **33,** 247-255.

Ahlenius, S., Heinmann, M. & Larsson, K. (1979): Prolongation of the ejaculation latency in the male rat by thioradazine and chlorimipramine. *Psychopharmacol.* **65,** 137-140.

Ahlenius, S., Larsson, K. & Svensson, L. (1980): Further evidence for an inhibitory role of central 5-HT in male rat sexual behaviour. *Psychopharmacol.* **68,** 217-220.

Al Satli, M. & Aron, Cl. (1981): Role played by serotonin in the control of estrous receptivity, ovarian activity and ovulation in the cyclic female rat. *Psychoneuroendocrinol.* **6,** 121-129.

Benkert, O. & Eversmann, T. (1972): Importance of the anti-serotonin effect for mounting behaviour in rats. *Experientia* **28,** 332-533.

Bertolini, A. (1971): Different type of sexual excitement produced in rats by intraliquoral ACTH and by intraperitoneal p-chlorophenylalanine. *Rivista di Pharmac. Terap.* **11,** 1023-1024.

Booth, J.E., van der Schoot, P. & Moleman, P. (1979): Parachlorophenylalanine and copulatory behaviour in neo-natally castrated male rats. *Psychol. Behav.* **23,** 701-707.

Borbely, A.A., Neuhaus, H.U. & Tobler, I. (1981): Effect of p-chlorophenylalanine and tryptophan on sleep EEG and motor activity in the rat. *Behav. Brain Res.* **2,** 1-22.
Breisch, S.T., Zemlan, F.P. & Hoebel, B.G. (1976): Hyperphagia and obesity following serotonin depletion by intraventricular p-chlorophenylalanine. *Science* **192,** 382-384.
Carter, C.S., Bahr, J.M. & Ramirez, V.D. (1978): Monoamines, estrogen and female sexual behaviour in the golden hamster. *Brain Res.* **144,** 109-121.
Colpaert, F.C., Niemegeers, C.J.E. & Janssen, R.A.J. (1979): *In vivo* evidence of partial agonist activity exerted by purported 5-hydroxytryptamine antagonists. *Europ. J. Pharmacol.* **58,** 505-509.
Cone, R.D., Davis, G.A. & Goy, R.W. (1981): Effects of ovarian steroids on serotonin metabolism within grossly dissected and microdissected brain regions of the ovariectomised rat. *Brain Res. Bull.* **7,**. 639-644.
Coscina, D.V., Daniel, J. & Warsh, J.J. (1978): Potential non-serotonergic basis of hyperphagia elicited by intraventricular p-chlorophenylalanine. *Pharmac. Biochem. Behav.* **9,** 791-797.
Creese, I., Burt, D.R. & Snyder, S.H. (1975): The dopamine receptor differential binding of d-LSD and related agents to agonist and antagonist states. *Life Sci.* **17,** 1715-1717.
Crowley, W.R., O'Donohue, T.L., Muth, A. & Jacobowitz, D.M. (1979): Effects of ovarian hormones on levels of luteinizing hormone in plasma and on serotonin concentrations in discrete brain nuclei. *Brain Res. Bull.* **4,** 571-574.
Dahlof, L.G. & Larsson, K. (1979): PCPA potentiates the effects of specific copulatory experience on the sexual behaviour of the pudentectomized male rat. *Pharmac. Biochem. Behav.* **11,** 701-704.
Dalhouse, A.D. (1976): Social cohesiveness, hypersexuality and irritability induced by p-CPA in the rat. *Physiol. Behav.* **17,** 679-686.
Da Prada, M., Carruba, M., O'Brien, R.A., Saner, A. & Pletscher, A. (1972): The effect of 5,6-dihydroxytryptamine on sexual behaviour of male rats. *Eur. J. Pharmac.* **19,** 288-290.
Davis, G.A. & Kohl, R. (1977): The influence of α-receptors on lordosis in the female rat. *Pharmac. Biochem. Behav.* **6,** 47-53.
Davis, G.A. & Kohl, R.L. (1978): Biphasic effects of the antiserotonergic methysergide on lordosis in rats. *Pharmac. Biochem. Behav.* **9,** 487-491.
Deguchi, T. & Barchas, J. (1972): Effect of p-chlorophenylalanine on tryptophan hydroxylase in rat pineal. *Nature* **235,** 92-93.
Edwards, D.J. & Blau, K. (1972): The *in-vivo* formation of p-chloro-ß-phenylethylamine in young rats injected with p-chlorophenylalanine. *J. Neurochem.* **19,** 1829-1832.
Eliasson, M. & Meyerson, B.J. (1977): The effects of lysergic acid diethylamide on copulatory behaviour in the female rat. *Neuropharmacol.* **16,** 37-44.
Eriksson, H. & Sodersten, P. (1973): A failure to facilitate lordosis behaviour in adrenalectomized and gonadoectomized oestrogen-primed rats with monoamine-synthesis inhibitors. *Hormones Behav.* **4,** 89-98.
Everitt, B.J., Fuxe, K. & Hokfelt, T. (1974): Inhibitory role of dopamine and 5-hydroxytryptamine on the sexual behaviour of female rats. *Eur. J. Pharmac.* **29,** 187-191.
Everitt, B.J., Fuxe, K. & Hokfelt, T. (1975*a*): Serotonin, catecholamines and sexual receptivity of female rats. Pharmacological findings. *J. Pharmac.* (Paris) **6,** 269-276.
Everitt, B.J., Fuxe, K. & Jonsson, G. (1975*b*): The effects of 5,7-dihydroxytryptamine pathways on the sexual and aggressive behaviour of female rats. *J. Pharmac.* (Paris) **6,** 25-32.
Everitt, B.J., Fuxe, K., Hokfelt, T. & Jonsson, G. (1975*c*): Role of monoamines in the control of hormones of sexual receptivity in the female rat. *J. Comp. Physiol. Psychol.* **89,** 556-572.
Everitt, B.J. & Fuxe, K. (1977): Serotonin and sexual behaviour in female rats. Effects of hallucinogenic indolealkylamines and phenylethylamines. *Neurosci. Lett.* **4,** 215-220.
Farabollini, F. & di Prisco, Ch. (1981): Modifications of brain steroidogenesis and plasma steroids after p-chlorophenylalanine-methyl-ester treatment. *Pharmacol. Biochem. Behav.* **14,** 911-914.
Ferguson, J., Henrickson, S., Cohen, H., Mitchell, G., Barchas, J. & Dement, W. (1970): Hypersexuality and behavioural changes in cats caused by administration of p-chlorophenylalanine. *Science* **168,** 499-501.

Foreman, M.M. & Moss, R.L. (1978*a*): Role of hypothalamic serotonergic receptors in the control of lordosis behaviour in the female rat. *Horm. Behav.* **10,** 97-106.
Foreman, M.M. & Moss, R.L. (1978*b*): Role of hypothalamic alpha and beta adrenergic receptors in the control of lordotic behaviour in the ovariectomised-oestrogen primed rats. *Pharmac. Biochem. Behav.* **9,** 235-241.
Franck, J.A.E. & Ward, I.L. (1981): Intralimbic progesterone and methysergide facilitate lordotic behaviour in estrogen-primed female rats. *Neuroendocrinol.* **32,** 50-56.
Fuller, R.W., Roush, B.W., Snoddy, H.D., Day, W.A. & Molloy, B.B. (1975): Norepinephrine-N-methyltransferase inhibition by benzamidines, phenylacetamidines, benzylyguanidines and phenylethylguanidines. *J. Med. Chem.* **18,** 304-306.
Gessa, G.L., Tagliamonte, A., Tagliamonte, P. & Brodie, B.B. (1970): Essential role of testosterone in the sexual stimulation induced by p-chlorophenylalanine in male animals. *Nature* **227,** 616-617.
Ginton, A. (19076): Copulation in noncopulators. Effect of PCPA in male rats. *Pharmac. Biochem. Behav.* **4,** 357-359.
Gold, M.S., Donabedian, R.K. & Redmond, D.E. (1978): Effect of piperoxane on serum prolactin: possible role of epinephrine-mediated synapses in the inhibition of prolactin secretion. *Endocrinol.* **102,** 1183-1188.
Gorzalka, B.B. & Whalen, R.E. (1975): Inhibition, not facilitation of sexual behaviour by PCPA. *Pharmac. Biochem. Behav.* **3,** 511-513.
Green, A.R., Hall, J.E. & Rees, A.J. (1981): A behavioural and biochemical study in rats of 5-hydroxytryptamine receptor agonists and antagonists with observations on structure-activity requirements for the agonists. *Brit. J. Pharmac.* **73,** 703-719.
Haigler, J.H. & Aghajanian, G.K. (1974): Peripheral serotonin antagonists: failure to antagonise serotonin in brain areas receiving a prominent serotonergic input. *J. Neurol. Trans.* **35,** 257-273.
Hamberger-Bar, R., Rigter, H. & Dekker, I. (1978): Inhibition of serotonin reuptake differentially affects heterosexual behaviour of male and female rats. *Life Sci.* **22,** 1827-1836.
Hansen, S., Stanfield, E.J. & Everitt, B.J. (1980): The role of ventral bundle noradrenergic neurons in sensory components of sexual behaviours and coitus-induced psuedopregnancy. *Nature* **286,** 152-154.
Humphries, C.R., O'Brien, M. & Paxinos, C. (1980): Effects on ejaculation, thermoregulation, salivation and irritability in rats. *Pharmac. Biochem. Behav.* **12,** 851-854.
Herndon, J.G. (1976): Effects of midbrain lesions on female sexual behaviour in the rat. *Physiol. Behav.* **17,** 143-148.
Hyyppa, M., Lehtinen, P. & Rinne, U.K. (1971): Effect of l-dopa on hypothalamic, pineal and striatal monoamines and on the sexual behaviour of the rat. *Brain Res.* **30,** 265-272.
Irving, S.M., Goy, R.W., Haning, R.V. & Davis, G.A. (1981): Prostaglandins, clonidine and sexual receptivity in the guinea-pig. *Brain Res.* **204,** 65-77.
Jacoby, J.H., Poulakos, J.J. & Bryce, G.F. (1978): On the central antiserotoninergic actions of cyproheptadine and methysergide. *Neuropharmacol.* **17,** 299-306.
Koe, B.K. & Weissman, A. (1966): P-Chlorophenylalanine: a specific depletor of brain serotonin. *J. Pharmac. Exp. Ther.* **154,** 499-516.
Kow, L.M., Malsburg, C.W. & Pfaff, D.W. (1974): Effects of progesterone on female reproductive behaviour in rats: possible models of action and role in behavioural sex differences. In *Reproductive behaviour,* eds Montagna, W. & Sadler, W.A. New York: Plenum Publishing Co. Pp 179-210.
Kow, L.M., Zemlan, F.P. & Pfaff, D.W. (1979): Attempts to reinstate lordosis reflex in estrogen-primed spinal female rats with neuroamine agonists. *Horm. Behav.* **13,** 232-240.
Ladisch, W. (1974): Effect of progesterone on regional 5-hydroxytryptamine metabolism in the rat brain. *Neuropharmacol.* **13,** 877-883.
Larsson, K., Fuxe, K., Everitt, B.J., Holmgren, M. & Sodersten, P. (1978): Sexual behaviour in male rats after intracerebral injection of 5,7-dihydroxytrypatime. *Brain Res.* **141,** 293-306.
Luttge, W.G. (1975): Stimulation of estrogen induced copulatory behaviour in castrated male rats with the serotonin biosynthesis inhibitor p-chlorophenylalanine. *Behav. Biol.* **14,** 373-378.
MacLeod, R.M. & Login, I.S. (1977): Regulation of prolactin secretion through dopamine,

serotonin and the cerebrospinal fluid. In *Advances in psychopharmacology,* Vol. 16, eds Costa, E. and Gessa, G.L. New York: Raven Press. Pp 147-158.
Malmas, C.O. & Meyerson, B.J. (1971): P-Chlorophenylalanine and copulatory behaviour in the male rat. *Nature* **232,** 398-400.
Marsden, C.A. & Curzon, G. (1976): Studies on the behavioural effects of tryptophan and p-chlorophenylalanine. *Neuropharmacol.* **15,** 165-171.
Matte, C.A. & Tornow, H. (1978): Parachlorophenylalanine produces dissociated effects on aggression 'emotionality' and motor activity. *Neuropharmacol.* **17,** 555-558.
McBride, W.J., Penn, P.E., Hyde, T.P., Lane, J.D. & Smith, J.E. (1976): Effects of p-chlorophenylalanine on the metabolism of serotonin from 5-hydroxy-tryptophan. *Neurochem. Res.* **1,** 437-449.
Meyerson, B.J. (1964): Central nervous system monoamines and oestrus behaviour in the spayed rat. *Acta Physiol. Scand.* **63,** Suppl. 1, 16-32.
Meyerson, B.J. & Lewander, T. (1970): Serotonin synthesis inhibition and oestrous behaviour in female rats. *Life Sci.* **9,** 661-671.
Miller, F.P., Cox, R.H., Snodgrass, W.R. & Maickel, R.P. (1970): Comparative effects of p-chlorophenylalanine, p-chloroamphetamine and p-chloro-N-methyl-amphetamine on rat brain norepinephrine, serotonin and 5-hydroxyindole-3-acetic acid. *Biochem. Pharmac.* **19,** 435-442.
Mitler, M.M., Morden, B., Levine, S. & Dement, W. (1972): The effects of parachlorophenylalanine on the mating behaviour of male rats. *Physiol. Behav.* **8,** 1147-1150.
Morin, L. (1977): Progesterone: inhibition of rodent sexual behaviour. *Physiol. Behav.* **18,** 701-715.
Nock, B. & Feder, H.H. (1979): Noradrenergic transmission and female sexual behaviour of guinea pigs. *Brain Res.* **166,** 369-380.
Ogren, S.O., Fuxe, K., Archer, T., Hall, H., Holm, A.C. & Kohler, C. (1981): Studies on the role of central 5-HT neurones in avoidance learning: a behavioural and biochemical analysis. In *Serotonin: current aspects of neurochemistry and function,* eds Haber, B., Gabay, S., Issidorides, M.R. and Alivisatos, G.S.A. New York: Plenum Publishing Co. Pp 681-705.
Parsons, B. & McEwen, B.S. (1981): Sequential inhibition of sexual receptivity by progesterone is prevented by a protein synthesis inhibitor and is not causally related to decreased levels of hypothalamic progestin receptors in the female rat. *J. Neurosci.* **1,** 527-531.
Perez-Gruent, J., Tagliamonte, A., Tagliamonte, P. & Gessa, G.L. (1971): Differential effect of p-chlorophenylalanine (PCPA) on sexual behaviour and on sleep patterns of male rabbits. *Rivista di Farmac. Terap.* **11,** 27-34.
Pujol, J.F., Keane, P., McRae, A., Lewis, B.D. & Renaud, B. (1978): Biochemical evidence for serotonergic control of the locus coeruleus. In *Interactions between putative neurotransmitters in the brain,* eds Garattini, S., Pujol, J.F. and Samanin, R. New York: Raven Press. Pp 410-419.
Reader, T.A. (1982): Catecholamines and serotonin in fat frontal cortex after PCPA and 6-OHDA: absolute amounts and ratios. *Brain Res. Bull.* **8,** 527-534.
Rodriguez-Sierra, J.F., Naggar, A.N. & Komisaruk, B.R. (1976): Monoaminergic mediation of masculine and feminine copulatory behaviour in female rats. *Pharmacol. Biochem. Behav.* **5,** 457-463.
Rodriguez-Sierra, J.F. & Davis, G.A. (1979): Tolerance to the lordosis facilitating effects of progesterone or methysergide. *Neuropharmacol.* **18,** 335-339.
Salis, P.G. & Dewsbury, D.A. (1971): P-chlorophenylalanine facilitates copulatory behaviour in male rats. *Nature* **232,** 400-401.
Segal, D.A. & Whalen, R.E. (1970): Effect of chronic administration of P-chlorophenylalanine on sexual receptivity of the female rat. *Psychopharmacologia* **16,** 434-438.
Segal, M. (1976): 5-HT antagonists in rat hippocampus. *Brain Res.* **103,** 161-166.
Sheard, M.H. (1969): The effects of p-chlorophenylalanine on behaviour in rats: relation to brain serotonin and 5-hydroxyindole acetic acid. *Brain Res.* **15,** 524-528.
Sietnieks, A. & Meyerson, B.J. (1980): Enhancement by progesterone of lysergic acid diethylamide inhibition of the copulatory response in the female rat. *Eur. J. Pharmac.* **63,** 57-64.

Sietnieks, A. & Meyerson, B.J. (1982): Enhancement by progesterone of 5-hydroxytryptophan inhibition of the copulatory response in the femalıe rat. *Neuroendocrinol.* **35,** 321-326.
Singer, J.J. (1972): Effects of P-chlorophenylalanine on male and female sexual behaviour of female rats. *Psychol. Rep.* **30,** 891-893.
Sloviter, R.S., Drust, E.G. & Connor, J.D. (1978): Serotonin agonist actions of p-chlorophenylalanine. *Neuropharmacol.* **17,** 1029-1033.
Sodersten, P., Larsson, K., Ahlenius, S. & Engel, J. (1976*a*): Sexual behaviour in castrated male rats treated with monoamine synthesis inhibitors and testosterone. *Pharmac. Biochem. Behav.* **5,** 319-327.
Sodersten, P., Larsson, K., Ahlenius, S. & Engel, J. (1976*b*): Stimulation of mounting behaviour but not lordosis behaviour in ovariectomized female rats by p-chlorophenylalanine. *Pharmac, Biochem. Behav.* **5,** 329-333.
Sodersten, P., Berge, O.G. & Hole, K. (1978): Effects of p-chloroamphetaime and 5,7-dihydroxytryptamine on the sexual behaviour of gonadectomized male and female rats. *Pharmac. Biochem. Behav.* **9,** 499-508.
Steigrad, P., Tobler, I., Naser, P.G. & Borbely, A.A. (1978): Effect of p-chlorophenylalanine on cerebral serotonin binding, serotonin concentration and motor activity in the rat. *N-S Archs Pharmacol.* **305,** 143-148.
Tagliamonte, A., Tagliamonte, M., Gessa, G.L. & Brodie, B.B. (1969): Compulsive sexual activity induced by P-chlorophenylalanine in normal and pinealectomised male rats. *Science* **166,** 1433-1435.
Valzelli, L., Bernasconi, S. & Garattini, S. (1981): p-Chlorophenylalanine-induced muricidal aggression in male and female laboratory rats. *Neuropsychobiol.* **7,** 315-320.
Van de Poll, N.E., van Dis, H. & Bermond, B. (1977): The induction of mounting behaviour in female rats by P-chlorophenylalanine. *Eur. J. Pharmac.* **41,** 225-229.
Ward, I.L., Crowley, W.R. & Zemlan, F.P. (1975): Monoaminergic mediation of female sexual behaviour. *J. Comp. Physiol. Psychol.* **88,** 53-61.
Whalen, R.E. & Luttge, W.G. (1970): p-Chlorophenylalanine methyl ester: an aphrodisiac? *Science* **169,** 1000-1001.
Wilson, C.A., Andrews, M., Hadley, J.C., Lemon, M. & Yeo, T. (:1977): The role of hypothalamic serotonin (5HT) before ovulation in immature rats treated with PMS. *Psychoneuroendocrinol.* **2,** 267-274.
Wilson, C.A., Bonney, R.C., Everard, D.M., Parrott, R.F. & Wise, J. (1982): Mechanisms of action of p-chlorophenylalanine in stimulating sexual receptivity in the female rat. *Pharmacol. Biochem. Behav.* **16,** 777-784.
Zemlan, F.P., Ward, I.L., Crowley, W.R. & Margules, D.L. (1973): Activation of lordotic responses in female rats by suppression of serotonergic activity. *Science* **179,** 1010-1011.
Zemlan, F.P., Trulson, M.E., Howell, R. & Hoebel, B.G. (1977): Influence of P-chloroamphetamine on female sexual reflexes and brain monoamine levels. *Brain Res.* **123,** 347-356.
Zitrin, A., Beach, F.A., Barchas, J.D. & Dement, W.C. (1970): Sexual behaviour of male cats after administration of parachlorophenylalanine. *Science* **170,** 868-870..

4

Endogenous opiates and the mechanisms of male sexual behavior

Michael R. MURPHY

Systems Research Laboratories, Inc., PO Box 35313, Brooks Air Force Base, Texas 78235, USA

Introduction

Endogenous opiates are chemicals that are produced by the body and have morphine-like effects. They are essentially 'the body's own morphine', hence their generic name of 'endorphins'. The stereospecific receptors for endogenous opiates were discovered in 1973 and two years later the first opiate peptides were isolated and identified. Since then, several endogenous, morphine-like, peptides have been found, including met-enkephalin, leu-enkephalin, beta-endorphin and dynorphin (see Olson *et al.*, 1979).

This recent discovery of endogenous opiates has led to increased interest in the effects of opiates on sexual function and to speculation that they may be involved in the regulation of sexual behavior and reproduction. The purpose of this paper is to discuss the relationship between endogenous opiates and the mechanisms of male sexual behavior. First, some of the literature which indicates that endogenous opiates are involved in sexual behavior will be reviewed and, secondly, four specific ways are suggested in which endogenous opiates might participate in the mechanisms of sexual function.

Evidence for endogenous opiate involvement in male sexual behavior

Effects of opiates on sexual behavior

Although the study of endogenous opiates is less than a decade old, the fact that opiate drugs affect sexual function has been known for centuries. In 1563 the Portuguese physician Garcia D'Orta wrote that he had heard of opium being used to enhance sexual pleasure but that, in his opinion, the drug only served to diminish sexual function and that its frequent use would lead to total impotence (Guerra, 1974).

More recent clinical observations and research have supported D'Orta's views, indicating that the use of opiate drugs by males can cause: depressed libido, impotence, delayed ejaculation, decreased sexual pleasure, absence of sexual dreams, and decreased nocturnal emissions (eg Cicero *et al.*, 1975; Cushman, 1972; Mintz *et al.*, 1974; Parr, 1976). The opinion that opiates are sometimes beneficial to sexuality can be traced to their ability to delay ejaculation, which might be helpful to those suffering from premature ejaculation.

Many of the effects of opiate addiction on male sexual behavior can be modeled by

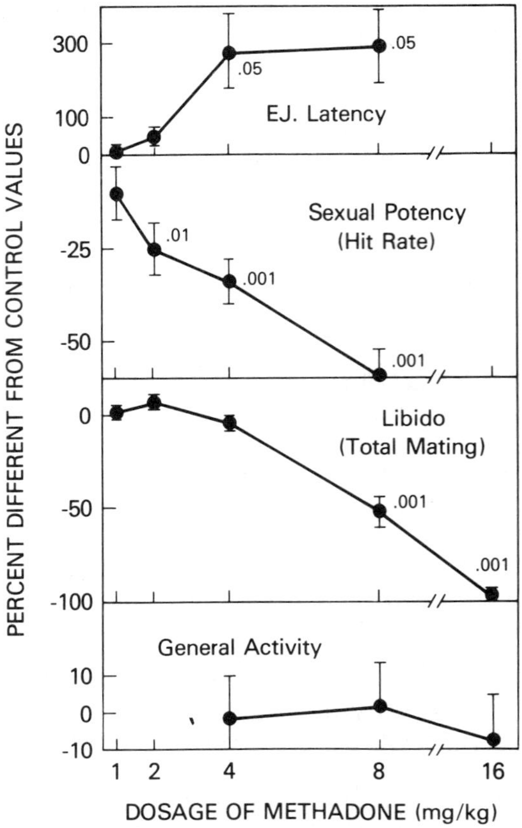

Fig. 1. *Effects of methadone on the sexual behavior of male hamsters.* Ejaculatory latency is the time between the first intromission and the first ejaculation. Sexual potency is measured by 'hit rate', which is computed as the per cent of correctly oriented mounts that result in penile intromission. Libido (total mating) is a summation of all time spent copulating, attempting to copulate and licking own or female's genitalia

the acute administration of opiates to experimental animals. For example, in male Syrian golden hamsters, methadone causes a dose-related increase in ejaculatory latency while decreasing both sexual potency and libido (Fig. 1). Sexual potency, here defined as the ability to gain penile erection and vaginal intromission, was reduced significantly by 2 mg/kg of methadone. Libido, however, defined as the total time engaged in mating activity, was only affected when the dose reached 8 mg/kg. Thus, as is also the case with alcohol, sexual performance is significantly more sensitive to opiate drugs than sexual motivation.

The ineffectiveness of methadone, even at the highest dose (16 mg/kg), on general activity (Fig. 1) indicates that its action on sexual behavior is somewhat specific. A similar conclusion can be inferred from the data shown in Fig. 2 in which the effects of methadone on two types of body manipulation are presented in graphical form. One of these activities, self-licking of the genitalia, is primarily a sexual activity, while the other, self grooming, is primarily non-sexual. As can be seen, with the higher doses of methadone sexual manipulation decreased, whereas non-sexual activity increased. Since both behaviors are forms of body manipulation involving the mouth and forepaws, this dissociation again indicates a specific effect of opiates on sexually related behaviors.

As with hamsters and man, the sexual behavior of other species is similarly debilitated by opiate drugs, and in the rat it has been shown that direct administration of opiate peptides into the ventricles of the brain eliminates sexual behavior without

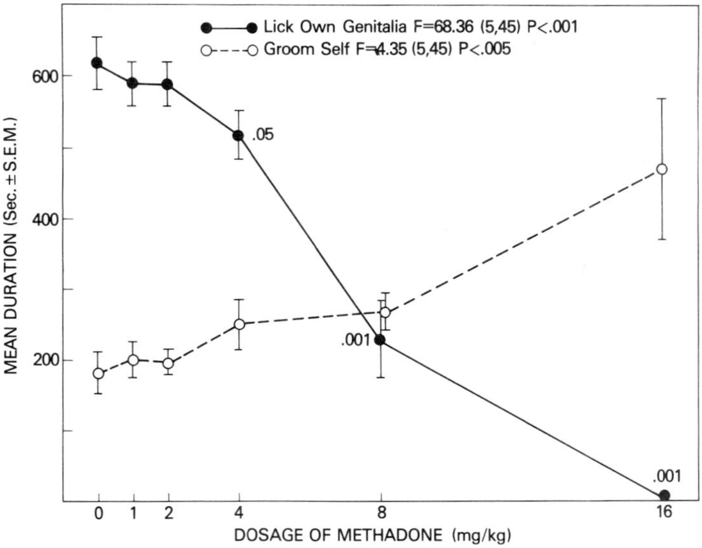

Fig. 2. *Effects of methadone on two aspects of body manipulation in the male hamster*

affecting motor, feeding or courtship behaviors (Meyerson & Terenius, 1977; Gessa *et al.*, 1979). Thus, there are considerable data from several species which show that sexual behavior is specifically sensitive to both exogenous and endogenous opiates.

Effects of opiate blockers on sexual behavior

In addition to the opiates themselves, another class of drugs that bind to opiate receptors are the opiate antagonists. These drugs compete with opiates at the receptor level and, therefore, depending on whether they are given before or after an opiate, will prevent or reverse its effect.

The ability of the opiate antagonist naltrexone to influence the sexual inhibiting effects of methadone in the Syrian hamster is significant. When methadone at 16 mg/kg was followed by an injection of saline, it completely eliminated all sexual behavior. However, when followed by naltrexone, 100% of the hamsters mated, with a mean latency of 120 seconds. If the saline control injection was given before the methadone, the sexual behavior was again eliminated; however, administration of naltrexone before methadone caused all animals to mate, with a mean latency of just 40 seconds. Similar results have been reported for the rat, and data have also been presented relating to the ability of opiate antagonists to reverse the sexual inhibiting effects of intraventricularly administered opiate peptides (Meyerson & Terenius, 1977; Gessa *et al.*, 1979).

The ability of opiate antagonists to transform an opiate-treated animal from one who is completely sexually apathetic into a vigorous copulator within a few seconds is quite dramatic. However, from a theoretical, mechanistic viewpoint, what is more important than this ability to interact with opiate drugs is the assumed ability of opiate antagonists to interfere with the functions of endogenous opiates. It would, thus, appear that by administering opiate antagonists to otherwise drug-free individuals one can examine the effects of inhibiting the action of endogenous opiates and thereby gain some understanding of their functions. While this rationale is by no means perfect (Sawynok *et al.*, 1979), it has been used extensively in studying the functions of endogenous opiates.

Opiate blocking drugs have been reported to have a variety of effects on male sexual behavior. They facilitate mating in the hamster and rat, primarily by decreasing the time and effort needed to achieve ejaculation (eg Murphy, unpublished data; Myers & Baum, 1979). They increase sexual potency in the hamster, apparently by a direct action on the ability to achieve erection (Murphy, 1980, 1981). In man and monkey, they elicit spontaneous erections in non-sexual situations (Braude & Morrison, 1976; Mendelson *et al.*, 1979) and in the hamster and rat they may delay the initiation of copulation and lengthen the post-ejaculatory interval (Murphy, 1980; Sachs *et al.*, 1981).

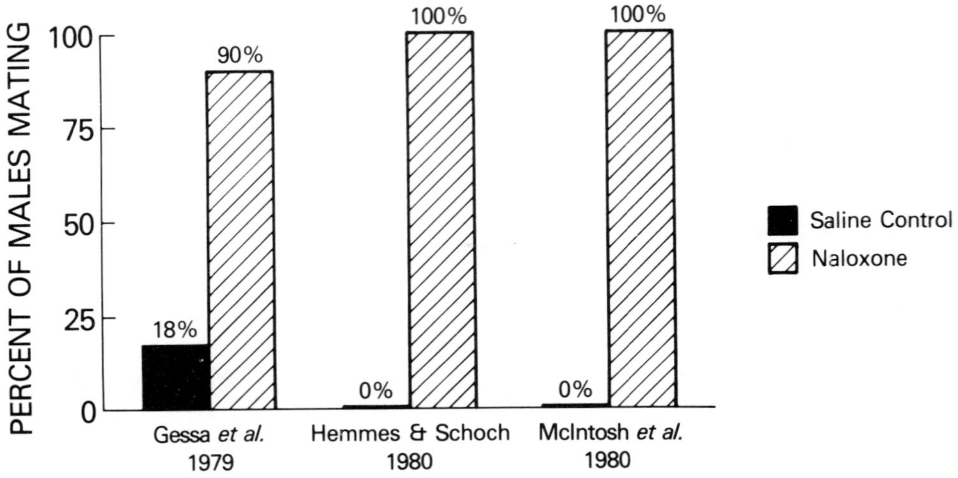

Fig. 3. *Summary of the results of three studies showing the stimulatory effect of naloxone on the mating bahavior of otherwise non-copulating male rats.*

Probably the most dramatic effect of an opiate antagonist on male sexual behavior is the ability of naloxone to elicit sexual behavior from non-copulatory male rats. The results of three studies have demonstrated this phenomenon (Fig. 3). In work reported by Gessa *et al.* (1979) and McIntosh *et al.* (1980), normal male laboratory rats were used. As is often the case with laboratory rats, some of the animals showed no interest in mating. However, after an injection of the opiate antagonist naloxone, almost every previously non-copulating rat started to mate. One week later, following a control injection of saline, these rats again failed to mate. In the study reported by Hemmes & Schoch (1980), a genetically obese strain of male rats was used. In addition to being overweight, this strain usually demonstrates a low interest in mating. However, these animals mated normally after an injection of the opiate blocker naloxone. An intriguing complement to this finding is that biochemical analysis has shown that rats of this specific obese strain have a chronically high level of beta-endorphin (Margules *et al.*, 1978; Gibson *et al.*, 1981). Although not yet tested, it is tempting to speculate that the failure of these obese rats, as well as of 'normal' non-copulatory male rats, to mate was due to an abnormally high level of an endogenous opiate that was suppressing sexual motivation and that the opiate antagonist elicitied mating by removing this inhibitory influence. Of course, it would also be of considerable interest to determine

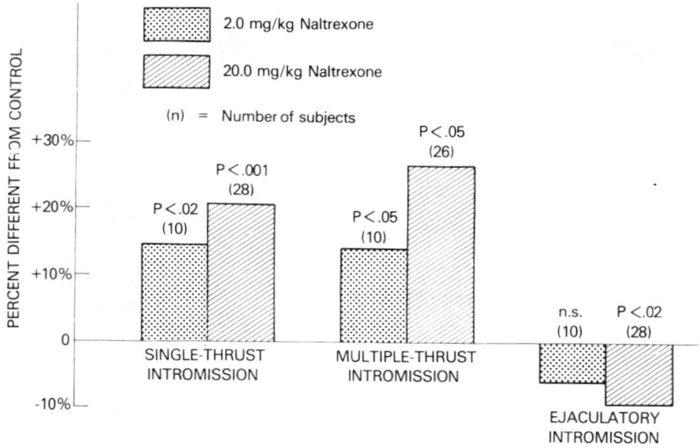

Fig. 4. *Effects of naltrexone on the average duration of three types of intromissions in the male hamster*

whether or not aberrant levels of endogenous opiates are responsible for any human sexual dysfunctions.

Another dramatic effect of opiate antagonists is the ability of naltrexone to increase the sexual potency of male hamsters. In contrast to the inhibitory effects of methadone (Fig. 1), naltrexone causes significnt improvement in relative sexual potency (Murphy, 1980, 1981). The suggestion that opiate antagonists are involved in mechanisms of penile erection is supported also by the analysis of the average duration of penile insertion in the hamster. The time that the male leaves his penis in the female reflects the quality of the erection. This time is decreased by methadone but is increased by the opiate antagonist naltrexone (Fig. 4) (Murphy, 1980, 1981).

Effects of copulation on endogenous opiates

A third area of research that relates endogenous opiates to sexual function is that of the effects of copulation on endogenous opiates. Three types of experiments have been carried out. First, serum levels of beta-endorphin-like immunoreactivity have been shown to increase during active copulation in the male hamster (Murphy *et al.*, 1979). Secondly, endogenous opiate systems have generally been found to be activated during copulation in the male rat (Szechtman *et al.*, 1981). And thirdly, a state of relative analgesia is produced during copulation in male rats (Szechtman *et al.*, 1981), hamsters (Noble, 1980) and humans (Kinsey *et al.*, 1953). This third point is important because it is well known that opiates produce analgesia, and it is assumed that the analgesia produced during copulation is mediated by endogenous opiates released during mating activity.

The effects of copulation on serum levels of an endogenous opiate are shown in more detail in Fig. 5. Under otherwise identical conditions, blood was collected from male hamsters that were not allowed to mate, from males immediately after their fifth ejaculation and from males that were approaching sexual exhaustion. It was found that levels of beta-endorphin-like immunoreativity were low in animals that did not mate, were increased significantly during active copulation, and then began to decline as the animals approach sexual exhaustion (Murphy *et al.*, 1979). Subsequent studies have indicated that the critical event for maintaining high levels of beta-endorphin is the stimulation of active copulation. When copulation ceases (for example, if the female hamster is removed), beta-endorphin levels decline.

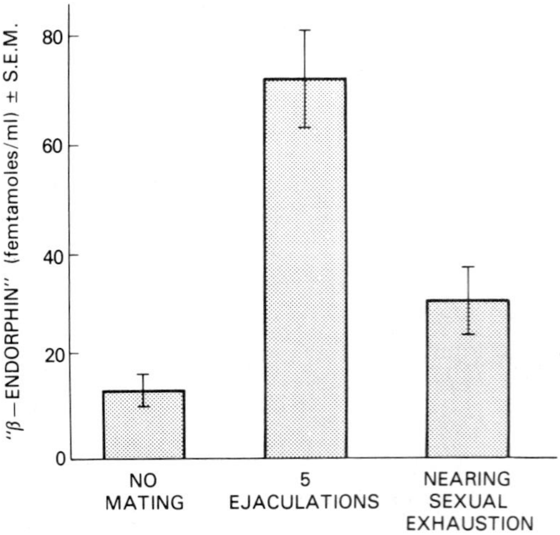

Fig. 5. *Effect of copulation on serum level of β-endorphin-like immunoreactivity in the male hamster*

Suggested mechanisms of endogenous opiate involvement in male sexual behavior

In the first part of this paper three types of evidence indicating that endogenous opiates are involved fundamentally in male sexual behavior were reviewed. These are that: opiates reduce sexual performance and motivation; opiate antagonists elicit and facilitate sexual behavior; and, copulatory activity releases endogenous opiates. In the second part of this paper, we propose and discuss four specific mechanisms by which such involvement might occur.

Opiates and the peripheral mechanisms of reproduction

The first hypothesis is that endogenous opiates are involved in the peripheral, or genital, mechanisms of sexual behavior. Endogenous opiates have been identified in human semen (Sharp & Pekary, 1981), in the prostate and in the seminal vesicle (Vaalasti *et al.*, 1980) and in rat testis, seminal vesicle and prostate (Sharp *et al.*, 1980). Opiate receptors have been found in the vas deferens of the rat and mouse (Huidobro-Toro & Way, 1981) and in the hamster seminal vesicle (Quirion, Murphy & Pert, unpublished observations, 1981). Since the effect of opiates *in vitro* is to inhibit the contractions of the vas deferens and seminal vesicle, it can be assumed that endogenous opiates would act to inhibit these same structures in the living organism. Considering the natural role of the accessory reproductive organs, it can further be hypothesized that one function of endogenous opiates is to regulate ejaculate volume and sperm count by inhibiting contractions of the vas deferens and the seminal vesicle, and perhaps, thereby, indirectly influencing the timing of ejaculation or other parameters of sexual behavior. This hypothesis has not been tested, but if it were substantiated it would suggest that opiates and opiate antagonists might be useful in controlling fertility. For example, opiate antagonists might be expected to increase sperm count and ejaculate volume.

Opiates and the hormonal control of sexual behavior

Another probable area or endogenous opiate involvement in reproduction is in the

Table 1. *Effects of opiate agonists and antagonists on serum levels of certain hormones (Meites et al., 1979)*

Hormone	*Drug effects*	
	Agonist	*Antagonist*
Testosterone	Decrease	Increase
LH	Decrease	Increase
FSH	Decrease	Increase
Prolactin	Increase	Decrease
GH	Increase	Decrease

hormonal control of sexual behavior. Table 1 summarizes the effects of opiates and opiate antagonists on several hormones (Meites *et al.*, 1979). The change in prolactin is of interest because hyperprolactinemia has been implicated in some forms of human impotence and, in many cases, such impotence has been alleviated by the prolactin-lowering drug bromocriptine (March, 1979). However, and probably more important for influencing sexual behavior, are the changes produced by opiate agonists and antagonists in testosterone and luteinizing hormone levels.

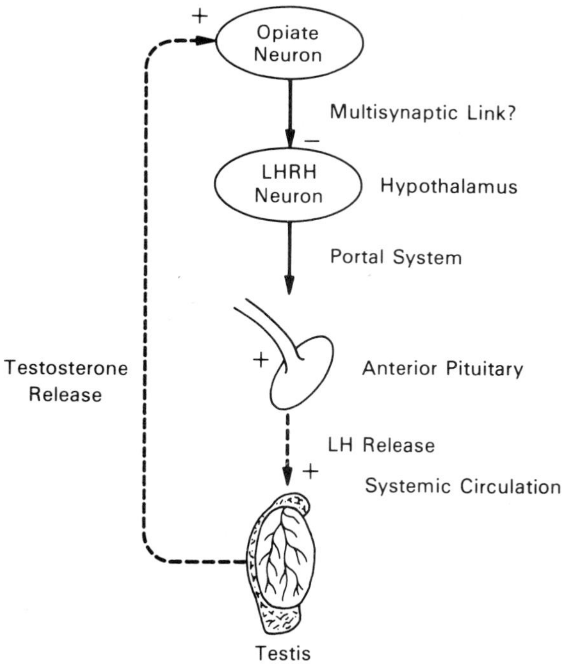

Fig. 6. *Cicero's model for opiate influence on the hypothalamic-pituitary-gonadal axis*

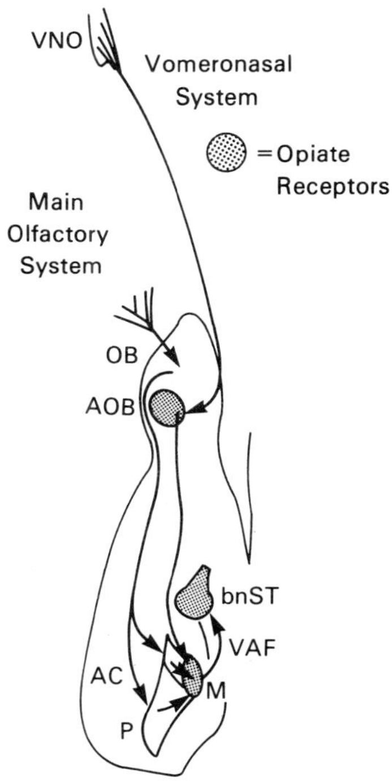

Fig. 7. *Ventral surface of a rodent brain showing nuclei and neural pathways that are critical to mating behavior in the male hamster.* Drawing is modified from Wysocki (1979). Additional anatomical detail based on Lehman *et al.* (1980*a*) and Kevetter & Winans (1981*a*, 1981*b*). Opiate receptor localization is based on Herkenham & Pert's work on the rat (1980)

Cicero and others (eg see Cicero *et al.*, 1980; Meites, 1980; Meites *et al.*, 1979, etc) have proposed a model for the role of endogenous opiates in the regulation of testosterone production which is shown in diagrammatic form in Fig. 6. The generally accepted theory is that luteneizing hormone releasing hormone (LHRH) which is produced in the hypothalamus is released into the hypothalamic-pituitary portal system and causes the anterior pituitary to release LH into the systemic circulation. The LH then acts on the testes to promote the production of testosterone, which then feeds back to inhibit further release of LHRH. What the new theory does is to interpose an opiate-containing neuron into the system. What is proposed is that instead of inhibiting the LHRH neuron directly, testosterone excites an opiate-containing neuron that then inhibits LHRH release. In this scheme, opiate drugs inhibit LHRH release by acting on the LHRH-containing neuron, mimicking the natural action of endogenous opiates. Opiate effects of endogenous opiates. If this hypothesis is correct, then endogenous opiates clearly play an important role in the hormonal regulation of sexual behavior, and it would seem that opiate antagonists might be useful in the treatment of some kinds of endocrine disorders. Cicero's theory certainly suggests a mechanism for the infertility and endocrine problems of opiate addicts (Cicero *et al.*, 1975).

Opiates and the central mechanisms of sexual motivation

A third possible role for endogenous opiates in sexual function is their possible involvement in the central mechanisms of sexual motivation. This role is suggested for several reasons: endogenous opiates or opiate receptors are found in high concentration in brain areas involved in the control of sexual behavior (for example, in the preoptic area, the amygdala, and the limbic system) (see Wamsley *et al.*, 1980; Cumming *et al.*, 1981; Finley *et al.*, 1981; Olson *et al.*, 1981); opiate receptors are often found in the same neuronal areas that contain LHRH and that concentrate androgen; opiate peptides eliminate sexual behavior in sexually active males, as was noted earlier in this paper, and, opiate antagonists elicit sexual behavior from non-copulatory males.

For a specific example of possible endogenous opiate involvement in the mechanisms of sexual arousal, the Syrian golden hamster will now be considered. Figure 7 is a diagram of the base of the rodent brain showing neuronal pathways and nuclei that are crucial for hamster mating behavior. Sexual arousal in the hamster is dependent on the sense of smell from two chemosensory channels, the main olfactory system and the vomeronasal system. Any procedure that eliminates both of these sensory channels also eliminates mating behavior in the hamster (Murphy & Schneider, 1970; Powers *et al.*, 1979). Also, lesions of brain areas that lie along the common tertiary and quaternary projections of these chemosensory systems, the medial amygdala and the bed nucleus of the stria terminalis, will eliminate hamster mating behavior. (Lehmen *et al.*, 1980*a*, 1980*b*; Lehman, personal communication, 1981). In the rat, both of these neuronal areas contain a high concentration of opiate receptors, as does the accessory olfactory bulb (Herkenham *et al.*, 1980). Hence, if high concentrations of opiate receptors exist in the same areas of the hamster brain, then endogenous opiates may be involved in the transmission and perception of sexually arousing olfactory stimuli, thereby affecting sexual motivation in this species. It is also significant that in the hamster the medial amygdala and the bed nucleus of the stria terminalis have been demonstrated to contain the peptide LHRH (Phillips *et al.*, 1980), and that neurons in these same areas concentrate androgen (Doherty & Sheridan, 1981).

Opiates and the 'sexual neurotransmitters'

As a fourth hypothesis, it is possible that endogenous opiates may affect sexual behavior by interacting with brain neurotransmitters. While endogenous opiates themselves may serve as neurotransmitters, they, as well as opiate drugs and opiate antagonists, affect other neurochemicals. Dopamine and serotonin may be referred to as 'sexual neurotransmitters' because a substantial body of evidence indicates that they are fundamentally involved in the control of sexual behavior, with dopamine being generally facilitatory and serotonin inhibitory (Gessa & Tagliamonte, 1975; Karczmar, 1980). This evidence is consistent with the hypothesis that endogenous opiates are involved in sexual behavior, since opiates have been shown to decrease the activity of the dopamine system and increase the activity of the serotonin system whereas opiate antagonists increase dopamine activity (Meites *et al.*, 1979). The similarity between the effects of naloxone, and dopamine agonists on the sexual behavior of male rats has been noted (McIntosh *et al.*, 1980; Pellegrini-Quarantotti *et al.*, 1979), and the possible role of serotonin in mediating the sexual effects of opiate antagonists has been discussed (McConnell *et al.*, 1981).

Recently, it has been demonstrated that opiate peptides have a direct inhibitory effect on the release of LHRH from hypothalamic neurons (Drouva *et al.*, 1981). Since LHRH has been shown to have an effect on sexual behavior that is similar, in part, to the effect of opiate antagonists (Myers & Baum, 1980), it is possible that endogenous opiates may modulate sexual behavior by influencing the release of LHRH. If this is the case, then it seems that LHRH other than that responsible for regulating LH levels must be involved, since there is no correlation between serum LH levels and the sexual effects of opiate antagonists (McConnell *et al.*, 1981).

Conclusion

At present, the ideas outlined above are merely hypotheses and have been subjected only to limited experimental examination and support. It should also be noted that the possible mechanisms which have been discussed are not mutually exclusive. For example, it has been suggested that opiate influence on prolactin levels may be mediated by either dopamine (Gold *et al.*, 1979) or serotonin (Spampinato *et al.*, 1979).

In keeping with the theme of this volume, we conclude by speculating on the possible significance of the endogenous opiates for the psychopharmacology of sexual disorders. Current data suggest that opiate or opiate blocking drugs may be useful in the treatment of such sexual dysfunctions as loss of libido, impotence, and premature or delayed ejaculation. By their action on the hypothalamic-pituitary axis, opiate antagonists may prove efficacious in treating some types of hormonal disorders. Lastly, such drugs, via their action on the genitalia, may be able to be used to affect fertility by influencing the ejaculate volume or the sperm count. All of these possibilities are still in the basic, experimental, stage and whether or not they come to fruition depends not only on the results of additional experiments, but also on the development of more selective drugs that can sucessfully and beneficially modify the sexual aspects of endogenous opiate systems while only minimally disturbing their other functions.

Acknowledgement — I thank Paul MacLean and John Eberhart of the NIMH for providing laboratory facilities for this work, Marvin Snyder and William Pollin of the NIDA for support and encouragement, and Jane Bupp, Paul MacLean, Janet Murphy, and Candace Pert for advice and comments on the manuscript.

References

Braude, M.C. & Morrison, J.M. (1976): Preclinical toxicity studies of naltrexone. In *Narcotic Antagonists: Naltrexone,* eds Julius, D. & Renault, P. NIDA Research Monograph 9, Rockville, Maryland: NIDA.

Cicero, T.J., Bell, R.D., Weist, W.G., Allison, J.H., Polakoski, K. & Robins, E. (1975): Function of the male sex organs in heroin and methadone users. *New Eng. J. Med.* **292,** 882-887.

Cicero, T.J., Meyer, E.R., Gabriel, S.M., Bell, R.D. & Wilcox, C.E. (1980): Morphine exerts testosterone-like effects in the hypothalamus of the castrated male rat. *Brain Res.* **202,** 151-164.

Cumming, R., Reaves, T.A. Jr & Hayward, J.N. (1981): Ultrastructural immunocytochemical localization of enkephalin in the goldfish preoptic nucleus. *Neurosci. Lett.* **27,** 313-318.

Cushman, P. (1972): Sexual behavior in heroin addiction and methadone maintenance. *N.Y. State J. Med.* **72,** 1261-1265.

Doherty, P.C. & Sheridan, P.J. (1981): Uptake and retention of androgen in neurons of the brain of the golden hamster. *Brain Res.* **219,** 327-334.

Drouva, S.V., Epelbaum, J., Tapia-Arancibia, L., Laplante, E. & Kordon, C. (1981): Opiate receptors modulate LHRH and SRIF release from mediobasal hypothalamic neurons. *Neuroendocrinology* **32,** 163-167.

Finley, J.C.W., Maderdrut, & Petrusz, P. (1981): The immunocytochemical localization of enkephalin in the central nervous system of the rat. *J. Comp. Neurol.* **198,** 541-565.

Gessa, G.L., Paglietti, E. & Pellegrini-Quarantotti, B. (1979): Induction of copulatory behavior in sexually inactive rats by naloxone. *Science* **204,** 203-205.

Gessa, G. & Tagliamonte, A. (1975): Role of brain serotonin and dopamine in male sexual behavior. In *Sexual Behavior: Pharmacology and Biochemistry,* eds Sandler, M. & Gessa, G. New York: Raven Press. Pp. 117-128.

Gibson, M.J., Liotta, A.S. & Krieger, D.T. (1981): The Zucker fa/fa rat: absent circadian corticosterone periodicity and elevated β-endorphin concentrations in brain and neurointermediate pituitary. *Neuropeptides* **1,** 349-362.

Gold, M.S., Redmond, D.E. Jr & Donabedian, R.K. (1979): The effects of opiate agonist and antagonist on serum prolactin in primates: Possible role for endorphins in prolactin regulation. *Endocrinology* **105,** 284-289.

Guerra, F. (1974): Sex and drugs in the 16th century. *Br. J. Addict.* **69,** 269-290.

Hemmes, R.B. & Schoch, R. (1980): Effects of high dosage testosterone and naloxone on the sexual behavior of genetically obese male Zucker rats. Program and Abstracts of the Eastern Conference of Reproductive Behavior, New York, p 55.

Herkenham, M. & Pert, C.B. (1980): *In vitro* autoradiography of opiate receptors in rat brain suggests loci of 'opiatergic' pathways. *Proc. Natl Acad. Sci.* **73,** 5532-5536.

Huidobro-Toro, J.P. & Way, E.L. (1981): Comparative study on the effects of morphine and the opioid-like peptides in the vas deferens of rodents: species and strain differences, evidence for multiple opiate receptors. *Life Sci.* **281,** 1331-1336.

Karczmar, A.G. (1980): Drugs, transmitters and hormones, and mating behavior. *Mod. Probl. Pharmacopsych.* **15,** 1-76.

Kevetter, G.A. & Winans, S.S. (1981*a*): Connections of the corticomedial amygdala in the golden hamster I. Efferents of the 'vomeronasal mygdala'. *J. Comp. Neurol.* **197,** 81-98.

Kevetter, G.A. & Winans, S.S. (1981*b*): Connections of the corticomedial amygdala in the golden hamster II. Efferents of the 'olfactory amygdala'. *J. Comp. Neurol.* **197,** 99-111.

Kinsey, A.C., Pomeroy, W.B., Martin, C.E. & Gebhard, P.H. (1953): *Sexual Behaviour in the Human Female.* Philadelphia: W.B. Saunders Co. Pp. 613-717.

Lehman, M.N., Winans, S.S. & Powers, J.B. (1980*a*): Medial nucleus of the amygdala mediates chemosensory control of male hamster sexual behavior. *Science* **210,** 557-560.

Lehman, M.N., Winans, S.S., Powers, J.B. & Slimp, J.C. (1980*b*): Neuroendocrine analysis of male hamster copulatory behavior. Program and Abstracts of the Eastern Conference on Reproductive Behavior, New York. p. 17.

March, C.M. (1979): Bromocriptine in the treatment of hypogonadism and male impotence. *Drugs* **17,** 349-358.

Margules, D.L., Moisset, B., Lewis, M.J., Shibuya, H. & Pert, C.B. (1978): β-endorphin is associated with overeating in genetically obese mice (ob/ob) and rats (fa/fa). *Science* **202,** 988-991.

McConnell, S.K., Baum, M.J. & Badger, T.M. (1981): Lack of correlation between naloxone-induced changes in sexual behavior and serum LH in male rats. *Horm. Behav.* **15,** 16-35.

McIntosh, T.K., Vallano, M.L. & Barfield, R.J. (1980): Effects of morphine, beta-endorphin and naloxone on catecholamine levels and sexual behavior in the male rat. *Pharmacol, Biochem. Behav.* **13,** 435-441.

Meites, J., Bruni, J.F., Van Vugt, D.A. & Smith, A.F. (1979): Relation of endogenous opioid peptides and morphine to neuroendocrine functions. *Life Sci.* **24,** 1325-1336.

Meites, J. (1980): Relation of endogenous opioid peptides to secretion of hormones. *Fed. Proc.* **39,** 2531-2532.

Mendelson, J.H., Ellingboe, J., Keuhnle, J.C. & Mello, N.K. (1979): Effects of naltrexone on mood and neuroendocrine function in normal adult males. *Psychoneuroendocrinology* **3,** 231-236.

Meyerson, B.J. & Terenius, L. (1977): Beta-endorphin and male sexual bahavior. *Eur. J. Pharmacol.* **42,** 191-192.

Mintz, J., O'Hare, K., O'Brine, C.P. & Goldschmide, J. (1974): Sexual problems of heroin addicts. *Archs Gen. Psychiat.* **31,** 700-703.

Murphy, M.R. (1980): Opiate agonist and antagonist effects on the sexual behavior of male hamsters. Program and Abstracts of the Eastern Conference of Reproductive Behavior, New York, p. 63.

Murphy, M.R. (1981): Methadone reduces sexual performance and sexual motivation in the male Syrian golden hamster. *Pharmacol. Biochem. Behav.* **14,** 561-567.

Murphy, M.R., Bowie, D.L. & Pert, C.B. (1979): Copulation elevates plasma beta-endorphin in the male hamster. *Soc. Neurosci. Abstr.* 9th Annual Meeting, Atlanta, Georgia. P 470.

Murphy, M.R. & Schneider, G.E. (1970): Olfactory bulb removal eliminates mating behavior in the male golden hamster. *Science* **167,** 302-304.

Myers, M.B. & Baum, M.J. (1979): Facilitation by opiate antagonists of sexual performance in the male rat. *Pharmacol. Biochem. Behav.* **10,** 615-618.

Myers, B.M. & Baum, M.J. (1980): Facilitation of copulatory performance in male rats by naloxone: Effects of hypophysectomy, 17 alpha-estradiol, and luteinizing hormone releasing hormone. *Pharmacol. Biochem. Behav.* **12,** 365-370.

Noble, R.G. (1980): Hamster sexual functioning: modulation by opiate agonists, opiate antagonists, and exercise. Program and Abstracts of the Eastern Conference of Reproductive Behavior, New York, p 18.

Olson, G.A., Olson, R.D., Kastin, A.J. & Coy, D.H. (1979): Endogenous opiates: through 1978. *Neurosci. Biobehav. Rev.* **3,** 285-299.

Olson, G.A., Olson, R.D., Kastin, A.J. & Coy, D.H. (1981): Endogenous opiates: 1980. *Peptides* **2,** 349-369.

Parr, D. (1976): Sexual aspects of drug abuse in narcotic addicts. *Br. J. Addict.* **71,** 261-268.

Pellegrini-Quarantotti, B., Paglietti, E., Bonanni, A., Petta, M. & Gessa, G.L. (1979): Naloxone shortens ejaculation latency in male rats. *Experientia* **35,** 524-525.

Phillips, H.S., Hostetter, G., Kerdelhue, B. & Kozlowski, G.P. (1980): Immunocytochemical localization of LHRH in central olfactory pathways of hamster. *Brain Res.* **193,** 574-579.

Powers, J.B., Fields, R.B. & Winans, S.S. (1979): Olfactory and vomeronasal system participation in male hamsters' attraction to female vaginal secretions. *Physiol. Behav.* **22,** 77-84.

Sachs, B.D., Valcourt, R.J. & Flagg, H.C. (1981): Copulatory behavior and sexual reflexes of male rats treated with naloxone. *Pharmacol. Biochem. Behav.* **14,** 251-253.

Sawynok, J., Pinsky, C. & LaBella, F.S. (1979): On the specificity of naloxone as an opiate antagonist. *Life Sci.* **25,** 1621-1632.

Sharp, B. & Pekary, A.E. (1981): Beta-endorphin (61-69) and other beta-endorphin-immuno reactive peptides in human semen. *J. Clin. Endocr Metabol.* **52**, 586-588.

Sharp, B. & Pekary, A.E. (1981): Beta-endorphin (61-91) and other beta-endorphin-immunoreactive peptides in human semen. *J. Clin. Endocr. Metabol.* **52,** 586-588.

Sharp, B., Pekary, A.E., Meyer, N.V. & Hershman, J.M. (1980): Beta-endorphin in male rat reproductive orrgans. *Biochem. Biophys. Res. Comm.* **95,** 618-623.

Spampinato, S., Locatelli, V., Cocchi, D., Vicentini, L., Bajusz, S., Ferri, S. & Muller, E.E. (1979): Involvement of brain serotonin in the prolactin-releasing effect of opioid peptides. *Endocrinology* **105,** 163-170.

Szechtman, H., Hershkowitz, M. & Simantov, R. (1981): Sexual behavior decreases pain sensitivity and stimulates endogenous opiods in male rats. *Eur. J. Pharmacol.* **70,** 279-285.

Vaalasti, A., Linnoila, I. & Hervonen, A. (1980): Immunohistochemical demonstration of VIP (Met5)- and (Leu5)-enkephalin immunoreactive nerve fibres in the human prostate and seminal vesicles. *Histochemistry* **66,** 89-98.

Wamsley, J.K., Young, W.S. III & Kuhar, M.J. (1980): Immunohistochemical localization of enkephain in rat forebrain. *Brain Res.* **190,** 153-174.

Wysocki, C,J, (1979): Neurobehavioral evidence for the involvement of the vomeronasal system in mammalian reproduction. *Neurosci. Biobehav. Rev.* **3,** 301-341.

5

Gonadal hormonal influences on aggressive behavior in male and female rats

N. E. van de POLL, N. J. BOWDEN, H. G. van OYEN, F. H. de JONGE and H. H. SWANSON

Netherlands Institute for Brain Research, Meibergdreef 33, 1105 A7 Amsterdam Zuidoost, THE NETHERLANDS

Introduction

Given the variety of responses falling under the heading 'aggression', and in view of the many classes of stimuli and experiential factors which characteristically influence these social interactions, it is self-evident that the 'biological mechanisms' implicated in the evocation and maintenance of aggression in all its forms are extremely complex. In the study of the influences of brain structures or neurohumoral factors on aggressive behavior, therefore, it is inevitable that only restricted classes and aspects of such social interactions can be studied. At the same time, rigorous demands have to be made for tests of behavior and for the validity of such tests. Unlike sexual behavior, the execution of aggressive behaviors varies widely depending upon the eliciting stimuli. Moyer (1976) discusses, as a most practical and useful approach to research on aggression, a variety of behaviors that may be subsumed in his definition of aggression: 'overt behavior involving intent to inflict noxious stimulation or to behave destructively towards another organism'. Such behavior can be as diverse as competitive fighting among males, a mother defending her young, and interspecies predation. Moyer distinguished several types of aggression and stressed the fact that not only are the stimuli and the repertoire of aggressive responses involved different, but that the underlying physiological mechanisms are also different. The present chapter offers a short review on the experimental analyses of gonadal hormonal influences on 'intermale' aggression in rats and the existence of sex differences in this form of aggression as an issue of dispute.

For the study of hormonal factors and sexual behavior, intermale aggression is an important category. This specific form of aggression is most commonly seen among males of the various species, and is involved in such diverse behavioral mechanisms important for reproduction as mate selection and the dispersion of conspecifics. For mice and rats, the species-typical behavior patterns of this form of aggression are fairly well described and it is now well known that specific stimulus factors of urinary origin, in which gonadal steroids play an important role, contribute to the selection of conspecifics which are aggressed upon more often than others. In this way, females and young animals are protected against this form of aggression. At the same time, gonadal steroids directly influence aggressive responses in the form of an activating influence. For the development of sex-specific behavioral patterns the important question is whether or not such behaviors can be activated to an equal degree in males and females, as a function of hormones present neonatally.

In this article, the term 'agonistic' behavior is used as a broad class of behaviors which, apart from aggression proper, also includes submissive behavior and the specific responses designed to avoid aggressive confrontations.

An important question for the measurement of aggression is the stability of the behavioral responses. Apart from contributing to the activation of aggressive tendencies by its present stimulus quality, the opponent also determines the further course of aggression by subtle changes in behavior, depending upon the outcome of the conflict. Since rather stable hierarchic relations result from such interactions, and the inhibition of aggression is an important aspect of agonistic behavior, it would be worthwhile developing tests specifically aimed at investigating these behavioral changes. At the same time, it should be noted that, for this very reason, an equal distribution of aggression among conspecifics can never be expected to be found. All responses subsumed under the heading 'aggressive behavior' are intimately entwined with other forms of social behavior, such as sexual and maternal behavior. The biological mechanisms influencing these behaviors will, therefore, partly overlap with many aspects of aggression. As a result, investigating the effects of gonadal hormones on specific social behaviors in principle asks for the selection of test situations where the responses are not confounded by other effects of the hormone. However, such an approach tends to result in well-investigated, isolated effects which can be very difficult to integrate into a clear picture of how hormones actually influence social behavior as a whole. Hence, in the present experiments due attention has been paid to aggressive and sexual responses of both opponents in an aggressive encounter. Two series of experiments are discussed, both of which aimed to investigate hormonal effects on the adult male's and adult female's aggressive responses. In the first series, an attempt was made to avoid experiential factors as a determinant of aggression, so that relatively 'naive' animals were chosen for experimentation. In the second series, we concentrated on the course of fighting and the effects of winning and losing on subsequent aggression in males and females.

Gonodal hormonal influences upon 'intermale aggression'

Gonadal involvement in the male

In by far the majority of mammalian species, including man, the male is the more aggressive sex (Moyer, 1976). The behavior patterns displayed by fighting males are characteristic of the species and have to be distinguished from aggressive behavior involved in predation or maternal defence. This category of 'intermediate aggression' specified by other workers as 'mate selection-related', 'territorial aggression' or 'social conflict' (Moyer, 1976; Brain, 1980; Brain, 1981) is one of the most frequently studied forms of aggression, although the experimental details of the procedures used may vary considerably. Specification of the stimulus dimension eliciting such aggressive responses indicates that the masculine characteristics are highly relevent for an animal to elicit this form of conflict (Mugford & Nowell, 1970, 1971; Mugford, 1974).

The significance of testosterone for intermale aggression has been investigated in many experiments. Fighting in male mice and rats as one indication of gonadal involvement generally does not occur until maturation (Seward, 1945; Lagerspetz & Talo, 1967), and prepubertal sexual and aggressive behaviors suggest that the males are predisposed to show more aggression. Castration of male mice and rats resulted in a reduction of fighting while testosterone restored this to preoperative levels (Beeman, 1947: Schuurman, 1980).

'Intermale' aggression in females?

The generally accepted phenomenon that intraspecific fighting occurs more often among males than among females has been related to the 'organization activation' model of gonadal hormonal influences. Initially, the presence of neonatal androgen as the so-called 'organizing' factor was thought to be a prerequisite for testosterone to activate fighting in adulthood (Edwards, 1969, 1970; Bronson & Desjardins, 1971). More recent experiments, also using mice, however, indiate that although the neural substrate which subserves the expression of fighting may be rendered more responsive to the activational property of testosterone by perinatal androgen, such behavior can still be observed in normally developed females when injected with testosterone in adulthood (Svare *et al.*, 1974; Barkley & Goldman, 1977). Therefore, only a thorough comparison of aggressive tendencies of males and females, necessarily including a specification of the stimulus factors involved, the topography of the responses and the relevance of hormonal factors, can answer the question as to whether the sexes differ in this aspect of behavior as well as identifying which aspects are affected by hormonal factors during development.

Metabolization of androgens and aggressive behavior

Much evidence now suggests that, in various species, estrogen as well as 5a-reduced androgen — especially dihydrotestosterone — as two important metabolites of testosterone, significantly contribute to the activation of sexual behavior (Larsson *et al.*, 1973; Parrott, 1975). It is suggested that androgens have to be aromatized, ie converted to estrogen, prior to having motivational effects upon the brain (Naftolin *et al.*, 1975). Dihydrotestosterone also derived from androgens in the context of this aromatization hypothesis would be of minor behavioral significance by affecting the qualitative aspects of masculine sexual behavior via its peripheral action, for instance, on the penile spines. There is also evidence in support of this theory being important for other androgen-mediated behaviors in a variety of species (Brain, 1977; Bowden, 1979). Estradiol has been proven to be highly effective in the restoration of aggressive behavior of castrated male rats (Christie & Barfield, 1979) and in the maintenance of aggression of mice (Brain & Bowden, 1978). A few studies on the effects of non-aromatizable androgens on aggression, however, argue against the relevance of this metabolism process for aggression. Thus, dihydrotestosterone restored aggressive responses in castrated male mice (Luttge, 1972; Brain, 1979) and in female mice (Schechter *et al.*, 1981).

For the comparison of behavioral effects of gonadal hormones in males and females, the aromatization hypothesis is of particular interest. Previous experiments in the organizing effects of testosterone on masculine and feminine sexual behavior in the rat indicate that the perinatal presence of androgens affects behavior either by inhibiting or facilitating feminine and masculine sexual responses *per se*, and by changing the activating effects of testosterone and estrogen (Whalen, 1968; Beach, 1971; van de Poll *et al.*, 1978). Androgens have been shown to be aromatized to estrogens in the male and female rat brain, although the rates of conversion were low (Naftolin *et al.*, 1972; Naes *et al.*, 1975). Aromatization has been shown to take place specifically in the preoptic area and anterior hypothalamus (Selmanoff *et al.*, 1977), a region of the brain that is involved in masculine and feminine sexual behavior (van de Poll & van Dis, 1979) and intermale aggression (Bermond, 1978). It seems especially relevant, therefore, to investigate the differential sensitivity of males and females to the activating effects of testosterone and estrogen on aggression and sexual behavior.

Methods and methodological considerations in hormonal studies of aggression in males and females

Gandelman (1981) rightly raised the question of whether the fighting behavior of chronically testosterone-exposed female mice is identical to that of males. The relevance of masculine pheromonal factors, as one of the principal stimuli that elicit fighting both in males and females, led him to conclude that females can react like males if injected with testosterone. For instance, it was found that like males, females preferentially attacked male but not female intruders (Svare *et al.*, 1974). In our studies on the hormonal influences on aggression in male and female aggression, we followed a comparable line of reasoning. In an experiment, to be summarized in this paper, aggression was studied in dyadic encounters of either males or females the relevance of the hormonal state of an animal as an opponent being assessed by injecting animals with either testosterone or with OIL. Because OIL-treated animals were also tested against each other, both the aggression-provoking effect and the aggression-promoting (activating) effect of testosterone (van de Poll *et al.*, 1981*a*,*b*) could be analysed.

Intermale fighting has frequently been shown to be intensified if the animals are isolated for a certain period of time (Scott & Fredericson, 1951). This enhancement of aggression, which in many procedures has been used to elicit stable levels of aggressive responses for study, entails specific problems for the comparison of males and females. Isolated and grouped animals are frequently shown to differ both in their hormonal status and in their brain chemistry (Brain, 1979). Interestingly, Lupo di Prisco *et al.* (1978) showed that isolation modified both plasma testosterone levels and brain aromatization in adult rats. Since these changes could be related to the predisposition to show aggressive behavior, and males and females can be expected to react differentially, it is of importance to avoid drastic isolation effects. In the experiments reported in this chapter, aggression was found to increase when animals were housed individually for 14 days in the company of a 'neutral' ovariectomized Wistar female.

A last procedural factor to be stressed when comparing hormonal studies of aggression is the distinction between 'initiated' and 'maintained' aggression. As we might expect, experiential factors are of great relevance to this kind of behavior and although hormonal factors may be highly relevant for the initiation of such behavior, its maintenance could depend on entirely different factors. Thus, it was shown in mice that experienced fighters persisted in the display of aggression following castration (Bevan *et al.*, 1960 unpublished results cited in Gandelman, 1981). In fact, this particular factor may acount for the high variability of behavioral results frequently found in studies of aggressive behavior. As gonadal hormones appear to be specifically involved in attack on a strange conspecific, the chances of experiential factors influencing aggression should be minimized: in our own experiments, males and females were tested once only after 24 h in isolated adaptation to the test cage.

Influences of testosterone and estrogen upon aggressive behavior in the male and female rat

In contrast to the many studies on aggressive responses in mice, the rat has not been used frequently for this kind of research. Wistar rats are notorious for their lack of aggressiveness under laboratory conditions, and this stimulated the use of other strains for this research. Barr *et al.* (1976), who used Sprague-Dawley rats, showed that the sex differences in the rat were associated with differences in circulating androgens during a brief postnatal period and also in adulthood. The results, however, suggested that only a restricted pattern of aggressive defensive behavior was influenced by testosterone administered in adulthood. In a study in our laboratory, three important aspects of intermale aggression of the S3-Tryon Maze-Dull rats were systematically compared in males and females: the activating effects of testosterone in two dosages; the relevance of the hormonal state of the opponent; and, the topography of the activated patterns of behavior. Five hundred μg and 100 μg/animal of testosterone propionate (TP) were injected for 14 days. In addition the effects of 10 μg estradiol benzoate were compared with testosterone injections and the effects of estrogen and testosterone (100 μg), as influencing the stimulus properties of the opponent, were additionally assessed. Masculine and feminine sexual responses, as they occur frequently in an aggressive context, were also scored. The experimental details and results have partly been published (van de Poll *et al.*, 1981*a,b*).

The results of 500 μg of testosterone on aggression are summarized in Fig. 1, representing the mean summed duration of aggressive paramaters. Analysis indicated that TP, as an activating factor increased aggression equally in males and females. TP treatment of the opponent was an additional factor which significantly increased aggression in both sexes. When a more detailed analysis of the aggressive interactions was attempted with a discriminant analysis of the aggression parameters no differences between males and females could be detected. Testosterone, at the lower dose, again activated equal levels of aggression in males and females (TP against TP in Fig. 1). This is an important finding, because it argues against a sex difference in sensitivity to testosterone which might be due to the organizing effects perinatally.

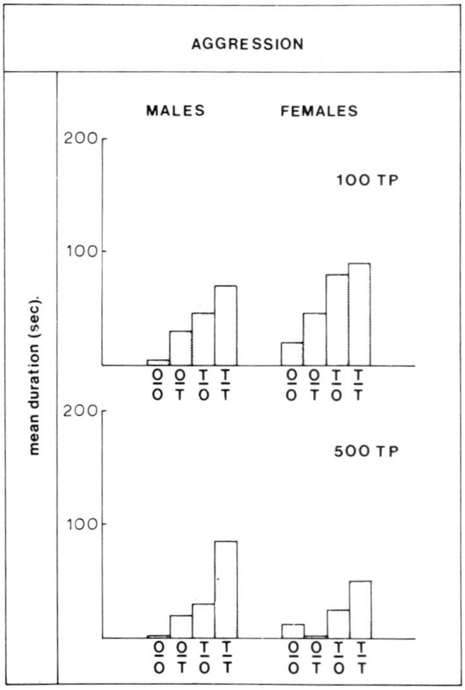

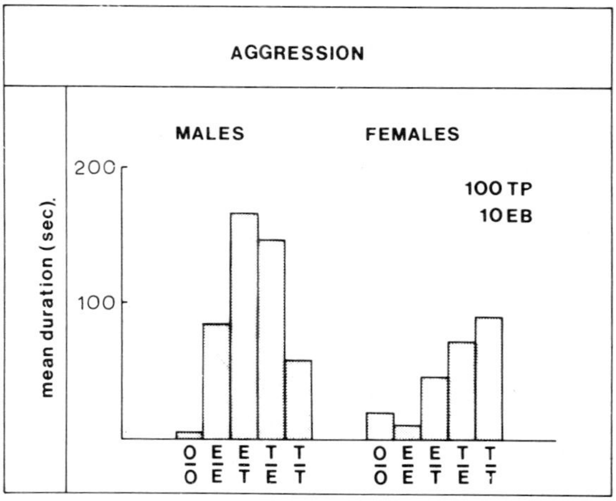

Fig. 1. (above, left). *Aggressive behavior in groups of male and female rats treated with OIL (O) or testosterone propionate (TP) (upper letter) and tested against OIL- or TP-treated opponents (lower letter).* Analysis indicated that both treatment and opponent's treatment increase aggression in males as well as in females. Because the effects of the two dosages were established in different experiments, the absolute values cannot be compared

Fig. 2. (above, right). *Aggressive bahavior in groups of male and female rats treated with OIL (O), estradiol benzoate (EB) or testosterone propionate (TP) (upper letter), and tested against OIL-, EB- or TP-treated opponents (lower letter).* Analysis indicated that in males both EB and TP activate comparable levels of aggression, whereas in females only testosterone activates aggression

The dose of 100 μg is considered to be low, since 750 μg was reported to restore baseline levels of testosterone and precastration aggression in castrated S3 rats (Schuurman, 1980). Estrogen substantially activated fighting in male rats, which was quantitatively and qualitatively similar to that of the TP-treated males. The females, by contrast, showed very low levels of aggression, especially when injected with EB and tested against EB-treated females. TP and EB in the females differed not only via the direct-stimulating effects but also via treatment of the opponents: apparently, TP-treated females were better aggression-provoking stimuli than estrogen-treated opponents of the same sex (Fig. 2).

Apart from aggression, estrogen-treated females, in contrast to males, also evinced high levels of feminine sexual response. This was particularly evident when these females were tested against TP-treated opponents. Apparently, a TP-treated female not only provoked aggression but was also an equally appropriate stimulus in eliciting feminine sexual responses of the EB-treated females. Both aggressive and sexual tendencies could be demonstrated in the same animal. This brings us to the interesting question of whether a possible relationship between sexual and aggressive behavior could provide an explanation for the low levels of aggression in the females compared to the males. Correlation coefficients calculated on the basis of the individual scores on aggression and lordosis or perceptive responses did not, however, reveal any such relationship. Apparently these behavior systems function relatively independently.

Testosterone, estrogen and dihydrotestosterone effects upon aggression in the male and female rat

In a further series of experiments, the effects of TP and EB were compared with those of dihydrotestosterone propionate (DHTP) added to estrogen alone, and with OIL. Adding DHTP to EB injections was found to inhibit feminine sexual response and to enhance masculine sexual behavior (Baum & Vreeburg, 1976). Such an experiment, comparing these effects with DHTP given alone, is obviously in line with many experiments on sexual behavior investigating the aromatization hypothesis. The methods employed in this experiment were basically the same as in previous studies. Groups of gonadectomized male and female rats were treated daily with TP (100 μg/animal), EB (2 μg/animal), EB + DHTP (1000 μg/animal) or DHTP or OIL for 14 days. Dyadic encounters between animals of the same sex were studied in confrontations with a TP-treated opponent (100 μg/animal) of the same sex.

As in all earlier tests for aggression, many sexual responses were observed. Mounts most frequently occurred in the females which, most probably, reflects the better stimulus properties of the female. Mounting occurred in all groups of females but was remarkably high in the EB + DTHP group (Fig. 3). Significant levels of lordosis were actually observed in the EB-treated females, whereas DHTP, when added to EB, completely suppressed female sexual response. Low, but reliable, levels of lordosis occurred in TP-treated females. Aggression in males and females was not very intensely activated by these low doses, although substantial levels of fighting were seen in all groups, the lowest being in the OIL-treated animals (Fig. 4).

In the males, the highest levels of aggression were seen in the EB + DHTP and DHTP groups. Further experiments now in progress reveal that when a higher dose of EB (10 μg) is combined with DHTP in females, aggression is lower in the EB and significantly higher in the EB + DHTP groups. Feminine sexual responses were then frequent in the EB and virtually absent in the EB + DHTP group of females.

It will be clear from the results presented thus far, that at least in the strain of rats used in our studies, no sex differences in testosterone-activated aggression were detected. Some evidence is in accordance with the hypothesis that the activating effects

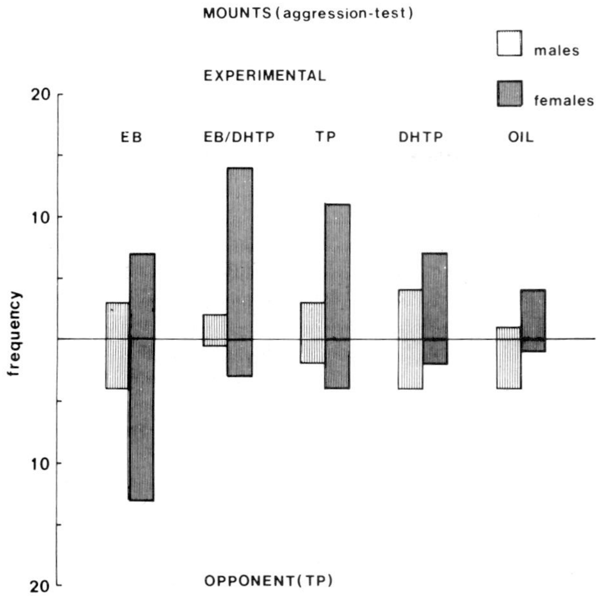

Fig. 3. *Mount frequencies observed in tests of aggression behavior of male or female rats treated with estradiol benzoate (EB), EB-dihydrotestosterone propionate (DHTP), testosterone propionate (TP). DHTP or OIL, all tested against TP-treated opponents.* Mount frequencies of the opponents are represented in the lower part of the figure

are derived from estrogenic stimulation. In the male a comparatively low dose of EB did indeed stimulate aggression to the same degree as TP injections. Moreover, EB, when combined with DHTP, increased aggression in males and in females at a higher dose of EB, in comparison to EB given alone. Whether this facilitating effect of DHTP is due to a direct central or peripheral effect or to an indirect effect via facilitation of masculine sexual behavior and/or inhibition of feminine sexual response in the animal remains to be determined.

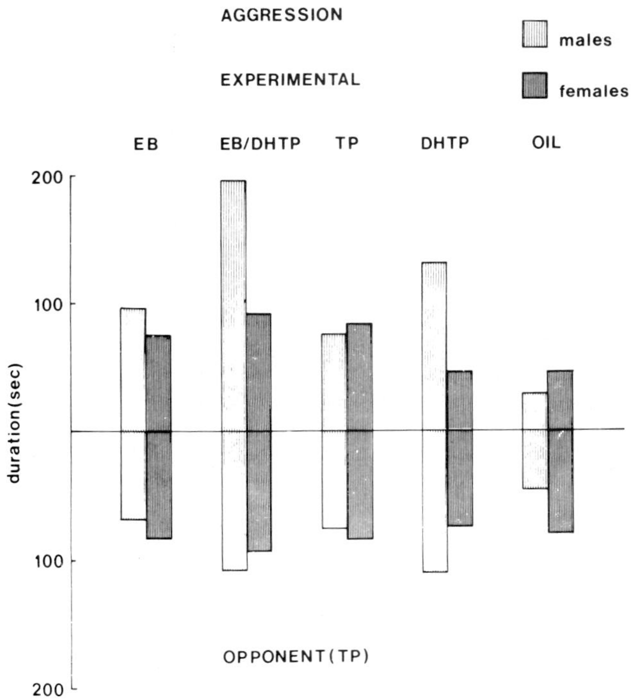

Fig. 4. *Aggressive behavior in groups of male and female rats treated with estradiol benzoate (EB), EB-dihydrotestosterone propionate (DHTP), testosterone propionate (TP), DHTP or OIL, all tested against TP-treated opponents.* Aggressive behavior of the opponents are represented in the lower part of the figure

Attack and submission: experiential factors in agonistic behavior

Like all social interactions, aggressive behavior typically involves two or more individuals, each contributing to the course of the interaction in its own manner. This offers problems which are only partly solved by rigorously standardizing test procedures and the quality of the opponent. Thus, fighting in mice was studied frequently using anosmic or prepuberally castrated conspecifics as opponents that sufficiently stimulate aggression but do not fight back when attacked (Brain & Pool, 1974; Brain, 1980). As a consequence, more is known about aggressive behavior in the dominant animal than about the factors affecting behavioral changes as a consequence of defeat and the development of submission. Therefore, concentrating on tests in which the effects of agonistic experiences are seen as confounding variables, in a way, rejects the good as well as the bad. Indeed, the presence of stable dominance relations within groups of conspecifics of a great variety of species, and the easily observed behavioral changes following winning or defeat, strongly point to the significnce of previous experience as a determinant of agonistic responses. Based upon such considerations, hypotheses about the involvement of hormones in agonistic behavior presuppose different mechanisms of action. On the one hand, 'pure activating' effects on the initiation of aggression are found in experiments already discussed in this chapter; on the other hand, hormonal reactions, contingent upon specific agonistic experiences, are supposed to assume control of behavior in a way recently described by Leshner as the 'hormonal feedback effect' (Leshner, 1979). Experiments on the conditioning of aggressive responses and the reinforcing aspects of aggressive behavior will lead to an incorporation of learning principles as a prominent basis for the plasticity of agonistic behavior. Concentrating on aspects of plasticity in agonistic behavior, instead of on aggression, as a relatively stable characteristic of an animal is, therefore, of the utmost importance to neurobiological research in this field. This latter aspect is, at the same time, of interest for the extrapolation of the often contradictory results in hormone and aggression research obtained in man.

The consequences of winning or losing on subsequent aggressive responses have been studied relatively frequently in mice (Scott & Fredericson, 1951; Lagerspetz, 1961). A highly persistent inhibition of fighting could be induced by the experience of being attacked on 4–6 consecutive days together with a rapid decline of motor activity and increased disorganized escape behavior (Kahn, 1951; Scott & Marston, 1953). More recently, the effects of defeat and complete or incomplete victory on subsequent aggression have been compared. Defeat, no matter how intense, led to decreased aggression, whereas only incomplete victory increased aggression. Earlier studies indicated that increased levels of aggression could result from success in fighting (Ginsburg & Allee, 1942; Fredericson, 1949; Bevan *et al.*, 1960; Tsai & Napier, 1968).

Systematic behavioral data on the effects of repeated testing on the outcome of conflict and the persistence of behavioral effects are virtually absent in the literature on aggression in the rat. Seward (1945, 1946), in a series of experiments on rats, systematically studied the results of the conditioning of submission and qualitatively described general characteristics, such as age and sex differences. It was reported that in male/male encounters the first fight was usually decisive in establishing a dominant/subordinate relationship. After a defeat, the loser tended to assume a submissive status in subsequent encounters, either with the same or with a different opponent. By contrast, although fights were just as frequent between females, they tended to be less violent and failed to have a decisive outcome. Females seemed to be less concerned with status and instead of being cowed, they often re-established contact with their opponent. Also, in subsequent encounters with new opponents, losing females did not automatically assume a subordinate position.

Effects of winning or losing upon subsequent behavior in rats

Recently, we developed a paradigm for the induction and study of the experience of winning or losing in the WEzob rat strain and studied the effects in intact male rats (van de Poll *et al.*, 1982). When tested against Tryon Maze Dull rats, WEzobs were always quickly defeated, whereas when tested against Wistar rats, WEzobs were the more aggressive strain and usually became dominant. After 3 days of confrontations either with an S3 or with a Wistar, the WEzob winners were tested against the losers on a fourth day, and were then retested after a period of 14 days. The behavior of losers in these encounters was characterized by a significant inhibition of aggression and social initiative along with an increase of freezing (Fig. 5).

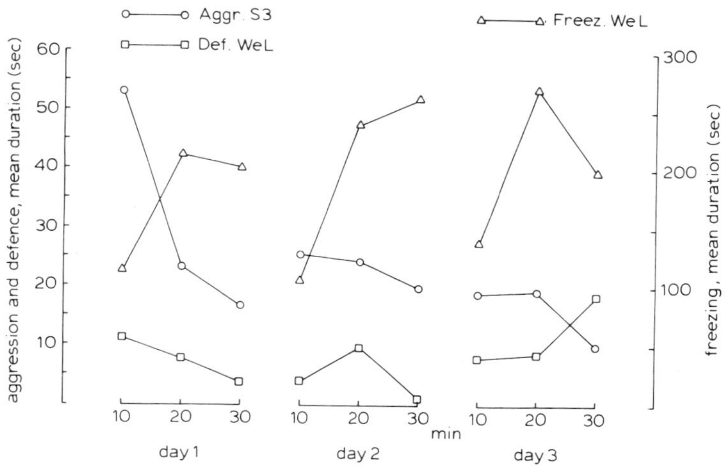

Fig. 5. *WEzob rats confronted with a highly aggressive S3 opponent: aggressive bahavior of the S3 (freezing and defence of the WEzob) presented as mean duration of 10-min periods of three 30 min tests on subsequent days.* Reproduced with permission (van de Poll *et al.*, 1982)

Winners, when confronted with losers, showed high levels of aggressive responses and more autogrooming. The localization in the test cage was clearly affected by the agonistic experiences, the winner being more often localized on the opponent's side of the cage, ie the side of the test cage this particular animal had been adapted to prior to testing. Finally, losers showed a significant decrease in body weight after 4 days of testing. The behavioral effects were still present 14 days later.

Further experiments using the same experimental procedure aimed to investigate whether there is a sex difference in the modification of agonistic responses by experience in the WEzob strain of rats (van de Poll *et al.*, 1982). To elucidate the effects of testosterone on this aspect of agonistic behavior, gonadectomized male and female WEzob rats, either treated with testosterone propionate (TP, 250 μg/animal) or with OIL, were used. From a general view on the effects of winning or losing, it became clear that males and females react totally differently to victory or defeat, and that the presence of testosterone is apparently a critical factor for this sex diference to become manifest. During the induction of winning or losing (the first three days of the

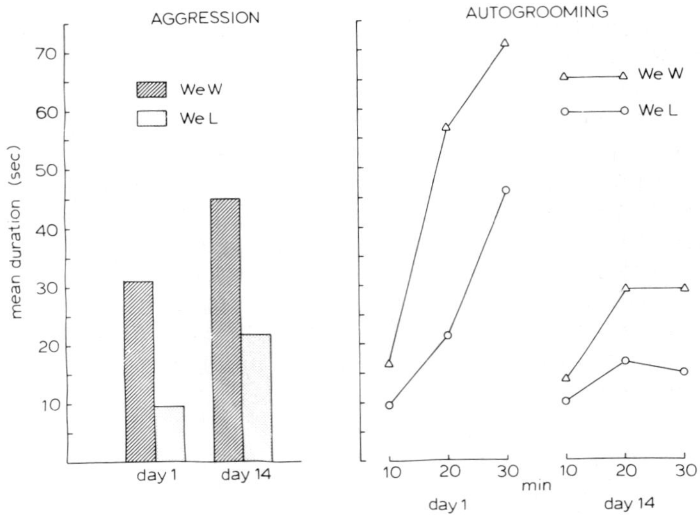

Fig. 6. *Aggressive behavior and autogrooming in WEzob winners and WEzob losers presented as mean duration of two tests with an interval of 14 days.* Aggressive behavior is presented as summed scores of each test, while autogrooming is presented in 3 10 min periods. Reproduced with permission (van de Poll *et al.*, 1982)

procedure), this was shown by observing the effects of experience on aggression of the different groups and this became especially clear with the results of the parameter 'approach'. Males and females reacted differently, depending on TP treatment; TP-treated male losers especially showed a marked inhibition of approach during three tests. In the confrontation of WEzob winners and losers, this sex difference and its dependence upon testosterone became even more clear. A permanent winner/loser effect on aggression, losers showing reduced levels of aggression, was only found in the TP-treated males. This effect was still present after 14 days (Fig. 6).

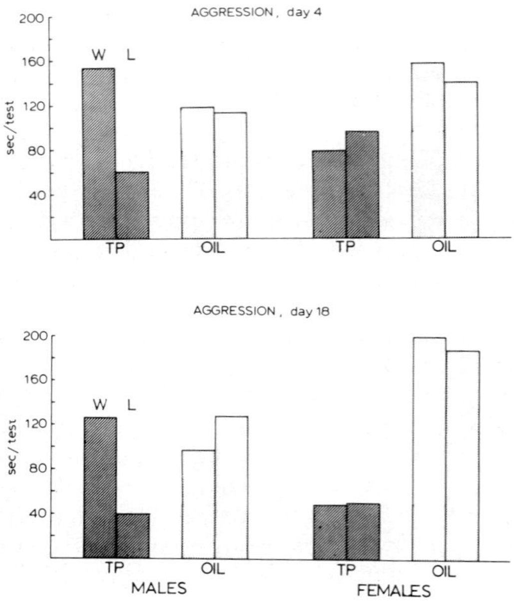

Fig. 7. *Aggressive behavior in confrontations of male or female WEzob winners and losers treated with testosterone propionate (TP) or OIL, at day 4, after 3 days of induction of winning or losing — upper part — and 14 days later.* Copyright (1982) by the American Psychological Association. Adapted by permission of the publisher and authors (van de Poll *et al.*, 1982: *J. Comp. Physiol. Psychol.* **96,** 893-903)

Similarly, only in this group was a reduction in locomotor activity noted in the losers and this sex- and hormone-dependent effect was expressed very clearly in the amount of time spent on the opponent's side of the cage: only TP-treated male losers showed a strong and permanent tendency to remain on their own side of the test cage, in contrast to male winners that had been treated similarly. The difference in the effects of defeat of the TP-treated males and the other groups was finally demonstrated by the marked effects on body weight: a significant weight loss occurred in TP-treated male losers as opposed to winners, and not in any of the other groups.

It should be noted that apparently intact males and gonadectomized males treated with testosterone react similarly to winning and losing. Aggression and defeat are known to affect endogenously produced levels of gonadal androgens but the behavioral significance of this phenomenon is a matter of dispute (Schuurman, 1980). The present results indicate that a relatively high and constant level of testosterone does not prevent the inhibition of aggression and the rise of submissive behaviors in losing animals. This interpretation is in agreement with earlier results on the effects of androgens on submission in mice (Leshner & Moyer, 1975; Leshner & Politch, 1979). Results comparable to the present findings were reported many years ago in a study on the role of age and sex in the aggressive behavior of rats (Seward, 1945, 1946). In spite of a difference in procedure, and the use of a small number of rats in the other studies, striking similarities occurred in several parameters with respect to the effects of winning or losing. For example, in this study, females mounted twice as much as males during aggressive encounters and, contrary to males, mounting behavior occurred in both winners and losers. In discussing his results, Seward noted that fights occurred among females but with less decisive effects on their subsequent reactions: 'The females were less concerned with their status' and were 'increasingly concerned with grooming to the mutual neglect of hostilities'. Seward hypothesized that the observed behavioral inhibition in males could be a function of the more intense and frequent fights in males which would result in more pain and subsequent avoidance of conflict. This hypothesis cannot be applied to the present results, as the aggression of the stimulus animals (S3s) during the induction phase was equally violent in both sexes.

The constellation of behavior patterns in males and females in tests in which they are confronted with novel stimuli has been interpreted as an indication that male rats are more fearful than females (Gray, 1971, 1979; Gray & Buffery, 1971). Previous work, performed by ourselves and others, demonstrated that sex differences in reaction to novel and aversive stimuli indeed fit in with the pattern of results observed after treatment affecting emotional reactivity (van Oyen *et al.*, 1980, 1981). It has been argued (Gray & Buffery, 1971) that sex differences in fearfulness are related to sex differences in aggressive behavior; males being the more fearful and aggressive sex in rodents. Indeed, male rats have been reported to display more dominance behavior and also more submissive behavior (Barnett, 1958; Grant & Change, 1958). However, if sex differences in the reaction to novel and aversive stimuli are actually linked to sex differences in the display of submissive behavior during aggressive encounters, one would expect the sexual dimorphism in agonistic behavior to only become manifest following the aversive experience of defeat. The present findings are unequivocally in favor of such a hypothesis and restrict the organizing effects of gonadal hormones with respect to aggression, if present at all, to this experiential aspect of agonistic behavior.

Conclusions

The absence of significant differences between males and females in testosterone-activated aggression in tests in which effects of experience are minimized together with findings of a pronounced testosterone-dependent sex difference in the assimilation of agonistic experience, lead to a complicated concept of gonadal hormone effects upon aggression. Apparently, attack and agonistic initiative are equally stimulated by testosterone in males and in females. This behavior is specifically directed against conspecifics which are under the influence of this hormone, by either pheromonal or behavioral mechanisms or both. At the same time, however, the susceptibility of the inhibition of aggressive tendencies and for the development of submissive behaviors is activated, but only in males. Therefore, the behavioral inhibition after defeat, at least in rats, is a specific characteristic of the male's agonistic repertoire. It is possible that this is programmed by the organizational action of androgens during development. Gonadal hormones, both as an organizing and as an activating factor, influence the occurrence of sexual response, which frequently occurs during agonistic interaction. The interdependence of sexual and aggressive behavior, therefore, deserves further study.

Traditionally, it is assumed that different social response systems can be accounted for relatively independently, and sexual and aggressive behavior are viewed as representatives of independent motivational systems. At the same time, however, a clear interrelationship can be found, both in behavioral terms and in terms of the underlying mechanisms. Physiologically, for instance, both of these behavioral systems are influenced by gonadal hormones. Behaviorally, the sexual status of the opponent clearly influences aggressive reactions. In heterosexual aggression, ie aggressive behavior between males and females, in a test situation that was very similar to the one used in the experiments described in this chapter, the overall levels of aggression were found to be very low on the day of estrus when the female was sexually receptive (Swanson *et al.*, 1982). Observations on male rats living in groups of 10 in a large 'enriched' cage indicated that when a single receptive female was introduced, only very few of these males were sexually active. The rank order in which these males initiated sexual activity was consistent, possibly as a result of an already existing dominance hierarchy. No increase in fighting was observed in these Wistar rats (Swanson & van de Poll, 1983). Gartner *et al.* (1980) showed that when an estrus female rat was placed in a cage containing 4 males for 5 minutes per day, a single individual was sexually most active and also sired most of the offspring.

It will be clear that human social interactions in all their complexity can only be fully appreciated by the study of the typically human antecedents of behavior, ie in terms of cognitive processes and the development of specific behavioral trials. It lies beyond the scope of this article to review, or even summarize, the often conflicting evidence of the gonadal hormonal involvement in human aggression (for a recent review see Benton, 1981). Yet, however far the aggression of rodents may be removed from conflict in man, the identification of specific biological mediating mechanisms remains imperative, since complex cognitive functioning must be expected to have its roots in the interaction of a wide variety of biological functions, each of which in itself will prove to be of minor significance.

Acknowledgements—The authors wish to acknowledge the award of a European Training Programme in Brain and Behavior Research Twinning Grant between the Netherlands Institute for Brain Research and the Zoology Department, University College, Swansea, Wales, which financed part of the work described. Our gratitude is also extended to Peter van Nieuwkoop for his assistance in the preparation of this paper.

References

Barkley, M.S. & Goldman, B.D. (1977): Testosterone-induced aggression in adult female mice. *Horm. Behav.* **9,** 76-84.

Barnett, S.A. (1958): An analysis of social behavior in wild rats. *Proc. Zool. Soc.* **130,** 107-152.
Barr, G.A., Gibbons, J.L. & Moyer, K.E. (1976): Male-female differences and the influence of neonatal and adult testosterone on interspecies aggression in rats. *J. Comp. Physiol. Psychol.* **90,** 1169-1183.
Baum, M.J. & Vreeburg, J.T.M. (1976): Differential effects of the anti-estrogen MER-25 and of three 5a-reduced androgens on mounting and lordosis behavior in the rat. *Horm. Behav.* **7,** 87-104.
Beach, F.A. (1971): Hormonal differentiation and ramstergig copulatory behavior. In *The biopsychology of development,* eds Tobach, E., Aronson, L.R. & Shaw, E. New York: Academic Press.
Beeman, E.A. (1947): The effect of male hormone on aggressive behavior in mice. *Physiol. Zool.* **20,** 373-405.
Benton, D. (1981): The extrapolation from animals to man: the example of testosterone and aggression. In *Multidisciplinary approaches to aggression research,* eds Brain, P.F. & Benton, D. Amsterdam: Elsevier/North Holland Biomedical Press. Pp 401-419.
Bermond, B. (1978): Neurohumoral regulation of aggressive and sexual behavior in the rat. Dissertation, University of Amsterdam.
Bevan, W., Daves, W.F. & Levy, G.W. (1960): The relation of castration, androgen therapy and pretest fighting experience to competitive aggression in male C57 BL/10 mice. *Anim. Behav.* **8,** 6-12.
Bowden, N.J. (1979): Studies on the manner in which sex steroids influence aggressiveness in Mus musculus. PhD Thesis, University of Wales.
Brain, P.F. (1977): *Hormones and aggression,* Vol. 1. Annual Research Reviews. Montreal: Eden Press.
Brain, P.F. (1979): *Hormones, drugs and aggression.* Vol. 3. Annual Research Reviews. Montreal: Eden Press.
Brain, P.F. (1980): Adaptive aspects of hormonal correlates of attack and defence in laboratory mice: a study in ethobiology. In *Adaptive capabilities of the nervous system,* eds McConnell, P.S. *et al.* Progress in Brain Research, Vol. 53. Amsterdam: Biomedical Press. Pp 391-413.
Brain, P.F. (1981): Differentiating types of attack and defence in rodents. In *Multidisciplinary approaches to aggression research,* eds Brain, P.F. & Benton, D. Amsterdam: Elsevier/North Holland.
Brain, P.F. & Poole, A. (1974): Some studies on the use of 'standard opponents' in intermale aggression testing in TT albino mice. *Behaviour* **50,** 100-110.
Brain, P.F. & Bowden, N.J. (1978): Studies on the blockade of testosterone or oestradiol-17b-maintained fighting in castrated aggressive mice. *J. Endocrinol.* **72,** 40-41.
Bronson, F.H. & Desjardins, C. (1971): Steroid hormones and aggressive behavior in mammals. In *The physiology of aggression and defeat,* eds Elefheriou, B.E. & Scott, J.P. New York: Plenum Press.
Christie, M.H. & Barfield, R.J. (1979): Effects of aromatizable androgens on aggressive behavior among rats (Rattus norvegicus). *J. Endocrinol.* **83,** 17-26.
Edwards, D.A. (1969): Early androgen stimulation and aggressive behavior in male and female mice. *Physiol. Behav.* **4,** 333-338.
Edwards, D.A. (1970): Post-neonatal androgenization and adult aggressive behavior in female mice. *Phsyiol. Behav.* **5,** 465-467.
Fredericson, E. (1949): Response latency and habit strength in relationship to spontaneous fighting in C57 black mice. *Anat. Rec.* **105,** 509.
Gandelman, R. (1981): Androgen and fighting behavior. In *The biology of aggression,* eds Brain, P.F. & Benton, D. Alphen a/d Rijn, The Netherlands: Sijthoff and Noordhoff.
Gartner, K., Dohler, K. & Rechenberg, I. (1980): Internal selection and hormonal balance in rat population. *Adv. Physiol. Sciences* **13,** 263-267.
Ginsburg, B. & Allee, W.C. (1942): Some effects of conditioning on social dominance and subordination in inbred strains of mice. *Physiol. Zool.* **15,** 485-506.
Grant, E.C. & Change, M.R.A. (1958): Rank order in caged rats. *Anim. Behav.* **6,** 183-194.
Gray, J.A. (1971): Sex differences in emotional behaviour in mammals including man: endocrine bases. *Acta Psychol.* **35,** 29-46.

Gray, J.A. (1979): Emotionality in male and female rodents: a reply to Archer. *Br. J. Psychol.* **70,** 524-440.

Gray, J.A. & Buffery, A.W.H. (1971): Sex differences in emotional and cognitive behaviour in mammals including man: adaptive and neural bases. *Acta Psychol.* **35,** 89-111.

Kahn, M.W. (1951): The effect of severe defeat at various age levels on the aggressive behavior of mice. *J. Genet. Psychol.* **79,** 117-130.

Lagerspetz, K. (1961): Genetic and social causes of aggressive behavior in mice. *Scand. J. Psychol.* **2,** 167-173.

Lagerspetz, K. & Talo, S. (1967): *Maturation of aggressive behaviour in young mice.* Reports from the Institute of Psychology, University of Turku, No. 28. 1-9.

Larsson, K., Sodersten, P. & Beyer, C. (1973): Sexual behavior in male rats treated with estrogen in combination with dihydrostesterone. *Horm. Behav.* **4,** 289-299.

Leshner, A.I. (1979): Kinds of hormonal effects on behavior: a new view. *Neurosci. Biobehav. Rev.* **3,** 69-73.

Leshner, A.I. & Moyer, J.A. (1975): Androgens and agonistic behavior in mice: relevance to aggression and irrelevance to avoidance-of-attack. *Physiol. Behav.* **15,** 695-699.

Leshner, A.I. & Politch, J.A. (1979): Hormonal control of submissiveness in mice: irrelevance of the androgens and relevance of the pituitary-adrenal hormones. *Physiol. Behav.* **22,** 531-534.

Lupo di Prisco, C., Lucarini, N. & Dessi-Fulgheri, F. (1981): Testosterone aromatization in rat brain is modulated by social environment. *Physiol. Behav.* **20,** 345-348.

Luttge, W.A. (1972): Activation and inhibition of isolation-induced intermale fighting behavior in castrated CD-1 mice treated with steroidal hormones. *Horm. Behav.* **3,** 71-81.

Moyer, K.E. (1976): *The psychobiology of aggression.* Harper's Physiological Psychology Series. New York: Harper and Row.

Mugford, R.A. (1974): Androgenic stimulation of aggression eliciting cues in adult opponent mice castrated at birth, weaning or maturity. *Horm. Behav.* **5,** 93-102.

Mugford, R.A. & Nowell, N.W. (1970): The aggression of male mice against androgenized females. *Psychon. Sci.* **20,** 191-192.

Mugford, R.A. & Nowell, N.W. (1971): Endocrine control over production and activity of the anti-aggressive pheromone from female mice. *J. Endocrinol.* **49,** 225-232.

Naess, O., Attramadal, A. & Asbjorn, A. (1975): Androgen binding proteins in the anterior pituitary, hypothalamus, preoptic area and brain cortex of the rat. *Endocrinol.* **96,** 1-9.

Naftolin, F., Ryan, K.J. & Petro, Z. (1975): Aromatization of androstenedione by the anterior hypothalamus of adult male and female rats. *Endocrinol.* **90,** 295-297.

Parrott, R.F. (1975): Aromatizable and 5a-reduced androgens: differentiation between central and peripheral effects on male rat sexual behavior. *Horm. Behav.* **6,** 99-108.

Schechter, D., Howard, S.M. & Gandelman, R. (1981): Dihydrotestosterone promotes fighting behavior of female mice. *Horm. Behav.* **15,** 233-237.

Schuurman, T. (1980): Hormonal correlates of agonistic behavior in adult male rats. In *Adaptive capabilities of the nervous system, Progress in brain research,* Vol. 53, ed McConnell, P.S., Boer, G.J., Romijn, H.J., van de Poll, N.E. & Corner, M.A. Amsterdam: Elsevier/North Holland. Pp 415-420.

Scott, J.P. & Fredericson, E. (1951): The causes of fighting in mice and rats. *Physiol. Zool.* **24,** 273-309.

Scott, J.P. & Marston, M.W. (1953): Nonadaptive behavior resulting from a series of defeats in fighting mice. *J. Abnorm. Soc. Psychol.* **48,** 417-428.
Scott, J.P. & Marston, M.W. (1953): Nonadaptive behavior resulting from a series of defeats in fighting mice. *J. Abnorm. Soc. Psychol.* **48,** 417-428.
Selmanoff, M.K., Brodkin, L.D., Weiner, R.T. & Siiteri, P.K. (1977): Aromatization and 5a-reduction of androgens in discrete hypothalamic and limbic regions of the male and female rat. *Endocrinology* **101,** 841-849.

Seward, J.P. (1945): Aggressive behavior in the rat. I. General characteristics, age and sex differences. II. An attempt to establish a dominance hierarchy. *J. Comp. Psychol.* **38,** 175-224.

Seward, J.P. (1946): Aggressive behavior in the rat. IV. Submission as determined by conditioning, extinction and disuse. *J. Comp. Psychol.* **39,** 51-76.

Svare, B., Davis, P.G. & Gandelman, R. (1974): Fighting behavior in female mice following chronic androgen treatment during adulthood. *Physiol. Behav.* **12,** 399-403.

Swanson, H.H. & van de Poll, N.E. (1983): Effects of an isolated or enriched environment after handling on sexual maturation and behaviour in male and female rats. *J. Reprod. Fertil.* **69,** 165-171.

Swanson, H.H., van de Poll, N.E. & van Pelt, J. (1985): Influence of the oestrous cycle on heterosexual aggression in two strains of rats (S3 and WEzob). *Horm. Behav.* (In press).

Tsai, L.S. & Napier, H.S. (1968): Social conditioning in the modification of dominance hierarchy in white rats. *J. Soc. Psychol.* **76,** 83-88.

van de Poll, N.E., de Bruin, J.P.C. & van Oyen, H.G. (1978): Gonadal hormones and the differentiation of sexual and aggressive behavior and learning in the rat. In *Maturation of the nervous system, Progress in brain research,* Vol. 48, eds Corner, M.A. *et al.* Amsterdam: Elsevier. Pp 309-325.

van de Poll, N.E., de Jonge, F., van Oyen, H.G., van Pelt, J. & de Bruin, J.P.C. (1981*a*): Failure to find sex differences in testosterone-activated aggression in two strains of rats. *Horm. Behav.* **15,** 94-105.

van de Poll, N.E., de Jonge, F., van Oyen, H.G. & van Pelt, J. (1982): Aggressive behaviour in rats: effects of winning or losing on subsequent aggressive interactions. *Behav. Processes* **7,** 143-155.

van de Poll, N.E., Smeets, J., van Oyen, H.G. & van der Zwan, S.M. (1982): Behavioral consequences of agonistic experience in rats. Sex differences and the effects of testosterone. *J. Comp. Physiol.* **96,** 893-903.).

van de Poll, N.E., Swanson, H.H. & van Oyen, H.G. (1981*b*): Gonadal hormones and sex differences in aggression in rats. In *The biology of aggression,* eds Brain, P.F. & Benton, D. The Netherlands: Sijthoff and Noordhoff.

van de Poll, N.E. & van Dis, H. (1979): The effect of medial preoptic-anterior hypothalamic lesions on bisexual behavior of the male rat. *Brain Res. Bull.* **4,** 505-511.

van Oyen, H.G., van de Poll, N.E. & de Bruin, J.P.C. (1980): Effects of retention interval and gonadectomy on sex differences in passive avoidance behavior. *Physiol. Behav.* **25,** 859-862.

van Oyen, H.G., Walg, H. & van de Poll, N.E. (1981): Discriminated lever press avoidance conditioning in male and female rats. *Physiol. Behav.* **26,** 313-317.

Whalen, R.E. (1968): Differentiation of the neural mechanisms which control gonadotropin secretion and sexual behavior. In *Perspectives in reproduction and sexual behavior,* ed Diamond, M. Bloomington: Indiana University Press. Pp 303-340.

6

The sexual side-effects of drugs

Domeena C. RENSHAW

Loyola University of Chicago, 2160 South First Avenue, Maywood, Illinois 60153, USA

Introduction

From time immemorial, sex and love potions have been linked in the mind of man. The search for magical sexual enhancers or inhibitors ('spells' in ancient times) continues at a more rational level in contemporary medicine. Some scientists seek to discover an instant, temporary erectant using animal experiments, then human volunteers. For the most part, however, clinicians attempt to understand and control distressing sexual symptoms that occur when medically indicated drugs are prescribed and ingested. The sexual effects of drugs are reviewed in this chapter using the following classification: commonly used illicit or non-prescribed drugs; placebos; fertility drugs; and, essential medications.

Commonly used illicit or non-prescribed drugs

Aphrodisiacs. Donkey's milk, dried salamander, powdered rhinocerous horn or elephant's foot, salted crocodile, shark's fin, bees' wings, yohimbine (tree bark), cantharides (crushed beetles), bat's blood, clams, ginseng, sheep gonads and many other unusual substances have been at some time in history, and up to the present day, been suggested and tried as virilizers or aphrodisiacs.

Aphrodite, the Greek goddess of love, alledgedly emerged from the sea bringing erotic ecstacy to mankind. Her cult persists today in our fervent worldwide contemporary search for aphrodisiacs, now specified as a 'two-hour erectant'. When in 1980 an article appeared regarding the use of bromocriptine in Italy, literally hundreds of phone calls were received by Chicago hospitals seeking the name of the Italian center so that wealthy executives might fly over for rapid restoration of their libido or potency.

As portrayed in old lyric operas (Holbrook, 1959), witch doctors, magicians and alchemists tell tales of potions sold to anxious men for themselves and also to obtain irresistable attraction from a desired lover. The sexual side-effects of ingested potions depended, then as now, on the gullibility of the subject and the prestige of the potion peddler (Weil, 1975). Anecdotes of success abound in magazine advertisements which still extract huge amounts of money from the public, knowing well that a dissatisfied customer will usually be too ashamed to make any legal claims because of the unwanted revelation of his/her sexual problem.

New myths abound today around the alleged unique special sexual joy obtained from certain youth culture drugs, particularly marijuana and cocaine (Chopra, 1969; Perlman & Adams, 1970; Zinberg, 1974; Gay *et al.*, 1975; Innes & Nickerson, 1975;

Labataille, 1975; Sigell *et al.*, 1978; Buffman *et al.*, 1981), scientific research in these areas is just beginning (Bell & Trethewan, 1969; Cushman, 1973; Mendelson *et al.*, 1974; Cicero *et al.*, 1975; Holister, 1975; Angrist & Gershon, 1976; Krevene, 1977; Patrick, 1977; Smith *et al.*, 1979). Since expectations are such an important part of personal experience, such claims of aphrodisia must be refuted or repeated by objective controlled comparative studies in order to be of value to the medical community.

Alcohol. Alcohol is a universally available and very popular legal over-the-counter liquid drug. Regarding its seductive value, Ogden Nash humorously said 'Candy is dandy, but liquor is quicker'. Many centuries ago, Shakespeare wrote accurately of alcohol's sexual side-effects, stating that 'it increaseth the desire but reduceth the performance' (Macbeth, Act II, Scene 3). In men, alcohol excess causes immediate and long-term sexual problems: partial erections, impotence and delayed ejaculation. Despite excellent advertising by the powerful alcohol industry that virility, vigor, sophistication and sexiness are all enhanced by the right brand, it is still safe to say that the most common cause of the first episode of impotence in men is related to excess alcohol, which is still widely overused as a social and sexual 'lubricant' to attain courage and comfort in interpersonal exchange (Renshaw, 1978*a*).

There are some recent scientific studies which go far beyond subjective reports (Lemere & Smith, 1973; Gordon *et al.*, 1976; van Thiel & Lester, 1976; Gordon *et al.*, 1979). The effects of acute alcohol intake on pituitary-gonadal hormones in men and women, although still inconclusive, have been documented (Shader *et al.*, 1970; Wilson & Lawson, 1976; Mendelson *et al.*, 1977). Long-range effects of hypogonadism and male feminization in chronic alcoholics have also been reported (Shader & Dimascio, 1970). Despite common myths, women alcoholics do not enjoy sex more than non-intoxicated women. However, they may be more compliant, often in order to obtain the alcohol upon which they have become dependent.

Marital problems may be profound when either male or female partner is the abuser. Fighting or withdrawal in the bedroom regarding past or present alcohol intake may interfere with pleasurable sexual exchange. Either sober or in a drinking state, verbal hostility or physical abuse may lead to pain and sensitivity to the point of a challenge: 'It's me or the drink, not both'. The bottle often wins immediately and divorce may follow some time later.

Marijuana. This today is a widely used 'recreational' street drug (Chopra, 1969). It is well known anecdotally that time perception is distorted in those who use tetrahydrocannabinol (THC), the active ingredient of 'pot', 'hash' or 'grass'. Whatever the subject's mood at the moment, when smoking or ingesting pot, it will be enhanced: for example, feeling blue may become tearful; wanting to be quiet may lead to marked withdrawal; feeling sexually neutral may become apathy; feeling sexually excited may become more so; anger may be sometimes aggravated to the point of violence. Therefore, those who feel sexy or anticipate fabulously long and great orgasms when smoking pot, may indeed have that feeling at a particular time when the drug is used. However, although multiple trials are made by some, the effect for that individual may, woefully, not be duplicated. Studies regarding testosterone levels and 'marijuana' are controversial (Chopra, 1969; Mendelson *et al.*, 1974; Zinberg, 1974; Buffman *et al.*, 1981).

Physicians should routinely ask about the use of 'pot' or other street drugs as they do about alcohol intake. Questions to ask are: Have you used marijuana? How frequently? Alone, or as a couple or in a group? For how many hours? What immediate subjective reactions? Are, or were there, domestic, work or sexual sequelae?

Stimulants. Both methylphenidate and amphetamine are thought to act centrally on the brain (Bell & Trethowan, 1964; Angrist & Gershon, 1976). They are available both legitimately and on the street where abuse potential is high (Patrick, 1977). Their sexual effects seems variable and relate to the sex, personality, extent and route of usage as well as to previous sexual experience, preferences and fears. Heightened or disturbed sexual response has been reported by acute and chronic ingesters.

A single white male aged 29 years was admitted to a Chicago Veteran's Hospital in 1969 after he had injected an unknown amount of self-mixed amphetamine into his left brachial artery; he developed sustained priapism and an acute toxic psychosis during which he agitatedly chopped off his penis and very nearly bled to death.

Most abusers who ingest the stimulant do not have such a dramatic reaction. Initially, they report high energy and a heightened sex drive which diminishes after a few days when exhaustion sets in. This is followed by irritability, anxiety, restlessness and paranoia.

Cocaine. Man's use of cocaine began with chewing coca (not cocoa) leaves in the Andes Mountains in South America. Early European explorers described the drug's effects on inhabitants there. Prolonged large doses over several days produced a toxic psychosis leading to frenetic hypersexuality which was insatiable and undifferentiated, giving no sexual relief to the exhausted individual who might attain climax after climax without any personal satisfaction. There was no selectivity in partner choice. In their sexual urgency, men were seen thrusting against a sack of hemp. The genitals were reported as swollen and mutilated at the end of a three day ritual festival.

The current wide social use of cocaine by upper contemporary urbanites is still poorly understood (Hollister, 1975; Buffman, 1981). It may be inhaled, ingested or injected. Nothing is known scientifically of the sexual side-effects, but there is much subjective lore about enhancement of sexual desire and performance (Patrick, 1977). As with pot and amphetamine, agitation, exhaustion and paranoia may occur in vulnerable individuals with a low dose, or in others with high doses or prolonged abuse.

Special caution is needed for persons who seek sexual rainbows with the use of non-prescribed drugs. The substances are often impure, and contaminants may be not only toxic but also lethal, especially when agricultural chemicals are sprayed to protect highpaying cash crops such as coca trees, but are not neutralized before processing for street sale.

Amyl nitrite, There are reports of death due to illicit inhalation of amyl nitrite capsules during sexual relations. These reports are poorly documented, since the licit drug is illicitly obtained to create a subjective sexual 'rush'. An altered state of consciousness allegedly occurs shortly after use, causing a tingling sensation in the head and whole body, while simultaneously producing visual scotomata (blind or dark spots) plus a feeling of faintness (Perlman & Adams, 1970; Sigell *et al.*, 1978). At times, there may be a tendency to lose the erection. After using amyl nitrite (Labataille, 1975) some men report relaxation of the anal sphincter for homosexual or anal intercourse or in a woman partner. The mind-altering effects seem to be enjoyed and sought after by a sizable number of homosexual men who use the drug recurrently and develop methemoglobinemia as a consequence. A fall in blood pressure may reduce available blood to the coronary arteries and so produce cardiac ischemia and infarct. Despite the wide use of nitrites, particularly in young men (both heterosexual and homosexual), scientific study is difficult. Therefore, there is, at present, little known of medical certainty.

Psychedelic drugs. Various kinds are available on the streets with much publicity as 'mind expanding' or 'mind destroying' agents. They have been promoted as recreational and defended by some pop psychologists as necessary for spiritual or religious experiences (Weil, 1975). Few physicians would agree. While the occasional psychedelic, such as lysergic acid, has been studied scientifically for cognitive, perceptual or therapeutic effects, none have been objectively studied regarding specific sexual side-effects. In terms of sexual functioning, inconclusive subjective reports range from 'no effect' to 'better intimacy' or 'worse'. Many hallucinogens produce a florid toxic psyhotic state where delusions have resulted in mutilating self-destruction or homicide.

Nicotine. When the West discovered and adopted tobacco smoking it was for men only and became a sign of machismo and opulence. In time, tobacco gradually became less scarce. In the 20th century, teenagers saw it as a rite of passage into the adult world. Since the 19th century, women smoked as an affirmation of their independence, sophistication, sexiness and freedom. Cigarette smoking in pregnancy has been associated with an increased rate of spontaneous abortion, perinatal mortality and decreased birthweight. This widespread practice is also a high risk factor for coronary disease in both men and women. In addition, smoking is associated with early menopause and cervical and pulmonary cancer. Its effect on testosterone levels, fertility and potency are unclear and inconclusive (Briggs, 1973; Jick *et al.*, 1977; Kline *et al.*, 1977; Pirani, 1978). Emphysema, as a complication of heavy smoking, may make the physical effort of intercourse more difficult as the increased rate of breathing of sex arousal may cause discomfort and distress to an anxious partner who may fear the terminal moment is upon her or him.

Other illicit drugs surface daily with great promises of general or sexual happiness. Each one will require careful evaluation of its effects on the user; its chemical content; the positive and the negative physical effects on the genital system plus the long-range side-effects. Science demands carefully controlled studies and comparisons, difficult enough with legitimate drugs and often impossible with illegal ones. However, unless these studies are carried out, we will be no further ahead than the African witchdoctors who dispense rhinocerous horn potions. In the 1980s, although there are as yet no magical aphrodisiacs for sexual joy, we are for the first time slowly coming to be aware of the physiological complexities of human sexual functioning. Currently, the perfume industry is attempting to isolate pheromones, the primate signal of estrus from human male sweat and vaginal lubrication. Irresistable aphrodisia is still the goal!

Placebos

Placebos have long been known to be powerful healers. Around the world, it is clinically noted that 30 per cent of subjects, when told reassuringly and enthusiastically that an inert substance or a gadget (which has no real therapeutic effect on the complaint) will help a symptom, obtain relief. The mechanism by which symptom reversal is obtained, as well as whether the use of placebos in medicine is deceitful or at times indicated and ethical, is controversial (Duncan & Laird, 1980). These same questions relate to sexual symptoms and the use of sexual aids, whether chemical or gimmicks: rings, straps, 'vacuum developers' for the penis (Holbrook, 1959).

Current placebo theories consider: the reassuring effects of the doctor-patient relationship (fear-reducing and a 'safety' signal); the predisposing effects of anxiety by the patient (better placebo response); an attitude of certainty of cure in the physician (more reassuring to an anxious patient); the patient's expectation-effect (positive or negative) of what will occur with the placebo; the personality of the patient: placebo effect more likely with a 'situation cuer' (one who looks to outside stimuli for his or her feeling orientation) and less likely with a 'self-cuer' (one who responds to cues from his or her own body like a frown, smile or muscle tension) (the self-cuer seems more prone to a reverse placebo effect with a worsening of symptoms); the patient's capacity for self-deception, eg analgesia through a placebo; and, the possible physiological release of endorphins (endogenous natural opiate-like brain peptides which seem to be synaptic transmitters or modulators of pain and emotions) when 'placebo-reassurance' occurs.

Whatever their mechanism(s) of action, even quack aphrodisiacs (powders, pomades, pills and potions) will be placebo-effective in one-third of the cases in which they are used when the sexual problem relates to underlying anxiety. Nevertheless if placebo reassurance from true or false newspaper testimonials, sex therapy or a minute amount of tranquillizer has attained physiological reversal of vaginismus or of impotence, then the art of healing (formal or informal) has served the patient well (for the time being, at least!). Unless the patient has the commonsense and personality strength to read and be reassured by the clear 'body language' of restored function, the placebo effect may be short-lived. Repeated symptom-free sexual expression may reinforce the new found self-confidence and lead to a true cure.

Fertility drugs

Even in overpopulated areas of the world, failure to conceive has, for thousands of years, been considered a calamity. Women have deemed barrenness a blight. Until the mid-nineteenth century, when scientific physiology began to supplement structural knowledge of the genitals, the actual process of conception was a total mystery. In the mid-1600s, the microscope allowed human spermatozoa and ova to be identified. Two centuries later, their union was observed microscopically in starfish and, much later, in humans.

In primitive times, the most urgent needs of man were to preserve life itself, the family, the tribe and the race. Infant and maternal mortality were exceedingly high. Religious and magical aids were sought to ensure fecundity. Prehistoric cave paintings and sculptures depict pregnant women and animals as if this could ensure the fertility of the tribe and the herds needed for food. Ritual festivals used genital images to invite, from the Gods, favors of abundant harvests and the children needed for the work and survival of the clan. Shame and ostracism resulted for barren women, but occasionally also for a sterile African Ashanti man who was ridiculed as having a 'wax penis'. East African Lango women not unusually commit suicide if they did not conceive soon after marriage. For orthodox Jews, a woman's failure to conceive after a certain time of marriage was considered sufficient grounds for divorce; the husband's fertility was not questioned until relatively recent times.

Besides prayers, magical spells and counter-spells, various medicines have been used formally and informally to cure sterility. Kiwai women ate spiders and their myriad eggs. Andamanese women ate a prolific frog. Some Polynesian men drank gallons of coconut milk since its vague resemblance to semen was said to enhance fertility. Codfish or salmon eggs have also been considered delicacies for the same reason.

Although there are a few tribes known who did not relate intercourse to conception (Trobrianders and Arunta, both Pacific islanders), most did; undoubtedly by observation of animal matings. However, there was still a mystery of why most human matings (not confined only to estrus) did not result in pregnancy. Supernatural powers, the phases of the moon, ancestral reincarnation, witchcraft, demon coitus (when the child was deformed) or special divine blessing have all been beliefs related to conception. The beliefs have, for obvious reasons, always been linked with potency in men and often with 'defects' in women, who were usually blamed both for infertility and for not bearing sons.

Scientific endocrinology is hardly a century old. With it came an understanding of the cycle of female ovulation-menstruation, the critical sperm count, and other physical barriers to conception. These parameters were medically utilized in infertility clinics and programs. Malformations or infections of the ovaries, fallopian tubes, uterus, cervix or vagina must be diagnosed and corrected. The husband's role has now been acknowledged in the literate West. His sperm count (more than 100 million sperm per ejaculate) is considered essential for impregnation. Causes of a low sperm count are varied: thyroid, adrenal or pituitary deficiency; infections (mumps, prostatitis); testicular abnormalities (congenital failure to descend or develop, irradiation, trauma); anemia; malnutrition; severe psychic stress; industrial or agricultural chemical toxins. Both partners are carefully studied; structurally (for anatomical patency of the reproductive organs) as well as physiologically. Remedial surgery may be indicated or medications prescribed, popularly known as fertility drugs, to stimulate ovulation or spermatogenesis.

In the past ten years, there has been unprecedented progress in understanding the complex hormonal factors involved in human reproduction (Murad & Gilman, 1975). Couples attending infertility clinics feel enormous pressures to 'succeed' and conceive, so much so that they have formed self-help groups to support each other. Improved technology has added ultrasound investigations of follicular development, human gonadotropins and anti-gonadotropins to the older anti-androgens, anti-estrogens and anti-prolactins, all adding astronomically to the cost of seeking pregnancy. Because of the newness of these drugs and procedures, long-term experience is limited. Careful data collection and reporting is, therefore, limited. In 1982 in Chicago, fertility treatment cost $3000 or more per menstrual cycle, and up to six or eight cycles of treatment might be required. This kind of financial strain may so increase the psychogenic pressure to conceive that the husband may become coitally impotent, at which stage, in some circumstances, artificial insemination of his ejaculate may be undertaken.

Little is mentioned of the arousal of women's sexual desire or of orgasm in the literature on fertility drugs since the medical goals of pregnancy or control of endometriosis are primary. Numerous gynecologists report that, clinically, their patients on fertility drugs did not report increased libido. It may be worth asking this question explicitly, since patients may not volunteer sexual information.

Some of the fertility drugs in use in the USA are:

Danazol (Danocrine). This compound is a synthetic androgen derived from ethisterone. The drug is used to suppress the pituitary-ovarian axis by inhibiting the output of pituitary gonadotropins. It is used for inducing fertility in women with endometriosis. It is also used for fibrocystic breast disease and for males or females with hereditary angioedema. The sexual effects are unknown, but there are isolated physician reports of heightened libido in women taking this drug.

Prednisone. This is a dihydrogenated analogue of cortisone and is somewhat more active; it is used in infertile women with high levels of androgen; its sexual effects are unknown.

Clomiphene citrate (Clomid). This is a non-steroidal synthetic compound, structurally similar to estrogen. In initial animal studies it gave surprising results: very slight estrogenic activity, moderate anti-estrogenic activity and striking inhibition of pituitary function with a potent contraceptive effect in both sexes. However, in humans, an increase in ovarian size with follicular maturation and ovulation was noted. In proper dose application, Clomid has been an effective agent for reversal of infertility in women with amenorrhea, the Stein-Leventhal syndrome or anovulatory cycles. There is a high incidence of multiple births with clomiphene treatment.

The mode of action of this drug is uncertain, but one theory is that clomiphene competitively binds to cytoplasmic estrogen receptors, diminishing the endogenous estrogen's inhibitory effect upon the pituitary. By preventing this natural 'feedback inhibition', there is increased secretion of LH-RH/FSH-RH and gonadotrophins. Many minor undesirable side-effects are noted: irritability, mood changes, cystic ovaries, hot flashes, gastric upset, skin rashes, visual disturbances, reduced cervical mucus and vaginitis. Major warnings are given regarding neoplasia, use during pregnancy (fetal abnormalities) and thrombotic disease (Murad & Haynes, 1980). The drug's sexual effects are unknown.

Clomiphene had also been used to treat infertile men in order to stimulate sperm formation by the anti-estrogen effect which theoretically frees the pituitary of endogenous estrogen inhibition, so that there is an increased production of luteinizing hormone to stimulate testicular Leydig cell production of testosterone. Theoretically, libido should, thus, be increased, but reports are sparse and the sexual effects unknown.

Bromocriptine mesylate. This non-hormonal peptide ergot alkaloid derivative is a dopamine receptor agonist that allegedly activates post-synaptic dopamine receptors. Secretion of prolactin from the anterior pituitary is inhibited by the administration of bromocriptine in women or men with hyperprolactinemia who then show a significntly reduced plasma level of prolactin after some weeks of treatment (Miller *et al.*, 1980; Buffman *et al.*, 1981). It has been approved for use in the USA for amenorrhea, galactorrhea and female infertility (Shader & DiMascio, 1970). It has also been used for hyperprolactinemic men, with or without pituitary pathology or infertility, on the theory that lowering plasma prolactin will increase testosterone secretion. The drug was available in Europe for at least six years before release in the USA, where, in the mid 1970s, bold newspaper headlines proclaimed the drug as the first scientific aphrodisiac, providing libido awareness for some women and men who had 'not had an erotic feeling in their lives'. In wide use in infertility clinics over the past two years, its sexual effects were stated to range from 'none in women and a temporary boost to some of the men'. Obviously, more definitive studies are needed.

Menotrophin. This compound contains FSH (follicle stimulating hormone) and LH (luteinising hormone) plus lactose for injection. This preparation of human gonadotrophins is from the urine of post-menopausal women. Chorionic gonadotrophin may be used in conjunction with menotrophin to induce ovulation in infertile women. On alternate days, post-injection, ultrasound tests are carried out in order to follow follicular development for optimal timing of coitus (or artificial insemination) for fertilization. The cost is roughly $3000 per cycle and, in some cases, six cycles of treatment are required before pregnancy occurs. The sexual effects of menotrophin are unknown.

Essential medications

While there are new horizons of knowledge relating to cerebral (central) as well as peripheral-genital neurohumoral connections and controls, much remains to be studied in sexual medicine.

More chemical aids are available, people are living longer, they read more and expect more answers from their physicians. There are few controlled studies of the pharmacodynamics and the sexual side-effects of needed medications, so there are still many unsolved riddles, particularly in women who are much less likely than men to complain to their physicians of sexual side-effects. Men immediately note a lack of erection and ejaculation and seek medical help to return to the active role of penetrator. Women are sexually receptive and may easily supplement lowered vaginal secretions by an artificial lubricant or saliva, and, therefore, they may continue to function sexually without a physician's help. Occasionally, however, a woman (like many men), when her libidinal or orgastic responses are suddenly affected by a new medication, may be non-compliant and discontinue treatment.

Hormones

Hormones produce sexual effects from the fetal stage onwards. Androgens cause sexual differentiation and dominance of male genitalia in the first trimester of pregnancy, while unopposed estrogen/progesterone acts on the embryonic female genitalia to enhance development and functioning.

In adolescence, estrogen and progesterone balance the menstrual cycle, while testosterone increases growth of male muscles, genitals and beard and causes voice changes. With abundant growth hormone, the combination results in an all-time high of new, sometimes overwhelming sexual feelings and genital responses for the teenager.

A newly studied congenital pseudohermaphroditism in Central America has led to the discovery of the enzyme 5-a-reductase which converts testosterone to active dehydrotestosterone in the embryo and again at puberty. It seems that when embryonic testosterone is non-responsive, the infant appears and is reared as a female, but at puberty differentiates as a male with hypospadias. This condition may yet provide a physiological key to understanding the complexities of virility.

Androgens. These compounds were first assayed and isolated in the 1930s. Gynecologists have for many years used microdoses of androgens empirically to stimulate the libido of female patients complaining of lowered sex interest, but their use for this purpose is highly controversial (Meyler, 1975; Goodman & Gilman, 1980; Renshaw, 1980). Some gynecologists insist that there is much more than a placebo effect in the monthly booster shots of methyltestosterone. The literature is threadbare on this prevalent gynecological practice, the results of which, endocrinologists say, spill over into their offices when the frightening virilizing signs appear. Real medical concern is needed regarding adverse side-effects of prescribed testosterone given orally or intramuscularly; 5 mg per day may result in irreversible beard growth, voice deepening and clitoral hypertrophy. In addition, cholestatic jaundice is a possible side-effect. When androgens are given during pregnancy, fetal abnormalities can occur.

There is undisputedly a definite place for the use of androgens in cases of adrenal insufficiency. We also know from rare cases that feminized hermaphrodites secreting large amounts of androgens may have a high libido and also a marked hypertrophy of the clitoris owing to their congenital mixed differentiation. The side-effects of inadequate vaginal cleft, voice, beard and pendulous clitoris all required correction. Sensitive sex education, life-long medical care and supportive counselling may be critical for long-term healthy life adjustment in those with birth defects of the genitalia.

Males seeking assistance with lowered libido or impotence actively seek 'hormone shots' from their physicians. If there is a lowered level of the active form of testosterone, dihydrotesterone replacement by testosterone enanthate (intramuscularly) or methyltestosterone (orally) is indicated. The intramuscular route is more effective than oral administration. Since the drug is detoxicated in the liver, cholestatic jaundice is a possible complication of treatment. Frequently, without the costly and complex assay of testosterone blood levels, men are given 'hormone shots' empirically. The known potential placebo success is 30 per cent. However, continued use may produce negative testosterone side-effects such as edema, gynaecomastia, acne, baldness and the risk of prostatic carcinoma.

Estrogens. When given therapeutically to postmenopausal women, estrogen opposes androgen action of the brain and genitals, maintains vaginal epithelium and lubrication and improves sexual functioning (Renshaw, 1980). Carcinogenic potential is of concern. Estrogens are used in the treatment of men with prostatic carcinoma but, by their anti-androgen effect, they reduce libido. Other estrogen side-effects in males may be loss of body hair and increased breast development.

Oral contraceptives. The relationship of these drugs to libido remains a matter of controversy, although millions of women have used them for thousands of days since the mid 1950s. For every study indicating that libido is decreased, another one points to its increase (Kurtner & Schwyhart, 1974; Murad & Gilman, 1975). In Ecuador, the results of a double-blind study of oral contraceptives versus placebo suggested that both decreased sexual desire by 30 per cent. In South Africa, a study by two gynecologists showed that medroxyprogesterone acetate resulted in an increase in libido in white women, but a decrease in black women. Pinkus, in the USA, in a double-blind study, found more negative side-effects with placebo than with the contraceptive pill. The results are very difficult to interpret (Kantor, 1977). Although progesterone-containing oral contraceptives may depress libido, some women report an increase (Kaplan, 1974). For some, the generalized and local edema may increase sensitivity of the clitoris and, therefore, sexual desire. For others, this group of drugs results in generalized irritability. Some women feel sexually liberated and no longer fear pregnancy, while others say that contraceptive safety 'takes the thrill of risk out of sex'. Recently, with media headlines being made by the potential hazards of the pill, carcinoma, cardiac disease, thrombosis, many women are returning to barrier contraceptives such as the diaphragm and spermicides. The Women's Liberation Movement has condemned the pill as a 'travesty on the body of women, invented by men'.

Synthetic steroids. Used in the treatment of allergic, inflammatory and other chronic diseases these drugs may, in both sexes, produce euphoria and improved general functioning and, therefore, improved sexual functioning. They may, however, have an anti-androgen effect and reduce libido (Cooper, 1972).

Thyroid hormone. Deficiency results in decreased libido as part of a general apathy. However, hyperthyroidism is not known to increase sexual desire.

Cyproterone acetate. This compound is a steroid that competes for dihydrotestosterone receptor sites. It is, therefore, a potent anti-androgen that 'impairs male sexual function'. It also suppresses gonadotrophins and is being used experimentally, in cases of compulsive sexual disorders, to assist men with 'irresistable impulses'. Some success has been reported in controlling unacceptable behavior in men with compulsive exhibitionism, pedophilia and fetishism. Feminizing side-effects soon occur. Within six weeks of treatment cessation, erections and deviant impulses recur, plus the driven sexual behavior (Bartholemew, 1968; Tennent, 1974; Byck, 1975).

Antibiotics

This group of drugs is widely used for a variety of general as well as local infections. Although resistant strains of organisms have developed, they have, of course, worked modern miracles in VD clinics since the late 1940s. Sexual effects of venereal diseases relate both to symptoms of local pain as well as to fear of general personal complications, partner infection, fetal damage (if the woman is pregnant), remorse, guilt and a cluster of anxieties about sinfulness, punishment, permanent contagion and future sterility.

Sexual effects of antibiotics *per se* are not known. Some, notably the tetracyclines, may cause women to have a distressing vaginitis by destroying normal vaginal organisms. Intercourse may then be uncomfortable and be avoided. This common side-effect can be avoided by telling the woman to eat unsweetened yoghurt daily, as well as to insert 5 cc of the same unsweetened yogurt into the vagina daily. Thus, new lactobacilli are introduced to restore the natural vaginal ecology.

Chemotherapeutic agents

Agents for cancer mitigation have been known to be associated with changes in adolescent boys and men and also menstrual changes in women and girls (some acute and reversible, others permanent) (Greenberg *et al.*, 1975; Guinan, 1976; Schilsky *et al.*, 1980). Sexual changes may relate to: general weakness; nutritional needs; effects of irradiation; disseminated malignancy; necessary but mutilating, surgery, eg mastectomy; the effects of chemotherapy: chlorambucil, vincristine or combinations with resultant nausea, amenorrhea, hair loss; the realization of having a life-threatening or terminal illness; fear of losing a marriage, loved ones and onself; fear of transmitting the cancer. Every cancer patient must be individually evaluated to establish the effect of the cancer and treatment on body image, the marital relationship and sexual functioning. The precancer sexual history must always be obtained (even in a teenager), so that the sexual effects of any drug given may be studied and understood in perspective.

With survival so important a goal, oncology research does not list sexual effects as a high priority for study. There also seems to be a marked reluctance on the part of oncologists to inquire about the sexual responses of cancer patients, who repeatedly complain in their self-help groups of being totally 'desexualized' by their physician's sexual silence and avoidance of this (to them) important part of their salvaged life and their adjustment to the post-cancer phase of rehabilitation.

With many young people recovering from leukemia, nephrotic syndrome and Hodgkin's disease, some information is beginning to appear in the literature relating to the fertility possibilities after chemotherapy, and reports of spermatogenesis are now being recorded.

Knowledge of increasing survival rates give hope of restored vitality to cancer patients. Women cancer patients, even those undergoing chemotherapy, approach nurses, asking questions about when coitus may be resumed. They say they hesitate to take up the physician's valuable time with sexual questions. Perhaps, they sense the physician's reluctance to deal with a sexual question, and find a nurse more sympathetic and open, but they do ask. Does the question mean the cancer patient has sexual desire, fear of losing her husband or a great need to be held by him and can only achieve this through intercourse? Until these questions are explicitly asked, we will not know.

Hypnotic drugs

These compounds are available over-the-counter in most countries to meet the perceived needs for 'instant sleep' in today's ovestimulated unrelaxed man and woman. Many commercial hypnotics are combinations of sedative and hypnotic drugs, some including analgesics. In 1853, bromide was the first of the 'modern sleeping pills'. Medically prescribed hypnotics, despite dangers of the development of dependency and abuse, still include barbiturates and sedating benzodiazepines. In 1976, an estimated one billion doses of hypnotics were dispensed on physician's orders. They are capable of widespread depression of central nervous system (CNS) function and cause drowsiness, ataxia, poor coordination, retrograde amnesia, and muscle relaxation which may persist the next day (Goodman & Gilman, 1980).

Since antiquity, sleeping potions have been used, some, according to folklore, surreptiously, for romantic or for sinister sexual seduction by producing stupor in a reluctant or unconsenting lady for what today would be regarded legally as rape. From sleep laboratory EEG studies, hypnotic drugs produce: increased REM (rapid eye movement) stage latency, ie from K spindle sleep to first REM burst; reduced total time in the REM stage; possible increase (late in the sleep segment) of cycles of brief REM. REM deprivation may result in anxiety, overeating, poor concentration, hypersexuality and vivid dream (more vivid, sexual and bizarre) (Karacan *et al.*, 1978; Karacan, 1982). The duration of the symptoms listed under this last heading is unknown, but what is known is that hypnotics very rapidly aggravate insomnia (Renshaw, 1977*b*; Williams, 1980).

Methaqualone. This compound is a hypnotic that has become widely abused with street drug salesmen contending there is a guaranteed aphrodisiac effect and instant uninhibited sexuality. 'Qualude', 'Sopers', 'Luders' are some of the street names coined by the non-medical users of methaqualone for sexual enhancement. A total body tingling is subjectively reported, especially in women, and the drug may work through a disinhibitory mechanism. In some men, it has a negative effect on both desire and erection. Regular abusers of methaqualone become ataxic and have leg weakness making going downstairs especially hazardous. Considered an inhibitor of spinal synapses, methaqualone could also result in impotence. Mild overdoses cause restlessness and excitation, rather than sedation, with myoclonic contractions and frank convulsions from both excess dosage as well as sudden withdrawal. Dialysis has not always been successful for treatment of an overdose.

Routine sexual questions for physicians to ask patients taking hypnotics relate to the frequency of intercourse, difficulties with desire, arousal, ejaculation, climax and satisfaction. For patients repeatedly requesting hypnotics, key questions relate to: underlying depressive illness with anorexia, weight loss and suicidal thoughts; marital conflict or a sexual dysfunction being handled by hypnotics to avoid sexual contact (Renshaw, 1977*b*).

Antihistamines

These are used for their capacity to compete for H_1 and H_2 histamine peripheral and CNS receptors. Since they may also interfere with serotonin and norepinephrine uptake, they are noted to have both sedative and stimulant effects (Innes & Nickerson, 1975). It was as recently as 1937 that histamine blocking activity was noted and the first antihistamine synthesized. Most H_1 blockers inhibit smooth muscle responses to histamine, thus protecting against bronchospasm, capillary permeability (reducing skin 'flare', itch and nasal congestion) and are effective treatment for allergic reactions. They may either stimulate the CNS causing restlessness and insomnia or produce sedation and sleepiness. H_1 blockers also exert an anticholinergic effect, peripherally and centrally, that may result in decreased libido, urinary difficulties and erectile problems. H_2 blockers were pursued for specific action on the hypersecretion of gastric acid leading to peptic ulcers, a prevalent modern stress disease.

Cimetidine. Two hundred and one systematic stepwise modifications of the histamine molecule finally led to a triumph of scientific chemistry in the early 1970s with the discovery of *cimetidine* which is generally well tolerated, of low toxicity and mostly excreted unchanged in 24 hours. Cimetidine reduces both the volume of gastric acid and its hydrogen ion concentration, and has proven value, therefore, in the treatment of duodenal ulcer, other gastric hypersecretory states and resistant urticaria. Despite its lack of anticholinergic action, men using it have complained of lowered libido, breast increase and impotence (Fave *et al.*, 1977; Hall, 1979; Peden *et al.*, 1979; van Thiel *et al.*, 1979; Winters *et al.*, 1979; Wolfe, 1979; Gifford *et al.*, 1980). The mechanisms of these sexual dysfunctions are unclear. In rat experiments cimetidine had anti-androgen effects. One woman developed galactorrhea. The possibility of a hypothalamic-pituitary-gonadal pathway of cimetidine affecting the seminiferous tubules is postulated for secondary hormonal changes. A very careful explicit pre-ulcer and pre-cimetidine sexual history must be taken by every family physician, internist and gastroenterologist before prescribing this newest popular drug. It is a tribute that seven papers in five years address the sexual effects of cimetidine. Does this mean a wide prevalence of sexual symptoms, better investigator questioning or more open patient voluntary reporting? These questions await further research reports.

Antihypertensive drugs

These drugs are divided into four groups: diuretics; sympatholytic or adrenergic effect on venous/arteriolar vessels; vasodilators; and, combinations of these three groups.

Untreated hypertensives have been noted to report impotency difficulties in 8-10 per cent of cases, more so with increasing age and severe hypertensive disease (Oaks & Mayer; Carver & Oaks, 1976). The effect of symptoms such as lassitude and severe headache may relate to sexual avoidance of lessened libido rather than impotence. Each man must be asked explicit questions.

Once antihypertensive treatment is initiated, the resultant sexual side-effects may instantly lessen medication compliance, with or without the physician being informed. Therefore, in order to ensure the use of needed medication through dose change or trials of an alternate drug (Shader, 1970; Seagraves, 1977; Renshaw, 1978*a*, 1980), on follow-up, each male or female patient should routinely be asked about their sexual desire and arousal, intercourse and masturbatory frequency, vaginal lubrication and also about ejaculation.

Diuretics. Diuretics alone are often used for milder degrees of hypertension to prevent retention of Na, Cl and water. Despite its not being mentioned as a side-effect in the Physician's Desk Reference (PDR), one group reported that 33 per cent of hypertensive men treated with diuretics alone, complained of erectile problems (Mroczek *et al.*, 1972). Scattered clinical vignettes report ejaculation problems, gynecomastia and hirsutism and menstrual irregularities indicating hormonal changes. Thiazides and spironolactone seem most likely to produce potency problems, often immediately (Viliet & Meyer, 1982). These complications are reversed when the drug is discontinued and this also holds true for combination antihypertensives containing diuretics. A switch to fluresmide, a derivative of anthirilic acid that acts specifically on renal tubules and Henle's loop, has been found sparing of sexual function. The mechanism of action is unclear.

If switching diuretic is not effective in reducing blood pressure, then either a switch in the timing of lovemaking or taking the diuretic at a different time can be discussed with the patient in order to attain optimum management.

Anti-sympathomimetic or anti-adrenergic antihypertensives. Methyldopa. This seems to be the most widely used drug in this group and is generally effective in lowering blood pressure. It is an inhibitor of dopa-decarboxylase. Although not yet conclusively demonstrated in humans, animal studies have shown tissue reductions in serotonin, dopamine, norepinephrine and epinephrine levels plus an elevation of serum prolactin. After ingestion, methyldopa is metabolized to alpha-methyl-norepinephrine which may, by fasle transmission, stimulate central inhibitory alpha-adrenergic receptors, thereby lowering the level of adrenergic transmitter. Whatever the site of action, methyldopa may cause up to 36 per cent impotency in hypertensive men. Inhibition of ejaculation and, at times, retrograde ejaculation into the bladder can also ensue. These side-effects are almost always reversed when the drug is discontinued. Ten normotensive men administered methyldopa were found to have no immediate erectile difficulty. Possible side-effects reported with long-term use of the drug are: breast enlargement in women: gynecomastia in men; and, in both sexes, galactorrhea and lowered libido. Two of the author's patients complained of partial erections and an inability to ejaculate, theoretically as a result of the drug's adrenergic effect. These symptoms reversed when the patients were switched to prazosin, a vasodilating hypotensive drug. Reports of comparative, double-blind studies are now appearing in the literature relating to this and other antihypertensives, such as clonidine, reserpine (central catecholamine depleting effect) which can also cause sexual problems (Horowitz, 1967; Kahn *et al.,* 1970; Masters & Johnson, 1970; Papadopoulous, 1972; Bullpit & Dollery, 1973; Greenblatt & Roch-Weser, 1973; Raftos *et al.,* 1973; Kaplan, 1974; Renshaw 1978; Hogan *et al.,* 1980).

Ganglion blocking hypertensives. Propranolol. This is a derivative of 'DCI', dichloroisoproterenol, a selective adrenergic receptor blocker. Since the mid 1970s, propranolol has enjoyed astronomical popularity in US medicine for the treatment of cardiac arrhythmias and angina as well as for hypertension and migraine. Dose levels have far exceeded PDR suggestions. Asthmatics and insulin-dependent diabetics are considered unsuitable candidates because of the drug's adverse effect on bronchodilation and glycogenolysis. However, some patients report emotional calming similar to that of the benzodiazepines.

Since the mechanisms of propranolol's therapeutic actions are still unclear, so are those of its adverse sexual effects. An extremely bright, alert 33 year old divorced male with a pacemaker (post-surgery for a congenital heart defect) whose therapeutic dose was at the high level of 600 mg per day could titrate his dose to 450 mg and enjoy good erections. He would return to 600 mg when extra systoles were experienced. He also reported 'withdrawal symptoms' of tremor, irritability, backache and restlessness when he titrated his dose below 400 mg, with all symptoms being reversed when he raised the dose to 600 mg. Other men report impotence on doses as low as 30 mg/day. Between 1-3 per cent report lowered libido as well as increased impotency (by up to 40 per cent). Although numerous reports have appeared in the literature relating to male sexual effects, no reports have yet appeared on the drug's sexual side-effects in women (Prichard & Gillam, 1969; Burnett & Chahine, 1975; Hollisfield *et al.,* 1976; Knarr, 1976; Warren *et al.,* 1976; Zacharias, 1976; Warren & Warren, 1977; Wagner & Green, 1980; Viliet & Meyer, 1982).

Nadolol is a related ß-blocker of more recent introduction, with impotency occurring more rapidly and at even lower doses than with propranolol. Restored sexual potency occurs on discontinuation of treatment.

Metoprolol is a selective ß-blocker not noted to be associated with sexual problems. Nevertheless, there are some implications (not yet understood or verified as causative) that are associated with Peyronie's disease.

Vasodilators. Hydralazine, discovered in 1950, is a phthalazine derivative which lowers blood pressure by reducing arteriolar resistance through peripheral smooth muscle relaxation. When used alone, no sexual dysfunction has been reported.

An incidence of 19–23 per cent impotence has been reported with the use of hydralazine with hydrochlorothiazide and or propranolol. Many combination drugs in everyday use, eg a hypertensive with an anti-epileptic or drugs used to treat psychosis or alcohol abuse have 'compound' sexual side-effects. The physician has the extra responsibility to adjust the dose or to obtain respected consultation (Meyler, 1975; Goodman & Gilman, 1980). 'Ask and believe the patient'. Substitutes are available and should be tried.

Hypolipemic agents

These are used to control hyperlipoproteinemia and may cause a surprising incidence of sexual dysfunction, for example 14 per cent with clofibrate, although 10 per cent of subjects in the same study also reported sexual dysfunction on placebo (Prichard & Gillam, 1969; Buffman *et al.*, 1980).

Antispasmodics

Methaneline, an anticholinergic, was surveyed for sexual side-effects (Schwatzer & Robinson, 1952; Shader & Greenblatt, 1972). Almost all men treated with this drug reported impotence directly after taking it. Sexual potency was restored on discontinuation. Large numbers of easily available over-the-counter drugs contain belladonna alkaloids and synthetic anticholinergics, producing similar sexual problems.

Anorexiants

Some women claim that they feel a greater sexual desire and increase their frequency of intercourse when taking anorexiant drugs which they generally obtain (in the USA) from their gynecologists. However, no scientific studies exist which substantiate these claims. It is possible that the expectation of being more attractive on losing weight has a great deal to do with their enhanced self-image and sexual activity. Youthfulness and activity are equated with slimness and, therefore, social response plays an important role in the greater sexual expectations of the subject, both from herself and from her partner.

Analgesics

These drugs may be prescribed for chronic disability that causes recurrent pain, eg arthritis, back problems, trigeminal neuralgia. Little is written or known about their adverse sexual side-effects. In practice, some people with arthritis say that they dislike lovemaking directly after taking analgesics, since it 'flattens' their sexual rsponse. They prefer coitus when rested in the morning and especially after a hot bath to free the joints. Others can only make love after two aspirin have lessened their discomfort. The physician who spends thirty minutes with a couple can greatly assist their general as well as their sexual adjustment by suggesting alternative comfortable coital positions.

Psychotropic drugs

Antipsychotic drugs. Phenothiazines may negatively affect sexuality by reducing libido or desire in both men and women. This is possibly a function of central dopamine blockade, hypothalamic-pituitary gonadal suppression, an effect on alpha-adrenergic innervation of the gonadal system, or to general drowsiness and slowed reactions (Beaumont *et al.*, 1974*a,b*). At times, *thioridazine* interferes more with ejaculation than with erection and as such has been discussed as a potential treatment in men with premature ejaculation (Singh, 1963; Mellgren, 1967; Dorman & Schmidt, 1976; Renshaw, 1977*a*, 1978*b*; Segraves, 1977). However, the critical dose for this effect is close to 75 mg which in a non-psychotic man may put him to sleep before he can complete coitus! Whether retrograde ejaculation occurs with thioridazine and other antipsychotics such as *haloperidol, benperidol* and *chlorprothixene* (which also interfere with ejaculation) is not yet known. Segraves (1977) theorizes that a central dopamine blockade may cause ejaculatory suppression.

Chlorpromazine, fluphenazine, perphenazine and *trifluoperazine* may occasionally result in the inability to achieve orgasm in both women and men (Goodman & Gilman, 1980). They have been used for the tretment of sex offenders, who usually discontinue medication on release from an inpatient setting (Bartholomew, 1968). These effects usually occur immediately, are dose-related and may subside with either lessened dosage or after about ten days of medication. Amenorrhea may result, galactorrhea may occur in either sex, and gynecomastia, all of which are, in themselves distressing effects.

Psychosis *per se* can make a sexual approach threatening. Muting the psychosis with antipsychotic drugs restores intimate contact, since the spouse may again be accepted as an ally.

In non-psychotic individuals with high anxiety due to entrenched nonorganic sexual dysfunction, very small doses of neuroleptic drugs are known to possibly affect sexuality, as a result of their calming effect. The patient, male or female, with reduced anxiety, may then participate more comfortably and effectively in a brief sex therapy program, using sex education and home exercises with reduced fear of failure.

Thioxene, 2 mg, or trifluoperaziune, 2 mg daily for 4-8 weeks, has been of great benefit as ancilliary to sex therapy at the Loyola Sex Clinic (Renshaw, 1977*a*, 1978*b*). Since these agents are long-acting, they may be used once a day at suppertime and they do not cause chemical dependence or drowsiness and may help a very tense of negativistic person to accept a sex self-help program.

Lithium. This is a valuable antipsychotic drug which is used in the manic phase of manic-depressive illness. It is also widely used to maintain stability, thereby reducing the psychotic cyclical highs and lows of this condition. Lithium does not increase sexual desire (Vinarova *et al.*, 1972). However, it reduces the distressing symptom of undifferentiated insatiable sexual urgency which occurs in men or women in the manic cycle of the illness. Unless carefully discussed, this very fact may occasionally result in non-compliance.

Antianxiety drugs. This group of compounds is blessed with the label 'minor' tranquillizer but cursed with addictive potential due to the rapid rush of good feelings which they produce. For this reason, *meprobamate* was banned in the USA for some years. Similar to *diazepam, chlordiazepoxide* and *tranxene, meprobamate* may interfere with internuncial neurons of the spinal cord, peripheral muscle relaxation and, thus, with sexual function, and in particular causing a delay in the second stage of ejaculation due to ineffective pubococcygenus contraction. Decreased libido may be dose- and limbic-system related (Usdin, 1960; Hughes, 1964; Kaplan, 1974; Viliet & Meyer, 1982). Despite excessive public usage of these drugs, almost no controlled or double-blind studies on their sexual effects are known to this author.

Antidepressants. When sexual desire disappears as a result of a clinical depression that lowers all appetites, for food, for sleep, for life and for sex, then adequate tricyclic antidepressant therapy, ie adequate dose *doxepin* or *amitriptyline* 50–250 mg at night, removes any need for an hypnotic for an appropriate period of time (6–12 weeks), and can and does reverse the depression with a return to pre-depressed level of sexual functioning by the fourth week of treatment (Clark, 1969; Renshaw, 1977*b*).

The negative sexual side-effects of antidepressant therapy are usually dose-related and reversible with reduction of dose or discontinuation of the drug. With the initially high therapeutic levels, women, as well as men, may complain that the sedation induced results in decreased sexual desire. However, this is rare on maintenance dose levels of the antidepressant (Renshaw, 1978*a*). The anticholinergic properties of tricyclic antidepressants may result in erectile and/or ejaculatory difficulties. This may also occur with monoamine oxidase inhibitors (MAO), despite their alleged lower anticholinergic activity. Ejaculatory delay (or retrograde ejaculation) may relate to alpha adrenergic antagonistic properties of the tricyclic antidepressants and/or to, as yet unknown, autonomic nervous system factors with the MAO inhibitors (Gordon *et al.*, 1976).

Summary

It may be categorically stated that while there are endless clinical anecdotes about the sexual side-effects of the thousands of drugs used daily by millions of people worldwide, there is a paucity of well designed research involving sufficient number of subjects on active drug treatment compared with age/sex matched controls. Knowledge of the pharmacodynamics of the sexual side-effects of abused and necessary drugs is rudimentary. Investigation is essential not only as a scientific (cognitive) luxury, but as an essential clinical tool: to refine the use of specific drugs so that their negative sexual effects do not cancel out their positive systemic ones, eg the antihypertensives. Also, such research may assist in solving some of the remaining riddles of the neurophysiology of human sexual response.

Today, newly developed tools, such as Doppler techniques and nocturnal penile tumescence (NPT) studies, although still unrefined, may nonetheless be applied to measure the vascular effects of the patient's penile blood flow, both awake and asleep, and before, during and after such medications as lithium and the antihypertensives. Vaginal lubrication must also be similarly well researched (Karacan *et al.*, 1978; Karacan, 1982). Sexual medicine can, indeed, be an important direction for scholarly inquiry and, in fact, there are many theses in need of presentation in this embryonic field of medicine in the 1980s.

References

Angrist, B. & Gershon, S. (1976): Clinical effects of amphetamine and L-dopa on sexuality and aggression. *Comp. Psychiat.* **17,** 715-722.

Bartholomew, A.A. (1968): A long-acting phenothiazine as a possible agent to control deviant sexual behaviour. *Am. J. Psychiat.* **124,** 917-922.

Bell, D.S. & Trethowan, W.H. (1961): Amphetamine addiction and disturbed sexuality. *Archs Gen. Psych.* **4,** 74-78.
Beaumont, P.J.V., Gelder, M.G., Frisen, H.G., Harris, G.W., MacKinnon, P.C.B., Mandelbrote, B.M. & Wiles, D.H. (1974*a*): The effects of phenothiazines on endocrine function: I. Patients with inappropriate lactation and amenorrhoea. *Br. J. Psychiat.* **124,** 413-419.
Beaumont, P.J.V., Corker, C.S., Friesen, H.G., Kolakowska, T., Mandelbrote, B.M., Marshall, J., Murray, M.A. & Wiles, D.H. (1974*b*): The effects of phenothiazines on endocrine function: II. Effects in men and post-menopausal women. *Br. J. Psychiat.* **124,** 420-430.
Briggs, M.H. (1973): Cigarette smoking and infertility in men. *Med. J. Aust.* **1,** 616-617.
Buffman, J., Moser, C., Apter, M., Buxton, M. & Davidson, J. (1981): Drugs and sexual function. In *Sexual problems in medical practice,* eds Lief, H. & Monroe, A.M.A. Wisconsin. Pp 211-242.
Bullpitt, C.J. & Dollery, C.T. (1973): Side-effects of hypotensive agents evaluated by a self-administered questionnaire. *Br. Med. J.* **3,** 485-490.
Burnett, W. & Chahine, R. (1979): Sexual dysfunction as a complication of propranolol therapy in men. *Cardiovas. Med.* **4,** 811-815.
Byck, R. (1975): Drugs and the treatment of psychiatric disorders. In *The pharmacological basis of therapeutics,* eds Goodman, L. & Gilman, A. New York: Macmillan Publishing Co., Inc. Pp 391-447.
Carver, J.R. & Oaks, W.W. (1976): Sex and hypertension. In *Sex and the life cycle,* eds Oaks, W.W., Melchiode, G.A. & Fisher, J. New York: Grune & Stratton.
Chopra, G. (1969): Man and marijuana. *Int. J. Addiction* **4,** 215-247.
Cicero, T.J., Bell, R.D., Wiest, W.G., Allison, J.H., Polakoski, K. & Robins, E., (1975): Function of the male sex organs in heroin and methadone users. *New Engl. J. Med.* **292,** 882-887.
Clark, F.C. (1969): The treatment of depression in general practice. *S. Afr. Med. J.* **43,** 724-725.
Cooper, A.J. (1972): Diagnosis and management of "endocrine impotence". *Br. Med. J.* **2,** 34-36.
Cushman, P. (1973): Plasma testosterone in narcotic addition. *Am. J. Med.* **55,** 452-458.
Dorman, B.W. & Schmidt, J.D. (1976): Association of priapism in phenothiazine therapy. *J. Urol.* **116,** 51-53.
Duncan, J. & Laird, J. (1980): "Placebos can be dangerous to health". *J. Personality Soc. Psychol.* **39,** 6.
delle Fave, G.F., Tamburrano, G., de Magistris, L., Natoli, C., Santoro, M.L., Carratu, R. & Torsoli, A. (1977): Gynecomastia with cimetidine. (Letter.) *Lancet* **1,** 1319.
Gay, G.R., Newmeyer, J.A., Eilon, R.A. & Wieder, S. (1975): Drug-sex practices in Haight Ashbury or "the sensuous hippie". In *Sexual behaviour: pharmacology and biochemistry,* eds Sandler, M. & Gessa, D.L. New York: Raven Press. Pp 63-79.
Gifford, L.M., Aeugle, M.E., Myerson, R.M. & Tannenbaum, P.J. (1980): Cimetidine postmarket outpatient surveillance program — interim report on phase 1. *J. Am. Med. Ass.* **243,** 1532-1535.
Gordon, G.G., Altman, K., Southern, A.L., Rubin, E. & Lieber, C.S. (1976): Effects of alcohol (ethanol) administration on sex-hormone metabolism in normal med. *N. Engl. J. Med.* **295,** 793-797.
Gordon, G.G. *et al.* (1979): Hypogonadism and feminization in the male: a triple effect of alcohol. *Alcoholism. Clin. Exper. Res.* **3,** 210-211.
Greenberg, H.R. (1965): Erectile impotence during the course of tofranil therapy. *Am. J. Psychiat.* **121,** 1021.
Greenberg, M.S. *et al.* (1979): Gynecomastia after chemotherapy. *Clin. Res.* **27,** 386A.
Greenblatt, D.J. & Roch-Wesrer, J. (1973): Gynecomastia and impotence complications of spironolactone therapy. *J. Am. Med. Ass.* **223,** 82.
Guinan, P.D., Sadoughi, W., Alsheik, H., Ablin, R.J., Alrenga, D. & Bush, I. (1976): Impotence therapy and cancer of the prostate. *Am. J. Surg.* **131,** 599-600.
Hall, W.H. (1976): Breast changes in males on cimetidine. (Letter.) *N. Engl. J. Med.* **295,** 841.
Hogan, M.J., Wallin, J.D. & Baer, R.M. (1980): Antihypertensive therapy and male sexual dysfunction. *Psychosomatics* **21,** 234-237.
Holbrook, S. (1959): *The golden age of quackery.* New York: Macmillan Publishing Co., Inc.
Hollifield, J.W., Sherman, K., van der Zwagg, R. & Shand, D.G. (1976): Proposed mechanisms of propranolol's antihypertensive effect in essential hypertension. *N. Engl. J. Med.* **295,** 68-73.

Hollister, L.E. (1975): The mystique of social drugs and sex. In *Sexual behavior: pharmacology and biochemistry,* eds Sandler, M. & Gessa, D.L. New York: Raven Press. Pp 85-92.
Horwitz, D., Pettinger, W.A., Orvis, H., Thomas, R.F. & Sjoesma, A. (1967): Effects of methyldopa in fifty hypertensive patients. *Clin. Pharm. Ther.* **8,** 224-234.
Hughes, J.M. (1964): Failure to ejaculate with chlordiazepoxide. *Am. J. Psychiat.* **121,** 610-611.
Innes, I.R. & Nickerson, M. (1975): Norepinephrine, epinephrine in the sympathomimetic amines. In *The pharmacological basis of therapeutics,* eds Goodman, L. & Gilman, A. New York: Macmillan Publishing Co., Inc.
Jick, H., Porter, J. & Morrison, A.S. (1977): Relation between smoking and the age of natural menopause. *Lancet* **1,** 1354-5.
Kahn, A., Camel, G. & Perry, H.M. (1970): Cloimidine (Catapres): a new anti-hypertensive agent. *Curr. Ther. Res.* **12,** 10-18.
Kantor, H.I. (1977): Sexual effects of oestrogen replacement. *Med. Aspects Hum. Sex.* **11,** 85-86.
Kaplan, H.S. (1974): *The new sex therapy.* New York: Bruner-Mazel. Pp 86-103.
Karacen, I., Ware, J.C., Dervant, B., Atinel, A., Thornby, J.,I., Williams, R.L., Kaya, N. & Scott, F.B. (1978): Impotence and blood pressure in the flaccid penis: relationship to nocturnal penile tumescence. *Sleep* **1,** 125-132.
Karacen, J. (1982): Nocturnal penile tumescence as a biologic marker in assessing erectile dysfunction. *Psychosomatics* **23,** 349-360.
Keverne, E. (1977): Pheromones and sexual behavior. In *Handbook of sexology,* eds Money, J. & Musaph, H. New York: Elsevier.
Kline, J., Stein, Z.A., Susser, M. & Warburton, D. (1977): Smoking a risk factor for abortion. *N. Engl. J. Med.* **297,** 793-796.
Knarr, J.W. (1976): Impotence from propranolol? (Letter.) *Ann. Intern. Med.* **85,** 259.
Kutner, S.J. & Schwyhart, W.R. (1974): Sexual adjustment to contraception. *Med. Aspects Hum. Sex.* **8,** 33-60.
Labataille, L.M. (1975): Amyl nitrite employed in homosexual relations. (Letter.) *Med. Aspects Hum. Sex.* **9,** 122.
Lemere, F. & Smith, J.W. (1973): Alcohol-induced sexual impotence. *Am. J. Psychiat.* **130,** 212-213.
Masters, W.H. & Johnson, V.E. (1966): *Human sexual response.* Boston: Little Brown.
Masters, W.H. & Johnson, V.E. (1970): *Human sexual inadequacy.* Boston: Little Brown. Pp 163-168.
Mellgren, A. (1967): Treatment of ejaculation praecox with thioridazine. *Psychother. Psychosom.* **15,** 459-460.
Mendelson, J.H. *et al.* (1974): Plasma testosterone levels before, during and after chronic marijuana smoking. *N. Engl. J. Med.* **291,** 309-310.
Mendelson, J.H., Mello, N.K. & Ellinghoe, J. (1977): Effects of acute alcohol intake on pituitary-gonadal hormones in normal human males. *J. Pharmacol. Exp. Ther.* **202,** 676-682.
Meyler's side-effects of drugs. (1975): Vol. 8. Amsterdam: Excerpta Medica.
Miller, J.B., Howards, S.S. & McLeod, R.M. (1980): Serum prolactin in organic and psychogenic impotence. *J. Urol.* **123,** 862-864.
Mroczek, W.J., Leibel, B.A. & Finnerty, F.A., Jnr. (1972): Comparison of clonidene and methyldopa in hypertensive patients receiving a diuretic: a double blind crossover study. *Am. J. Cardiol.* **29,** 712-717.
Murad, F. & Gilman, A.G. (1975): Estrogens and progestins. In *The pharmacological basis of therapeutics,* eds Goodman, L. & Gilman, A. New York: Macmillan Publishing Co., Inc.
Murad, F. & Haynes, E.C., Jnr. (1980): Estrogens and progestins. In *The pharmacological basis of therapeutics,* eds Goodman, L. & Gilman, A. New York: Macmillan Publishing Co., Inc. Pp 1432-1433.
Oaks, W.W. & Moyyer, J.H. (1972): Sex and hypertension. *Med. Aspects Hum. Sex.* **6,** 128-137.
Papadopoulous, C. (1980): Cardiovascular drugs and sexuality: a cardiologist's review. *Archs Intern. Med.* **140,** 1341-1345.
Patrick, R.L. (1977): Amphetamine and cocaine: biological mechanisms. In *Psychopharmacology: from theory to practice,* eds Barchas, J.D. *et al.* New York: Oxford University Press.
Peden, N.R., Cargill, J.M., Browning, M.C.K., Saunders, J.H.B. & Wormsley, K.G. (1979): Male sexual dysfunction during treatment with cimetidine. *Br. Med. J.* **1,** 659.

Perlman, J.T. & Adams, G.I. (1970): Amyl nitrite inhalation fad. (Letter.) *J. Am. Med. Ass.* **212,** 160.
Pirani, B.B.K. (1978): Smoking during pregnancy. *Ob. & Gynec. Survey* **3,** 1-13.
Prichard, B.N. & Gillam, P.M. (1969): Treatment of hypertension with propranolol. *Br. Med. J.* **1,** 7-16.
Raftos, J., Bauer, G.E., Lewis, R.G. *et al.* (1973): Clomidine in the treatment of severe hypertension. *Aust.* **30,** 786-793.
Renshaw, D.C. (1975): Sexuality and depression in adults and elderly. *Med. Aspects Hum. Sex.* **9,** 40-62.
Renshaw, D.C. (1976): The symptom of insomnia. *Cont. Ed.* 103-112.
Renshaw, D.C. (1977*a*): Psychotropics in treatment of sexual dysfunction. *Med. Aspects Hum. Sex.* **11,** 6-9.
Renshaw, D.C. (1977*b*): A guide to sex counselling. *Female Patient* **2,** 46-48.
Renshaw, D.C. (1978*a*): Impotence: some causes and cures. *Am. Fam. Phys.* **17,** 143-146.
Renshaw, D.C. (1978*b*): Premature ejaculation. *Consultant* **18,** 143-146.
Renshaw, D.C. (1980): Pharmacotherapy and female sexuality. In *Modern problems of pharmopsychology*. 15. Basel: Karger. Pp 145-157.
Schilsky, R.L., Lewis, B.J., Sherins, R.J. & Young, R.C. (1980): Gonadal dysfunctions in patients receiving chemotherapy for cancer. *Ann. Intern. Med.* **93,** 109-114.
Scheider, J. & Kaffarnik, H. (1975): Impotence in patients treated with clofibrate. *Atherosclerosis* **21,** 455-457.
Schwartz, N.H. & Robinson, B.D. (1952): Impotence due to methantheline bromide. *N.Y. St. J. Med.* **52,** 1530.
Segraves, R.T. (1977): Pharmacological agents causing sexual dysfunction. *J. Sex. Marital Ther.* **3,** 157-176.
Shader, R.I. (1970): Ejaculation disorders. In *Psychotropic drug side effects, clinical and theoretical perspectives*, eds Shader, R.I. & DiMascio, A. Baltimore: Wilkins & Wilkins.
Shader, R.I. & DiMascio, A. (1970): Galactorrhea and gynecomastia. In *Psychotropic drug side effects, clinical and theoretical perspectives,* eds Shader, R. I. & DiMascio, A. Baltimore: Wilkins & Wilkins.
Shader, R.I., Giller, D.R. & DiMascio, A. (1970): Hypothalamic pituitary adrenal axis. In *Psychotropic drug side effects, clinical and theoretical perspectives,* eds Shader, R.I. & DiMascio, A. Baltimore: Wilkins & Wilkins.
Shader, R.I. & Greenblatt, D.J. (1972): Belladonna alkaloids and synthetic anticholinergics: uses and toxicity. In *Psychiatric complications of medical drugs,* ed Shader, R.I. New York: Raven.
Sigell, L.T., Kapp, F.T., Fusaro, G.A., Nelson, E.D. & Falck, R.S. (1978): Popping and snorting volatile nitrites: current fad for getting high. *Am. J. Psychiat.* **135,** 1216-1218.
Singh, H. (1963): Therapeutic use of thioridazine in premature ejaculation. *Am. J. Psychiat.* **119,** 8.
Smith, D.E. *et al.* (1979): Amphetamine abuse and sexual dysfunctions: clinical and research considerations. In *Amphetamine use, misuse and abuse,* ed Smith, D.E. Cambridge, Ma: G.K. Hall.
Tennent, G., Bancroft, J. & Cass, J. (1974): The control of deviant sexual behavior by drugs: a double-blind controlled study of benperidol, chlorpromazine, and placebo. *Archs Sex. Behav.* **3,** 261-271.
Usdin, G.L. (1960): Preliminary report on Librium, a new psychopharmacologic agent. *J. La. Med. Soc..* **112,** 142-147.
van Thiel, D.H. & Lester, R. (1976): Sex and alcohol: a second peek. *N. Engl. J. Med.* **295,** 835-836.
van Thiel, D.H., Gavaler, J.S., Smith, W.I., Jnr. & Paul, G. (1979): Hypothalamic-pituitary-gonadal dysfunction in men using cimetidine. *N. Engl. J. Med.* **300,** 1012-1015.
Vinarova, E., Uhlir, O., Stika, L. & Vinar, O. (1972): Side effects of lithium administration. *Activ. Nerv. Suppl.* (Praha) **14,** 105-107.
Vliet, L.W. & Meyer, J.K. (1982): Erectile dysfunction: progress in evaluation and treatment. *Johns Hopks. Med. J.* **151,** 246-258.
Wagner, G. & Green, R. (1981): *Impotence — physiological, psychological, surgical diagnosis and treatment.* New York: Plenum Press. Pp 47.

Warren, S.G., Brewer, D.L. & Oregin, F.S. (1976): Long-term propranolol therapy for angina pectoris. *Am. J. Cardiol.* **37,** 420-426.
Warren, S.G. & Warren, S.G. (1977): Propranolol and sexual impotence. (Letter.) *Ann. Intern. Med.* **86,** 112.
Weil, A. (1975): The love drug. *J. Psychedel. Drugs* **8,** 335-337.
Williams, R. (1980): Sleeping pill insomnia. *J. Clin. Psychiat.* **4,** 153-154.
Wilson, G.T. & Lawson, D. (1976): Effects of alcohol on sexual arousal in women. *J. Abnorm. Psychol.* **85,** 489-497.
Winters, S.J., Banks, J.L. & Loriaux, D.L. (1979): Cimetidine is an antiandrogen in the rat. *Gastroenterology* **76,** 504-508.
Wolfe, M.M. (1979): Impotence on cimetidine treatment. (Letter.) *N. Engl. J. Med.* **300,** 94.
Zacharias, F.J. (1976): Patient acceptability of propranolol and the occurrence of side effects. *Postgrad. Med. J.* **52** (Suppl. 4), 87-89.
Zinberg, N.E. (1974): Marijuana and sex. (Letter.) *N. Engl. J. Med.* **291,** 309-310.

7

Pharmacological aspects of sexual dysfunction caused by drugs of abuse

H. SCHNIEDEN and J. M. H. REES

Department of Pharmacology, Materia Medica and Therapeutics, University of Manchester, MANCHESTER M13 9PT

Introduction

The most important aspects of sexual dysfunction caused by drug abuse concerns those drugs that act on the brain, and it is on those drugs that we concentrate in this short review. However, any drug taken unnecessarily, in excess or habitually, is a drug of abuse and such drugs may have indirect effects on sexual function (eg vitamins).

The interpretation of sexual dysfunction caused by psychotropic drugs is fraught with difficulty and some of these problems have been recently outlined (see Horowitz & Goble, 1979; Griffin, 1981; Rees, 1983). The problems are greatly compounded when psychotropic drugs are abused for the following, additional, reasons. First, in only a few instances are single drugs taken, and this makes it difficult to associate an identifiable effect with a causative agent. This problem is further complicated by an ignorance of the dose of drug(s) taken, and a reluctance on the part of the patient to disclose the duration and nature of drug-taking. A brief consideration of the potential effects on prolactin secretion of opiates, amphetamines, barbiturates and alcohol individually or in combination, at unknown doses, for indeterminable lengths of time illustrates the point well.

Any reviewer discussing the illicit drug usage must stress the difficulty in establishing the dose of the compound the subject has taken. Moreover, formulations can vary, especially since many drugs of abuse are taken in their raw state and adulteration is commonplace. For instance, it is known that two active constituents of marijuana are Δ^9-tetrahydrocannabinol (Δ^9-THC) and Δ^6-tetrahydrocannabinol (Δ^6-THC). Marijuana from Thailand contains about 4 per cent whilst that from Mexico has one per cent (Koff, 1974). In addition, drugs available on the street are of variable purity and may be diluted with any powder which may or may not possess pharmacological activity. The rate of administration may also modify response. The drug can be inhaled or ingested in the form of cookies or brownies. The time courses of action and plasma concentrations will be different by these two routes. Moreover, it should not be assumed that administration of a potent constituent alone (eg Δ^9-THC) exactly mimics the effects of the crude preparation.

Excessive drug consumption is also likely to be accompanied by secondary physiological disturbances, eg the nutritional deficiency characteristic of alcohol and other addictions.

The physiology of sexual excitation is still not well understood. Whilst it is now appreciated that parasympathetic and sympathetic pathways are involved in the completion of the sexual act, the initiating stimuli to these pathways is still a matter of conjecture. Suffice to say that by some process or processes as yet ill-defined, information from tactile, visual, auditory and olfactory stimuli are assessed by the brain and this can lead to a heightening of sexual excitement.

In the initial stages of a relationship between two people there can be periods when either partner is unsure, hesitant or anxious. Drugs which help to depress such inhibitions can thereby ease the relationship and presumably, within a dose range, all central nervous system depressants can achieve this. Expectation in relation to existing mores can also affect the sexual relationship. In addition, the setting in which the event takes place can modify the response. Soft lights and sweet music are well-known aids; and many commercial industries depend (at least in part) on the imagination and its effect on sexual response to sell their goods.

It can, thus, be seen that anyone attempting to set up a trial to evaluate the effects of drugs on sexual response may encounter a number of confounding variables. A further problem is that in the majority of instances, the sexual act is undertaken in private and that if one is attempting to obtain information from individuals taking drugs of dependence, the information is not always reliable. Bearing all these factors in mind, it is no wonder that for the same drug contrasting effects have been reported.

To summarise, sexual response depends on the personality, medical history, attitude, mood, character and expectations of the drug-user and the setting in which the drug experience takes place, as well as on the pharmacolgy of the drug. As Fort (1976) so aptly stated, 'the mind is the main sex organ'.

Physiological factors

Libido depends on a number of factors, some of which are endocrinological or involve the activities of neurotransmitters in the central and peripheral nervous systems. Testosterone is an important factor in the male. Lowered testosterone concentrations can be associated with a diminution of libido and anti-androgenic agents have been used to diminish hypersexual drive. A second important hormone is prolatin. High prolactin concentrations are associated with amenorrhea and excess prolactin secretion can cause loss of sexual potency, oligospermia or aspermia, signs of androgen failure, low androgen production and galactorrhea (Horowski & Gräf, 1979; Besser & Thorner, 1976).

In animals, the role of the neurotransmitters dopamine and 5-HT appear to be of importance. A fall in central 5-HT concentration produced by *p*-chlorophenylalanine is associated with increased sexual activity, and an increase in mounting behaviour has been reported following treatment with levodopa (Sheard, 1969; Benkert *et al.* 1973; Gessa & Tagliamonte, 1974). Sicuteri (1974) has claimed that *p*-chlorophenylalanine enhances human sexual activity.

The autonomic nervous system controls penile erection and ejaculation. Erection is under the control of the parasympathetic nervous system. The parasympathetic outflow arises from the pelvic nerves. The transmitter released is acetylcholine and its receptors are muscarinic. Weiss (1972) has discussed the physiology of human penile erection and comments that whilst sacral centres are of importance, other locations, such as the thoracic spinal level and the central nervous system, also have important parts to play. Ejaculation is under the control of the sympathetic nervous system. Sympathetic fibres from the lumbar spinal chord synapse at the mesenteric ganglia. Noradrenaline released following stimulation of the postganglionic sympathetic nerve fibres acts on α-adrenoceptors in the vas deferens causing contraction.

Marijuana: preparations and extracts of Cannabis sativa

The attitude towards and extent of drug usage are of importance in the analysis of sexual behaviour in persons taking marijuana. Burdsal *et al.* (1975) administered a questionnaire on sexual attitudes, behaviour, family relationships and marijuana usage to 358 undergraduates at a university in the United States. Using factor analysis, they noted 12 factors related to sexual behaviour. These were: liberal versus conservative attitudes; age-experience; symbolic sexual preoccupation; romantic love versus cynicism; experience linked drug effects; affectual dependence; mature satisfaction; conservative versus liberal sexual practices; high versus low sexual activity; sexual revolution; sex; and, traditional versus cynical love roles.

They found, as might have been anticipated, that liberal views on sex were associated with liberal marijuana views, and individuals who were high on this dynamic tended to have a high use of marijuana. With regard to experience-linked drug effects, the persons who used marijuana tended to feel that both marijuana and alcohol had beneficial effects on sexual intercourse.

Dawley *et al.* (1979) have also looked at the effects of marijuana on sexual enjoyment by students. Eighty-four students participated in the study. The students fell into three categories: those who had sexual experience while under the influence of marijuana (33 experienced smokers); non-experienced smokers (26 in number) (those who had smoked marijuana but who had little sexual experience); and 25 non-smokers. The majority of the experienced smokers held the view that marijuana increased sexual pleasure and sensations in addition to increasing the intensity of orgasm. Sixty-one per cent of the group considered marijuana to be aphrodisiac. Non-experienced smokers and non-smokers did not consider marijuana to be an aphrodisiac.

Bouquet (1950) noted that in Egypt and North Africa there is a strong belief that marijuana increases sexual satisfaction and Chopra & Chopra (1967) reported that out of 1200 users of the drug, approximately 10 per cent claimed increased sexual excitation as a cause that led to the use of cannabis.

Koff (1974) looked at the effect of the dose of marijuana on sexual activity among university students. Following the use of marijuana, sexual desire was said to increase in just under 50 per cent of those questioned. Looking at dose effect, 61 per cent of individuals who smoked one joint or less had an increase in sexual drive. Women were more affected than men: 71 per cent of women noted an increase compared with 51 per cent of men. For people who smoked two or more joints, 50 per cent of the women noted an increase in sexual drive compared with 35 per cent of the men. This suggests that as the dose increases, the tendency to an increase in sexual desire wanes. The author estimated that when smoked and shared between two people, a joint leads to between 3.75–5.00 mg of tetrahydrocannabinol in the blood stream. The author noted in his survey that cases of secondary impotence among men and situationally non-orgasmic women followed the use of marijuana. He suggests that marijuana, if taken at relatively low doses together with appropriate psychological and sociological conditioning, can release inhibitions to the extent of being called an aphrodisiac, but at higher doses this effect disappears. The influence of set and setting is well illustrated in the following remarks from one of the female students who answered the questionnaire: 'Marijuana itself does not in any way increase sexual desire, it is merely the atmosphere in which the drug is used, combined with the drug . . . a darkened room with candlelight, incense burning possibly, often just the two alone, which actually promotes sexual desire.'

There have been a number of suggestions on how marijuana can enhance sexual enjoyment. One possibility is that marijuana can induce a change in time perception thus giving the feeling of a prolonged orgasm (Tart, 1971). Another explanation is that an enhancement of tactile sensitivity occurs (Traub, 1977).

There have been many investigations of the endocrinological effects of cannabis. In 1974, Kolodny *et al.* reported a depression of plasma testosterone levels after chronic and intensive use of marijuana in 20 men who had smoked marijuana at least four times a week for the previous six months. Following drug abstinence, there was a rise in plasma testosterone levels. The Leydig cells in marijuana drug users were able to respond to human chorionic gonadotrophin. Testosterone levels rose by over 100 per cent.

Other workers have not been able to confirm the work of Kolodny and his colleagues. Schaefer *et al.* (1975) found no significant change in plasma testosterone levels between men given placebo or Δ^9-tetrahydrocannabinol (Δ^9-THC). Mendelson *et al.* (1974) also studied plasma testosterone levels in chronic marijuana users. Their study was in three parts: baseline measurements were made for the first five days; for the next 21 days subjects smoked marijuana; and in the final five days of the study marijuana was not used. No significant changes in testosterone levels were found between the three phases of the study. Neither was any significant difference in testosterone levels noted between 'casual' or 'heavy' marijuana smokers. Cushman (1975) compared plasma testosterone levels in 13 non-smokers with 25 marijuana smokers who were taking five marijuana cigarettes per week for about three years on average. No significant differences were noted.

The weight of evidence in man, therefore, is in favour of marijuana having no marked effects on plasma testosterone levels.

In animals, several studies have shown that marijuana causes inhibition of sexual behaviour. Merari *et al.* (1973) noted that Δ^9-THC inhibited the copulatory activity of male rats. Following ip injection of 2–3 mg/kg of the drug, an increase occurred in the latency to mounting and to ejaculation. Cutler *et al.* (1975) noted that in mice cannabis resin caused a significant reduction both in male mounts and in attempted male mounts. Corcoran *et al.* (1974) also noted that hashish resin when injected ip decreased male sexual behaviour. In contrast, Δ^9-THC given daily to monkeys for 3–18 months did not appear to affect sexual behaviour.

In mice, Dixit and his colleagues (Dixit *et al.*, 1974; Dixit & Lohiya, 1975) have shown that high doses of cannabis can cause arrest of spermatogenesis and regression of Leydig cell tissue. Jakubovic *et al.* (1979) showed that a number of water soluble cannabinoids inhibited human chorionic gonadotrophin and dibutyryl-cAMP stimulated testosterone production from rat testicular Leydig cell preparations. This inhibition was produced by concentrations of cannabinoids which were in the same order of magnitude as those previously found in the rat testis after the rat had been exposed to the smoke of a [^{3}H] THC-containing cigarette for 15 minutes.

There have been some studies on the effect of marijuana smoking on human sperm count. Kolodny *et al.* :1974) noted that six out of 17 marijuana users had sperm counts of less than 30 million per ml. Hembree and his colleagues (Hembree *et al.*, 1976, 1980) monitored the sperm count in chronic marijuana users who participated in the three-part trial. Sperm counts were noted and in an initial period or 2–4 weeks of non-smoking. During the next few weeks, the subjects smoked marijuana and then this was followed by a period of abstinence for 2–4 weeks. In both studies, sperm count fell in the first two weeks after smoking ceased. The authors suggest that the fall in sperm count was due to a direct suppressant effect of the cannabinoids on germinal epithelium but the short time between exposure and effect makes this unlikely bearing in mind the length of spermatogenesis in man. In animals, cannabinoids have been shown to interfere with protein synthesis in rat testis Leydig cells (Jakubovic *et al.*,

1980). In the rat, Δ^9-THC has been shown to inhibit suckling-induced prolactin release in the lactaating rat (Bromley *et al.*, 1978). Kramer & Ben-David (1974) also reported suppression of prolactin secretion in male rats following acute administration of Δ^9-THC. However, other workers have reported increases in serum prolactin levels in male rats (Daley *et al.*, 1974). Thus, perhaps the explanation for the fall in sperm count lies in endocrine modulation of the testis either locally or centrally.

Hembree *et al.* (1980) noted no untoward effects of marijuana on sperm motility in the single subject studied. However, more recently, Hong *et al.* (1981) have reported that Δ^9-THC inhibits human sperm motility *in vitro.* Motility is reduced by about 40 per cent when sperm were incubated with a concentration of 0.5 mM Δ^9-THC for two hours.

In ancient times, there were two opposing views on the actions of marijuana. In the Middle East, it was credited with aphrodisiac properties. An Arabic poem mentions:

> *'Abdu'l Haylukh deflowered in one night*
> *Eighty virgins in a rigid rite*
> *After smoking hashish.'* (Quoted in *Abel, 1981.*)

Dioscorides mentions that the juice of the marijuana seed was useful for treating diminished sexual desire. Galen, however, warned that over-indulgence in marijuana seeds could cause impotence (Abel, 1981). In the twentieth century, the acute observations of these physicians appear vindicated depending on dose, set and setting. The mechanism(s) by which they are produced is still unclear in spite of evidence from animal studies that the drug can interfere with testicular function.

Opiates

In the interesting article by Francisco Guerra in 1974 entitled 'Sex and drugs in the 16th century' reference is made to the effect of opium on sexual performance. The 16th Century physician, Cristobal Acosta, a native of the Cape Verde Islands spent considerable time in the East Indies and wrote:

> *'The use of opium is widespread in those regions (using it) . . . they can for a time free themselves of all anxieties . . . it is also used for venereal purposes. Although contrary to reason, it is used so widely for this purpose, indeed to such an extent, that it is the most common and ordinary remedy used by the vile children of Venus. It is believed not only by our own physicians but also by other physicians, Arabs, Parsees, Turks, Caracens, Sundas, Malaysians, Chinese and Malabars . . . that the use of opium (by reason of its stupefying and narcotic quality) causes impotence in addicts and this is confirmed by our reasoning and experience. But the imagination of common folk is so powerful that it can transform impotence into potency, and they commonly employ it to increase their lascivious carnal pleasures.'*

Another 16th century physician, Garcia d'Orta wrote as follows:

> *'The imaginative virtue plays a great part in carnal lust and it is stronger than the expulsive virtue that follows it. Hence the Act of Venus is completed all the more rapidly. And because the imaginative virtue is so powerful dominates the expulsive one forcing into the testicles the genital seed and the greater the imagination the more rapid the emission of the seed. And as those who take Amfian (opium) have lost control, they actually complete this venereal act much later. And because many females do not give away the seed that quickly, and when the man is also slow she completes the act of Venus much later the act of conception ends exactly at the same time in both of them and taking Amfian is here a help. It also assists to complete the venereal act more slowly . . .'*

It can be seen that these physicians were aware that a tranquilising drug could be of value in the treatment of premature ejaculation and that opium could cause impotence.

Weiland & Younger (1971) have reported that opiates can cause decreased libido, decreased fertility and a tendency to become impotent. Bai *et al.* (1974) noted that 63 per cent of heroin-addicted women had amenorrhea and that in spite of the lack of contraception and frequent sexual contacts, only 4.5 per cent of the heroin-dependent women became pregnant.

Cushman (1972) interviewed four groups to obtain information on their sexual life. These were controls who were normal male volunteers, the majority of whom were graduate students or hospital employees. The subjects were 13 active heroin addicts, 13 former heroin addicts and 27 methadone-maintained former narcotic addicts. The study revealed a high incidence of disturbed sexual performance in active heroin addicts. The most common problem was a delay in ejaculation time beyond 25 minutes. Reduction in libido was also reported as well as erectional insufficiency. Addicts on the methadone-maintained programme also reported sexual problems. Two of this group said, however, that on occasions the heroin 'high' may have enhanced their sexual desires. Although the methadone-maintained patients as a group still had sexual problems, they were reported to be less than when the same patients were taking heroin, though in this small series this was not significant.

There have been a number of studies on the effect of methadone on sexual performance. Goldstein (1972) considered that interference with normal sexual function was one of the most aggravating side effects of the methadone maintenance therapy programme. In another study (Hanbury *et al.*, 1977), 33 per cent of those involved in a methadone-maintained programme reported sexual dysfunction. In 50 per cent of these individuals, onset occurred within one month of the initiation of methadone therapy. Individuals on heroin had a higher prevalence of inadequate sexual function, approximately 70 per cent being affected.

Langrod *et al.* (1981) asked 102 male patients on a methadone maintained programme in New York about the physical complaints that they attributed to taking methadone. Sweating was the most common complaint in both long-term patients (those treated for at least two years) and new patients (those treated for five months or less), and it caused problems for about 89 per cent of patients. In contrast, sexual problems, defined as a delay in ejaculation and/or impotence, were less common; at the time of interview, only 21 per cent of 'new' and 33 per cent of long-term patients were concerned by such problems.

Effect of opioids on the endocrine system. A number of studies have revealed that opioid use can modify sex hormone secretion. Mendelson *et al.* (1975) noted a significant dose-dependent fall in plasma testosterone in narcotic addicts given known doses of heroin. Mendelson *et al.* (1979*a*) also noted a fall in plasma testosterone levels following acute heroin administration. They also reported that heroin-induced suppression of plasma testosterone and luteinizing hormone levels following a 10 day period of self administration was less than the degree of suppression following initial acute dosage with heroin. This suggested that tolerance had developed. One of the most dramatic effects was the rise in prolactin concentration following both acute and chronic heroin administration. Again tolerance appeared to have developed.

Bolelli *et al.* (1979) examined hormone levels in 16 male and three female addicts who, in the year prior to the study, had been taking heroin in doses higher than 150 mg/day. All subjects had sexual problems, including difficulty in achieving erection, delayed ejaculation or amenorrhea. Using radioimmunoassay procedures, they assessed the plasma levels of heroin, testosterone, dihydrotestosterone, androstenedione, luteinizing hormone and follicle stimulating hormone. They found a significant fall in plasma testosterone and dihydrotestosterone levels concomitant with higher plasma levels of heroin but no relevant changes in the other hormones measured. A fall in heroin concentration was associated with a rise in testosterone and dihydrotestosterone levels. It is of interest that Cushman (1975) who also measured plasma luteinizing hormone had come to the conclusion that the inhibitory effects of heroin use on sexuality did not appear to involve resting levels of plasma luteinizing hormone.

Lafisca *et al.* (1981) studied hormone levels in 25 males who were on a methadone-maintained programme. All had received 30 mg/day methadone orally for at least two months. Plasma levels of luteinizing hormone (LH), follicle stimulating hormone (FSH), 17-β-estradiol (E_2), estrone (E_1), testosterone (T), dehydroepiandrosterone sulphate (DS), androstenedione (A), dehydrotestosterone (DHT), progesterone (P) and prolactin (PRL) were estimated. All the subjects had a history of sexual problems.

FSH values were mainly below the normal range. The levels of E_1, E_2, P and LH were always within normal values, whilst A, DS and PRL were noticeably increased in many subjects. In some cases, the values of T and DHT were below normal. Thus, with this dose of methadone, some abnormalities in plasma hormone levels were detected but the effects were not as marked as those reported in some patients taking heroin.

Narcotic antagonists have been reported to affect hormone levels and sexual activity. Naltrexone, a narcotic antagonist which is more potent than naloxone and which has a longer duration of action (Verebely & Mulé, 1975) caused a significant rise in integrated plasma luteinizing hormone concentrations in seven subjects given 50 mg of the drug orally. Three subjects reported spontaneous penile erections one to three hours after administration of the drug. This was accompanied by dysphoric sexual ideation (Mendelson *et al.*, 1979*b*). Delitala *et al.* (1981) gave a met-enkaphalin analogue or naloxone to post-menopausal women by intravenous infusion. The met-enkaphalin analogue induced a fall in circulating luteinizing hormone (LH). Following naloxone, a significant rise in LH occurred. Naloxone increased the frequency and amplitude of spontaneous LH secretion. It had similar effects in normal males. In healthy women, naloxone caused a reduction in plasma prolactin levels. Interestingly, no significant effect of naloxone on plasma prolactin levels was found in men (Steardo *et al.*, 1981). Brady & Bianco (1980) tried intravenous naloxone therapy in three women with low sexual arousability but found no evidence of it enhancing sexual arousal in this small study.

In animals, injections of naloxone to untreated sexually inactive rats produced copulatory behaviour (Gessa *et al.* 1979). Myers & Baum (1980) suggest, from studies in male rats, that the facilitatory effects of naloxone on sexual performance results in part from drug-induced release of luteinizing hormone releasing hormone (LHRH). Ixart *et al.*, (1980) reported that in rats, naloxone (1 mg/kg sc) increased plasma baseline levels by a factor of six for ACTH, by a factor of 17 for corticosterone, by a factor of two for testosterone and by a factor of three for LH. The cholinergic agonists physostigmine, pilocarpine and nicotine inhibited the prolactin release by morphine in the rat (Muraki *et al.* 1973). It is interesting to speculate that if high prolactin plasma levels are an important factor in sexual dysfunction in addicts, then perhaps through nicotine the addict has a potent antidote in his hands.

The mechanisms by which opioids alter sexual functions are not known. Among the possibilities is that their effect on monoaminergic systems may be of importance. For instance, opioids can influence 5-HT turnover (Van Loon & de Souza, 1978) as well as the release of other putative neurotransmitters such as dopamine (Subramanian *et al.*

1977). As indicated earlier, the central dopamine 5-HT balance may be of importance in relation to sexual function.

Testosterone is also of importance and the Leydig cell is under the control of luteinizing hormone. The fluctuations in hormonal levels produced by opioids could be due to the action of such drugs on hypothalamic receptors, transport proteins or at peripheral sites where sex hormones are produced or metabolised. Intraventricular injection of β-endorphin has been shown to inhibit mounting frequency in rats and since this effect is inhibited by naltrexone, central opiate receptors may be involved in modifying sexual behaviour in the rat (Myerson & Terenius, 1977).

Nicotine

Ganglion blocking drugs such as hexamethonium and mecamylamine have been reported to produce impotence (Griffin, 1981). Nicotine in low doses stimulates autonomic ganglia, but in high doses it is a ganglion blocking agent. In animals, nicotine administration or the inhalation of cigarette smoke by rats and hamsters has resulted in testicular degeneration. Moerover, exposure to cigarette smoke has been shown to decrease the percentage of mobile and normal spermatozoa and to lower blood testosterone levels (Viczian, 1968; Briggs, 1973; Dontenwill *et al.* 1973; Patra *et al.* 1979). Biswas & Patra (1981) reported that whilst nicotine treatment reduced spermatogenesis in immature rats and decreased the weights of the secondary sex organs, subsequent testosterone therapy was able to reverse these effects suggesting that endogenous pituitary gonadotrophin release is inhibited by nicotine (Biswas, 1969; Biswas & Deb, 1970; Biswas *et al.* 1979). Cigarette smoke diminishes Leydig cell function possibly by action on enzymes such as Δ^5-3β hydroxysteroid dehydrogenase.

Nebe & Schirren (1980) surveyed patients attending the andrological department at the University of Hamburg. When they studied patients who were smokers, they came to the conclusion that, in general, nicotine increased the motility of sperm and caused a reduction in the number of malformed spermatozoa. Also, there was an age-dependent increase in the number of pathological tail changes, although they pointed out that the same findings could occur as a purely age-dependent phenomenon without reference to nicotine.

LSD and the hallucinogens

Hallucinogenic agents can also affect sexuality. In the rat, pretreatment with lysergic acid diethylamide (LSD) has been shown to decrease sexual dominance behavior in the male rat (Uyeno, 1967).

In man, LSD can produce inconsistent effects in sexuality. Some users report that the sexual act is more pleasurable under LSD, with orgasm prolonged and heightened in intensity (Ludwig & Levine, 1965). Others are so concerned with their inner experience that normal sexual relationships are inhibited although mental eroticism can occur. Stories of 'hundreds' of orgasms under LSD are probably the product of a distorted imagination whilst under the drug's influence (Hofmann, 1975).

Cocaine, amphetamine and the sympathomimetics

To a pharmacologist, cocaine and amphetamine are quite different drugs. They differ clearly in their chemical structure their neurochemical mechanisms of action and in their erstwhile clinical use.

In terms of abuse, however, they are very similar. Subjects dependent on cocaine cannot distinguish between its subjective effects and those of amphetamine under laboratory conditions (Fischman *et al.*, 1976). The acute and chronic toxicities of the two drugs are similar. What differences exist are more likely to be explained in terms of differing routes of administration (oral, nasal, injection) and duration of action (some of the effects of amphetamines are particularly prolonged).

The sympathomimetics have a euphoriant action which has been likened to orgasm. Users of these drugs claim that sexual perception is enhanced and orgasm prolonged in both sexes (Kramer *et al.*, 1967). This is difficult to confirm objectively, and more difficult to explain particularly in terms of their peripheral mechanisms of action. Both drugs will enhance peripheral sympathetic activity, which is incompatible with delayed ejaculation. Blockade of α-adrenoreceptors prevents ejaculation.

A more likely mechanism of action is central in origin. Amphetamine releases dopamine and there is scope for sexual dysfunction mediated in this way. The neuroleptic drugs which antagonise dopamine decrease the satisfaction of orgasm in women (Kotin *et al.*, 1976).

A decrease in sexual activity might be expected of amphetamine in men in view of the report that the drug is capable of causing gynaecomastia (Tooley & Lack, 1949). However, this observation is characteristically difficult to explain because it is the dopamine antagonists that are commonly associated with this side effect mediated via prolactin release. Emphasis has been placed on the difficulty in identifying causative agents in sexual dysfunction among those who are taking drugs illicitly and/or excessively because of the likely 'cocktails' taken, the scope for drug interactions, and the likely concurrent consumption of the ubiquitous alcohol.

It is, therefore, more helpful to consider reports of sexual dysfunction caused by drugs related to the sympathomimetics that are used clinically, and are hopefully more controlled, namely the anorectic agents and some of the inhibitors of monoamine oxidase.

Both fenfluramine and mazindol have been reported to decrease libido in women, and this is of interest since the two drugs are representative of anorectic agents with different pharmacological profiles and which are likely to have differing mechanisms of central action (Garattini, 1980). The depressant action of fenfluramine on libido can be particularly marked (Pinder *et al.*, 1975). This action of mazindol is far more rare (about 0.06 per cent of cases, personal communication from Wander Pharmaceuticals), and at variance with the single (albeit spectacular) report of mazindol-induced aphrodisia in a woman (Friesen, 1976).

Diethylpropion, which shares a similar mechanism of anorectic action with amphetamine and mazindol, has been shown to cause gynaecomastia and the mechanism of this may be due to release of luteinizing hormone (Bridgman & Buckler, 1974).

The monoamine oxidase inhibitors like phenelzine that possess a hydrazine group in place of the amine characteristic of the sympathomimetics have also been shown to cause orgasmic failure in women, and failure of ejaculation in men (Blackwell, 1981). Interestingly, this has not been shown for the non-hydrazine derivatives such as tranylcypromine, although it possesses many of the pharmacological properties of amphetamine. Emphasis must again be placed on the difficulties in interpreting these reports because of the range of actions of these drugs (enhancing tryptaminergic systems, for instance) and the additional sexual complication in patients suffering from depression.

Ethyl alcohol

Whilst it is true that in the past society's ambivalent attitude to alcohol and alcohol-related problems has not received appropriate attention, the same cannot be said today.

Among the drugs capable of disturbing sexual function none is so legendary as alcohol. It is, therefore, surprising that in many texts of alcohol and alcoholism, impotence is not commonly indexed and mention of 'sex' usually refers to sexual differences in drinking habits. The most commonly cited reference is that attributed in 1606 to a porter in the region of Inverness.

During recent years, an intense amount of research has been carried out on the molecular mechanism of action of alcohol, and numerous studies of its biochemical actions on various enzyme systems have appeared. Interference with various central neurotransmitters has been postulated, including links with the endorphins and the hypotheses of a common basis of alcohol and opioid dependence (Lancet, 1982). These have all tended to detract from the fact that alcohol is a non-specific depressant of brain function, and its pharmacology is that of a weak general anaesthetic.

The parasympathetic component of autonomic control is more susceptible to depression by alcohol than the sympathetic division. In this way, doses of 0.4 to 1.6 g/kg in dogs impaired erection while somewhat higher doses were necessary to impair ejaculation (Gantt, 1952, 1957). Gantt also showed that sexual reflexes could be improved by alcohol in 'neurotic' dogs.

Both Rasmussen (1953) and Dewsbury (1967) showed that alcohol caused a dose dependent inhibition of all components of copulatory behaviour in male rats. For obvious reasons, female animals have been less extensively studied, though Hart (1968) noted that 'interest' in receptive female dogs was undiminished following doses that in males delayed or abolished ejaculation.

In male volunteers, low doses of alcohol increased arousal elicited by viewing erotic films as measured by penile size, while higher doses were inhibitory (Farkas & Rosen, 1976).

In addition to accompanying causes of impotence not directly due to alcohol (eg taking other drugs, nutritional deficiency), another potential mechanism for impotence is endocrinological in origin. Disturbance of hypothalamic-pituitary function in alcoholic men is well documented, and is manifested as a decrease in FSH and LH and an increase in prolactin (Van Thiel *et al.*, 1974; 1975). Feminization occurs in male alcoholics (eg gynaecomastia). The mechanism of this may have two components. First, liver damage may result in increased oestrogen and decreased testosterone production. Secondly, the well-known effect of alcohol in inducing hepatic enzymes could result in an accelerated metabolism of testosterone.

One of the best known endocrinological effects of alcohol is inhibition of the release of the antidiuretic hormone. In the same way, oxytocin is similarly inhibited. In those species in which oxytocin is released during coitus (eg the rabbit), alcohol can inhibit release thereby preventing fertilisation (Chaudhury & Matthews, 1966). In addition, the uterine effects of oxytocin are also inhibited by ethanol even to the extent of the drug being tried in premature labour (Luukkainen *et al.*, 1967).

The incidence of sexual impotence in alcoholism is difficult to quantify. Lemere & Smith, 1973) estimated it at about eight per cent from their experiences of treating many thousands of patients. They stress that in about half these cases, impotence was irreversible. They attribute the mechanism to widespread destructive effects of alcohol on all planes of the central nervous system and in the periphery, and equate it with the impotence seen in diabetics due to nervous system damage. Although the consequences of this small proportion become important taken in the context of the growing incidence of ethanol addiction in the West, perhaps the greatest problem posed by this drug is related to its central action in depressing inhibition.

The most cursory examination of the more popular press emphasises the role of alcohol in crime and violence. In our opinion, it is clear that aggressive perversions are exposed by the drug leading to a significant incidence of physical and mental damage. Allen (1969) has stressed the importance of this aspect. Perhaps Shakespeare had his priorities wrong.

Other sedatives and the anxiolytics

Pharmacologically, these drugs — including the barbiturates, the so-called 'non-barbiturate' sedatives and hypnotics, organic solvents and the benzodiazepine anxiolytics — have qualitatively similar actions, and are potentially drugs of abuse, although the potential for abuse differs widely within the group.

Theoretically, these compounds are capable of disturbing sexual function in a manner similar to alcohol. However, their potential for so doing differes because of differing patterns of abuse, routes of administration and durations of action.

Abuse of other organic solvents, either as such (eg petrol) or as constituents of glues and paints reaches intermittent epidemic proportions. By virtue of their inhalational route of administration, they are unlikely to have any sexual effects since the duration of action will be too short, but, like alcohol, their propensity to depress inhibition makes them particularly worrying.

Barbiturate abuse was common in the UK until recently. Like alcohol, all planes of the central nervous system are depressed, and in higher doses peripheral neurotransmission can also be inhibited (notably at sympathetic ganglia), and microsomal enzymes induced. Individuals dependent on these drugs favour the shorter acting drugs such as pentobarbitone, since the experience is more intense thereby making any sexual dysfunction immaterial.

Up to a point this also applies to the benzodiazepines. These have become the most widely prescribed drugs, with between one in five and one in ten of the adult population of the UK taking them. Many of those who are in this category have been taking the drugs for several years, and dependence is clearly established. There are at least two populations of dependent patients. The first is the individual who has been prescribed an anxiolytic, and continues taking the drug for a long period using supplies that are prescribed. The second is the group with a history of illicit drug taking who take anxiolytics in addition to opiates or barbiturates by means of 'topping up'.

The former group would not be considered dependent by themselves, nor perhaps by their physicians, and the appearance of tremor or restlessness on drug withdrawal will be interpreted as a return to the original anxiety rather than as a withdrawal syndrome.

Like any sedative drug, benzodiazepines will depress sexual activity if taken in excess. A much quoted case history of ejaculatory failure caused by chlordiazepoxide is that of Hughes (1964). In this patient, ejaculatory failure was quite clearly linked to two separate periods of chlordiazepoxide treatment since function returned between the two periods, and was quite reversible following final discontinuation of the drug. But it is clear that this is a very rare event. Hughes has not seen a similar case since (personal communication) and we are unaware of any other reports. Taken in the context of the millions of prescriptions dispensed annually for the fourteen currently available benzodiazepines this side effect seems of little concern. Of far greater importance are the drugs' value in the management of sexual problems.

Cooper (1972) considered that of all the causes of sexual dysfunction, 95 per cent of them are due to psychogenic factors. This perspective is somewhat paradoxical in view of the widespread use and abuse of drugs that can alter sexual function by so many different ways. We believe it may not be uncommon that one of the above drugs may depress sexual function as an acute effect, eg failure of erection, and that the distress so caused may then precipitate the more permanent sexual dysfunction, the mechanism of which is psychogenic.

Acknowledgement — We are grateful to Dr Griffith Edwards, Editor of the British Journal of Addiction, and to the Longman Group for their permission to quote the passage above.

References

Abel, E.L. (1981): Marihuana and sex: a critical survey. *Drug Alcohol Depend.* **8,** 1-22.

Allen, C. (1969): In *A textbook of psychosexual disorders,* 2nd edition, London: Oxford University Press, Pp 127-128, 245, 270.

Azizi, F., Vagenakis, A.G., Longcope, C., Ingbar, S.H. & Braverman, L.E. (1973): Decreased serum testosterone concentration in male heroin and methadone addicts. *Steroids* **22,** 467-472.

Bai, J., Greenwald, E., Caterini, H. & Kaminetzky, H.A. (1974): Drug-related menstrual aberrations. *Obstet. Gynecol.* **44,** 713-719.

Benkert, O., Renz, A. & Matussek, N. (1973): Dopamine, noradrenaline and 5-hydroxytryptamine in relation to motor activity fighting and mounting behaviour. *Neuropharmacol.* **12,** 187-193.

Besser, G.M. & Thorner, M.O. (1976): Bromocriptine in the treatment of the hyperprolactinaemia-hypogonadism syndrome. *Postgrad. Med. J.* **52,** 64-70.

Biswas, N.M. (1969): Δ^5-3β-hydroxysteroid dehydrogenase in toad testis: synergistic action of ascorbic acid and leuteinizing hormone. *Endocrinology* **85,** 981-983.

Biswas, N.M. & Deb, C. (1970): *In vitro* studies of the effect of ascorbic acid and dehydroascorbic acid on Δ^5-3 β-hydroxysteroid dehydrogenase in toad testis. *Endocrinology* **87,** 170-173.

Biswas, N.M. & Patra, P.B. (1981): Role of testosterone propionate on spermatogenesis following chronic nicotine administration in immature rats. *Indian J. Exp. Biol.* **19,** 604-606.

Biswas, N.M., Patra, P.B., Sanyai, S. & Deb, C. (1979): Andrenogonadal interactions in nicotine-induced alterations of steroidogenesis in male rat. *Andrologia* **11,** 227-233.

Blackwell, B. (1981): Antidepressant drugs. In *Side effects of drugs annual,* ed Dukes, M.N.G. Amsterdam: Excerpta Medica, Pp 19-20.

Bolelli, G. Lafisca, S., Flamigni, C., Lodi, S., Franceschetti, F., Filicori, M. & Mosca, R. (1979): Heroin addiction: Relationship between the plasma levels of testosterone dihydrotestosterone, androstenedione, LH, FSH and the plasma concentration of heroin. *Toxicology* **15,** 19-29.

Bouquet, J. (1950): Cannabis. *Bull. Narc.* **2,** 14-20.

Brady, J.P. & Bianco, F.C. (1980): Endorphins: naloxone failure to increase sexual arousal in sexually unresponsive women: a preliminary report. *Biol. Psychiat.* **15,** 627-631.

Bridgman, J.F. & Buckler, J.M.H. (1974): Drug-induced gynaecomastia. *Br. Med. J.* **ii,** 520-521.

Briggs, M.H. (1973): Cigarette smoking and infertility in men. *Med. J. Aust.* **1,** 616-617.

Bromley, B.L., Rabii, J., Gordon, J.H. & Zimmerman, E. (1978): Δ^9-tetrahydrocannabinol inhibition of suckling-induced prolactin release in the lactating rat. *Endocr. Res. Commun. 5,* 271-278.

Burdsal, C., Greenberg, G., Bell, M. & Reynolds, S. (1975): A factor-analytic examination of sexual behaviours and attitudes and marihuana usage. *J. Clin. Psychol.* **31,** 568-572.

Chaudhury, R.R. & Matthews, M. (1966): Effect of alcohol on the fertility of female rabbits. *J. Endocrinol.* **34,** 275-276.

Chopra, R.N. & Chopra, G.S. (1967): The use of cannabis drugs in India. In *Book of grass,* eds, Andrews, G. & Vinkenoog, S. New York: Grove Press. P 138.

Cooper, A.J. (1972): The causes and management of impotence. *Postgrad. Med. J.* **48,** 548-552.

Corcoran, M.E., Amit, Z., Malsbury, C.W. & Daykin, S. (1974): Reduction in copulatory behaviour of male rats following hashish injections. *Res. Commun. Chem. Pathol. Pharmacol.* **7,** 779-782.

Cushman, P. (1972): Sexual behaviour in heroin addiction and methadone maintenance. *N. Y. State J. Med.* **72,** 1261-1265.

Cushman, P. (1975): Plasma testosterone levels in healthy male marihuana smokers. *Am. J. Drug Alcohol Abuse* **2,** 269-275.

Cutler, M.G., Mackintosh, J.H. & Chance, M.R.A. (1975): Cannabis resin and sexual behaviour in the lab mouse. *Psychopharmacologia* **45,** 129-131.

Daley, J.D., Branda, L.A., Rosenfeld, J. & Younglai, E.V. (1974): Increase of serum prolactin in male rats by (n)-trans-Δ^9-tetrahydrocannabinol. *J. Endocrinol.* **63,** 415-416.
Dawley, H.H., Winstead, D.K., Baxter, A.S. & Gay, J.R. (1979): An attitude survey of the effects of marihuana on sexual enjoyment. *J. Clin. Psychol.* **35,** 212-217.
Delitala, G., Giusti, M., Devilla, L., Mazzocchi, G., Lotti, G. & Giordano, G. (1981): Effect of a met-enkephalin analogue and naloxone infusion on gonadotrophin secretion in man. *Acta Eur. Fertil.* **12,** 287-288.
Dewsbury, D.A. (1967): Effects of alcohol ingestion on copulatory behaviour of male rats. *Psychopharmacologia* **11,** 276-281.
Dixit, V.P. & Lohiya, N.K. (1975): Effect of cannabis extract on the response of accessory sex organs of adult male mice to testosterone. *Indian J. Physiol. Pharmacol.* **19,** 98-100.
Dixit, V.P., Sharma, V.N. & Lohiya, N.K. (1974): The effect of chronically administered cannabis extract on the testicular function of mice. *Eur. J. Pharmacol.* **26,** 111-115.
Dontenwill, W., Chevalier, H.J., Harke, H.P., Lofrenz, U., Reckzeh, G. & Schnieder, B. (1973): Experimental investigations of the effect of cigarette smoke exposure on testicular function of Syrian golden hamsters. *Toxicology* **1,** 309-320.
Farkas, G.M. & Rosen, R.C. (1976): Effect of alcohol on elicited male sexual response. *J. Stud. Alcohol* **37,** 265-272.
Fischman, M.W., Schuster, C.R., Rosnekov, L., Schick, J.F.E., Krasnegor, N.A., Fennell, W. & Freedman, D.X. (1976): Cardiovascular and subjective effects of intravenous cocaine administration in humans. *Archs Gen. Psychiat.* **33,** 983-989.
Fort, J. (1976): Youth: drugs, sex and life. *Curr. Probl. Pediat.* **6,** 1-42.
Friesen, L.V.C. (1976): Aphrosdisia with mazindol. *Lancet* **ii,** 1974.
Gantt, W.H. (1952): Effect of alcohol on the sexual reflexes of normal and neurotic male dogs. *Psychosom. Med.* **14,** 174-181.
Gantt, W.H. (1957): Acute effect of alcohol on autonomic (sexual, secretory, cardiac) and somatic responses. In *Alcoholism. Basic aspects and treatment* ed Himwich, H.E., Publication No. 47. Washington: American Association for the Advancement of Science. Pp 73-89.
Garattini, S. (1980): Recent studies on anorectic agents. *Trends Pharmacol. Sci.* **1,** 354-356.
Gessa, G.L., Paglietti, E. & Quarantotti, B.P. (1979): Induction of copulatory behaviour in sexually inactive rats by naloxone. *Science* **204,** 203-205.
Gessa, G.L. & Tagliamonte, A. (1974): Role of brain monoamines in male sexual behaviour. *Life Sci.* **14,** 425-436.
Goldstein, A. (1972): The pharmacological basis of methadone treatment. In *Proceedings of the fourth national conference on methadone treatment,* New York: NAPAN, Pp 27-32.
Griffin, J.P. (1981): Drug-induced sexual dysfunction. In *Iatrogenic Diseases.* Update to 2nd edition, eds D'Arcy, P.F. & Griffin, J.P., London: OUP. Pp 197-204.
Guerra, F. (1974): Sex and drugs in the 16th century. *Br. J. Addict.* **69,** 269-290.
Hanbury, R., Cohen, M. & Stimmel, B. (1977): Adequacy of sexual performance in men maintained on methadone. *Am. J. Drug Alcohol Abuse* **4,** 13-20.
Hart, B.L. (1968): Effects of alcohol on sexual reflexes and mating behaviour in the male dog. *Q. J. Stud. Alcohol* **29,** 839-844.
Hembree, W.C., Zeidenberg, P. & Nahas, G.G. (1976): Marihuana's effects on human gonadal function. In *Marihuana: chemistry, biochemistry and cellular effects,* ed Nahas, G.G., New York: Springer Verlag. Pp 521-532.
Hembree, W.C., Nahas, G.G., Zeidenberg, P. & Huang, H.F. (1980): Changes in human spermatozoa associated with high dose marihuana smoking. In *Marihuana: biological effects,* eds Nahas, G.G. & Paton, W.D.M., Oxford: Pergamon Press. Pp 429-439.
Hoffman, F.G. (1975): In *A handbook on drug and alcohol abuse. The biochemical aspects,* London: OUP. Pp 11, 157.
Hong, C.Y., Chaput de Saintonge, D.M. & Turner, P. (1981): Δ^9-tetrahydrocannabinol inhibits human sperm motility. *J. Pharm. Pharmacol.* **33,** 746-747.
Horowitz, J.D. & Goble, A.J. (1979): Drugs and impaired male sexual function. *Drugs* **18,** 206-217.
Horowski, R. & Gräf, K.J. (1979): Neuroendocrine effects on neuropsychotropic drugs and their possible influence on toxic reactions in animals and man. *Archs Toxicol.* (Berlin) Suppl 2, 93-104.

Hughes, J.M. (1964): Failure to ejaculate with chlordiazepoxide. *Am. J. Psychiatry* **121,** 610-611.

Ixart, G., Szafarczyk, A., Malval, F., Nouguier-Soule, J & Assenmacher, I. (1980): Résponses au stress des systemes ACTH-corticostérone et LH-testosterone chez le rat male sous naloxone. *C. R. Acad. Sc.* (Paris) **291,** 265-270.

Jacubovic, A., McGeer, E.G. & McGeer, P.L. (1980): Biochemical alterations induced by cannabinoids in the Leydig cells of the rat testes *in vitro.* Effects on testosterone and protein synthesis. In *Marihuana: biological effects,* eds Nahas, G.G. & Paton, W.D.M., Oxford: Pergamon Press. Pp 251-263.

Koff, W.C. (1974): Marihuana and sexual activity. *J. Sex. Res.* **10,** 194-204.

Kolodny, R.C., Masters, W.H., Kolodner, R.M. & Toro, G. (1974): Depression of plasma testosterone levels after chronic intensive marihuana use. *N. Engl. J. Med.* **290,** 872-874.

Kotin, J., Wilbert, D.E., Verberg, D. & Soldinger, S.M. (1976): Thioridazine and sexual dysfunction. *Am. J. Psychiat.* **133,** 82-85.

Hughes, J.M. (1964): Failure to ejaculate with chlordiazepoxide. *Am. J. Psychiatry* **121,** 610-611.

Ixart, G., Szafarczyk, A., Malval, F., Nouguier-Soule, J. & Assenmacher, I. (1980): Résponses au stress des systemes ACTH-corticostérone et LH-testosterone chez le rat male sous naloxone. *C. R. Acad. Sc.* (Paris) **291,** 265-270.

Jacubovic, A., McGeer, E.G. & McGeer, P.L. (1979): Effects of Cannabinoids on testosterone and protein synthesis in rat testis Leydig cells *in vitro. Mol. Cell. Endocrinol.* **15,** 41-50.

Jacubovic, A., McGeer, E.G. & McGeer, P.L. (1980): Biochemical alterations induced by cannabinoids in the Leydig cells of the rat testes *in vitro.* Effects on testosterone and protein synthesis. In *Marihuana: biological effects,* eds Nahas, G.G. & Paton, W.D.M., Oxford: Pergamon Press. Pp 251-263.

Koff, W.C. (1974): Marihuana and sexual activity. *J. Sex. Res.* **10,** 194-204.

Kolodny, R.C., Masters, W.H., Kolodner, R.M. & Toro, G. (1974): Depression of plasma testosterone levels after chronic intensive marihuana use. *N. Engl. J. Med.* **290,** 872-874.

Kotin, J., Wilbert, D.E., Verberg, D. & Soldinger, S.M. (1976): Thioridazine and sexual dysfunction. *Am. J. Psychiat.* **133, 82-85.**

Kramer, J. & Ben-David, M. (1974): Suppression of prolactin secretion by acute administration of Δ^9-tetrahydrocannibinol in rats. *Proc. Soc. Exp. Biol. Med.* **147,** 482-484.

Kramer, J.C., Fischman, V.S. & Littlefield, D.C. (1967): Amphetamine abuse. *J. Am. Med. Ass.* **201,** 305-309.

Lafisca, S., Bolelli, G., Franceschetti, F. Filicori, M., Flamigni, C. & Margio, M. (1981): Hormone levels in methadone-treated drug addicts. *Drug. Alcohol Depend.* **8,** 229-234.

Lancet, (1982): Salsolinol and alcoholism. (Editorial.) *Lancet,* **ii,** 80-81.

Langrod, J., Lowinson, J. & Ruiz, P. (1981): Methadone treatment and physical complaints: a clinical analysis. *Int. J. Addiction* **16,** 947-952.

Lemere, F. & Smith, J.W. (1973): Alcohol induced sexual impotence. *Am. J. Psychiat.* **130,** 212-213.

Ludwig, A.M. & Levine, J. (1965): Patterns of hallucinogenic drug abuse. *J. Am. Med. Ass.* **191,** 92-96.

Luukkainen, T., Vaisto, L. & Jarvinen, P.A. (1967): The effect of oral intake of ethyl alcohol on the activity of pregnant human uterus. *Acta Obstet. Gynaecol. Scand.* **46,** 486-488.

Mendelson, J.H., Ellingboe, J., Kuehnle, J. & Mello, N.K. (1979*a*): Heroin and naltrexone effects on pituitary-gonadal hormones in man: tolerance and supersensitivity. *Nat. Inst. Drug Abuse Res. Monogr. Ser.* **27,** 302-308.

Mendelson, J.H., Ellingboe, J., Kuehnle, J.C. & Mello, N.K. (1979*b*): Effects of naltrexone on mood and neuroendocrine function in normal adult males. *Psychoneuroendocrinology* **3,** 231-236.

Mendelson, J.H., Kuehnle, J., Ellingboe, J. & Babor, T.F. (1974): Plasma testosterone levels before, during and after chronic marihuana smoking. *N. Engl. J. Med.* **291,** 1051-1055.

Mendelson, J.H., Mendelson, J.E. & Patch, V.D. (1975): Plasma testosterone levels in heroin addiction and during methadone maintenance. *J. Pharmacol. Exp. Ther.* **192,** 211-217.

Merari, A., Barak, A. & Plaves, M. (1973): Effects of Δ^1-(2)-tetrahydrocannabinol on copulation in the male rat. *Psychopharmacologica* **28,** 243-246.

Myerson, B.J. & Terenius, L. (1977): β-Endorphin and male sexual behaviour. *Eur. J. Pharmacol* **42,** 191-192.

Muraki, T., Tokunaga, A., Nakadate, T. & Kato, R. (1979): Inhibition by cholinergic agonists of the prolactin release induced by morphine. *Naunyn-Schmiedeberg's Archs Pharmacol.* **308,** 249-254.

Myers, B.M. & Baum, M.J. (1980): Facilitation of copulatory performance in male rats by naloxone: effects of hypophysectomy, 17α-estradiol and luteinizing hormone releasing hormone. *Pharmacol. Biochem. Behav.* **12,** 365-370.

Nebe, K.H. & Schirren, C. (1980): Statistiche untersuchungen bei andrologischen Patienten. iii Nikotin und Ejakulatparameter. *Andrologia* **12,** 493-502.

Patra, P.B., Sanyal, S. & Biswas, N.M. (1979): Possible α-adrenergic involvement in nicotine-induced alteration of spermatogenesis in rat. *Andrologia* **11,** 273-278.

Pinder, R.M., Brogden, R.N., Sawyer, P.R., Speight, T.M. & Avery, G.S. (1975): Fenfluramine: a review of its pharmacological properties and therapeutic efficacy in obesity. *Drugs* **10,** 241-323.

Rasmussen, E.W. (1953): Alkohol problemet belyst ved eksperimentelle dyreforsok. In *Forhandlingar, Nordiska Psykologmötet i Helsingfors.* Pp 249-256.

Rees, J.M.H. (1983): Sexual dysfunction and prescribed psychotropic drugs. In *Psychopharmacology of sexual disorders,* ed Wheatley, D. London: OPU. Pp 138-147.

Schaefer, C.F., Gunn, C.G. & Dubowski, K.M. (1975): Normal plasma testosterone concentrations after marihuana smoking. *N. Engl. J. Med.* **292,** 867-868.

Sheard, M.H. (1969): The effect of p-chlorophenylalanine on behaviour in rats: relation to brain serotonin and 5-hydroxyindole acetic acid. *Brain Res.* **15,** 524-528.

Sicuteri, S. (1974): Serotonin and sex in man. *Pharmacol. Res. Commun.* **6,** 403-411.

Steardo, L., Monteleone, P., Buscaino, G.A., Maj, M., Zizolfi, S. & Kemali, D. (1981): Naloxone-induced decrease of plasma prolactin in healthy women. *Acta Neurol.* **36,** 379-383.

Subramanian, N., Mitznegg, P., Sprügel, W., Domschke, W., Domschke, S., Wünsch, E. & Demling, L. (1977): Influence of enkephalin on K^+-evoked efflux of putative transmitters in rats brain. *Naunyn-Schmiedeberg's Archs Pharmacol.* **299,** 163-165.

Tart, C.T. (1971): In *On being stoned* Palo Alto, CA: Science & Behaviour Books. Pp 141-151.

Tooley, P.H. & Lack, C. (1949): Gynaecomastia during treatment with amphetamine. *Lancet* **i,** 650-651.

Traub, S.H. (1977): Perceptions of marihuana and its effects: A comparison of users and non users. *Br. J. Addict.* **72,** 62-74.

Uyeno, E.T. (1967): Lysergic acid diethylamide and sexual dominance behaviour of the male rat. *Int. J. Neuropsychiat.* **3,** 188-190.

Van Loon, G.R. & De Souza, E.B. (1978): Effect of β-endorphin on brain serotonin metabolism. *Life Sci.* **23,** 971-978.

Van Thiel, D.H., Gavaler, J.S. & Lester, R. *et al.* (1975): Plasma estrone, prolactin, neuro-physin and sex-steroid-binding globulin in chronic alcoholic men. *Metabolism* **24,** 1015-1019.

Van Thiel, D.H., Lester, R. & Sherins, R.J. (1974): Hypogonadism in alcoholic liver disease: evidence for a double defect. *Gastroenterology* **67,** 1188-1199.

Verebely, K. & Mulé, S.J. (1975): Naltrexone pharmacology, pharmacokinetics and metabolism: current status. *Am. J. Drug Alcohol Abuse* **2,** 357-363.

Viczián, M. (1968): The effect of cigarette smoke inhalation on spermatogenesis in rats. *Experientia* **24,** 511-513.

Weiland, W. & Younger, M. (1971): Sexual effects and side effects of heroin and methadone. In *Proceedings of the third national conference on methadone treatment,* Washington DC: US Government Printing Office, Pp 50-53.

Weiss, H.D. (1972): The physiology of human penile erection. *Ann. Intern. Med.* **76,** 793-799.

8

Neuroleptics and sexual behavior of male schizophrenics

Thomas A. BAN, William GUY and William H. WILSON

Vanderbilt University, Department of Psychiatry and Clinical Research Service, Tennessee Neuropsychiatric Institute, Nashville TN, USA

Introduction

Throughout this century, the sexual behavior of schizophrenics has been characterized by ambiguity and controversy. Echoing the then prevalent view, Krafft-Ebbing (1965) stated that sexual excesses, in particular onanism, were among the important factors leading to insanity. Although stated less emphatically, this view concerning the contribution of sexual activity to the development of, as well as the prolongation of recovery in, schizophrenia continued to be held by a significant number of psychiatrists (Pinderhughes *et al.*, 1972, etc).

In contrast, Freud (1911) felt that the main factor in the development of schizophrenia was the withdrawal of libido from relationships with other people. Rado (1962) similarly emphasized the schizophrenic's apparent lack of interest in sexual activity and suggested that it might be due to their inability to experience pleasure (anhedonia), a view particularly supported about chronic schizophrenics by the later work of Stein & Wise (1971) and Harrow *et al.* (1977). Thus, aberrant sexuality has been cited as the cause of, a consequence of, or interactive with the development and course of schizophrenic illness. Unfortunately, most of these hypotheses have been put forward on the basis of individual case studies, and only infrequently on the basis of controlled clinical data.

Even controlled clinical trials, which are rare relative to the voluminous number of annual citations relating to schizophrenia, are often ambiguous in their findings. Lukianowicz (1963) compared 100 male inpatient schizophrenics with 100 normal males and 100 depressed patients and found that, during the first two years of their illness, there was a marked increase in sexual activity, particularly autoerotic activity. He suggested that, in these early phases of their illness, schizophrenics retain their premorbid sexual level. In contrast, Rozan *et al.* (1971) suggested that the onset of psychiatric illness was associated with a significant lowering of sexual activity, while Akhter *et al.* (1977) indicated that schizophrenics were less sexually active than patients with other psychiatric diagnoses. Nestoros *et al.* (1980) found that the sexual functioning of drug-treated chronic schizophrenics differed from normal controls in most respects, that the differences existed in the patient's premorbid state and that patients tended to become progressively worse with increasing age. Perhaps the most consistent finding is that patients with a history of reasonably adequate premorbid heterosexual adjustment tend to be those with a good response to neuroleptics.

Given the conflicting findings on schizophrenic sexual behavior in general, it is difficult to formulate a defensible position on neuroleptic-induced sexual changes in male schizophrenics. Supporting the common contention that neuroleptics interfere with sexual function, one especially reflective outpatient schizophrenic (Ban, 1972) on prolonged neuroleptic treatment stated that, prior to his illness, he had experienced preoccupations since adolescence, which would focus primarily on a premature ejaculation pattern. With neuroleptics, the situation was reveresd and went to the other extreme. More importantly, Ban (1972) observed that no active olfactory, visual or tactile simulation could elicit an erection. Erection was only obtained by persistent passive stimulation, ie the partner stimulating him, and that ejaculation, in these circumstances, was achieved by friction without any of the psychological/emotional concomitants of orgasm. Although he was preoccupied with sex and was able to perform to the satisfaction of his partner, he was unable to achieve any pleasure or satisfaction himself. This loss of the feeling of pleasure (anhedonia) in schizophrenics is not unique to this patient. Long before the psychopharmacological era, Holderlin (as referred to by Jaspers, 1962), who had himself experienced it, wrote the expressive verse:

'June and July and May
I have gone so far away
I have no more to give
I do not want to live.'

(Free translation by H. E. Lehmann)

The role of sex hormones

In a group of drug-free schizophrenics, Brambilla & Penati (1970) demonstrated significant reductions in total gonadotrophin secretion. In a group of 22 chronic schizophrenics treated with haloperidol, total urinary gonadotrophin secretion was raised to normal levels within 15 days of initiating treatment and, after withdrawal of the drug, returned to low, pretreatment, values. These authors further reported that a significant percentage of these patients exhibited low androgen secretion as measured by levels of 17-ketosteroids. Tourney & Hatfield, (1973) found significant reductions of plasma dehydroepindrosterone, produced primarily in the adrenal cortex rather than the testis, in a group of drug-free schizophrenics. These findings, however, contrast with those of Matsumoto *et al.* (1966) who found higher urinary levels of 17 ketosteroids in drug-free chronic schizophrenics than in a normal control group.

The role of histamine

Because the patient referred to above gave an account of premature ejaculation prior to being placed on neuroleptics, the possibility of a relationship between premature ejaculation and schizophrenia is raised. In this context, the findings of Pfeiffer *et al.* (1973) are of particular importance. In the course of exploratory studies, this group of workers found that approximately 50 per cent of schizophrenic patients were histapenic (H−) and about 20 per cent were histadelic (H+). Histapenic patients were characterized by a low blood histamine level (below 40 mg/ml), a low basophil count (below 0.4 per cent of WBC's), prevalent paranoid symptoms, a low incidence of allergies, rare head colds and delayed ejaculation or organism. In contrast, histadelic patients were characterized by high histamine levels, a high basophil count, prevalent depressive symptoms, a high incidence of allergies, frequent head colds, and premature ejaculations.

The role of dopamine

Considerably more convincing than the association between blood histamine levels in schizophrenia is the relationship between schizophrenia and dopaminergic functions. Dopaminergic mechanisms appear to occupy a strategic position in those functions which are disturbed in schizophrenia and the inhibition of central dopamine functions appears to be the common pathway of action for all neuroleptic drugs (Meltzer & Fang, 1976; Carlsson, 1978). In fact, there is substantial evidence that a good correlation exists between the clinical antipsychotic potency of neuroleptics and their potency to bind stereospecifically with postsynaptic dopamine receptors (Creese *et al.*, 1976).

Much evidence exists suggesting that dopamine plays an excitatory role in the sexual behavior of animals and man. Dopamine agonists and treatments which elevate brain dopamine, such as L-dopa, stimulate sexual behavior; while dopamine antagonists suppress this behavior (Gessa & Tagliamonte, 1975). Angrist & Gershon (1976) in their studies on the effects of L-dopa in schizophrenic male patients showed that its administration increased sexual delusions as well as overt sexual behavior. The arousal of sexual feelings was also found in non-schizophrenic patients. Given these findings, one should not ignore the possibility that schizophrenic episodes might be associated with increased sexual activity and that this increase may be counteracted by the administration of neuroleptic drugs.

Central mechanisms

Sexual behavior is a complex interrelationship between central mechanisms mediated, in part, by central monoamines and the sexual organs controlled by peripheral autonomic input. Neuroleptics, as well as antidepressants and stimulants, produce both central and peripheral effects (Petrie, 1980).

A large volume of literature on sexual behavior in animals has linked the central effects of dopamine, norepinephrine and serotonin to this behavior (Karczmur, 1980). The facilitatory effects of dopamine on animal behavior can also be seen following the administration of parachlorophenylalanine (PCPA), a serotonin synthesis inhibitor. This effect is potentiated by the addition of MAOI and can be abolished by administering 5-hydroxytryptophan (5-HTP). Data such as these indicate that increased sexual activity may be associated with increased dopamine activity and decreased seratonin activity, and vice versa.

Luteinizing hormone (LH) is the major direct stimulus for the control of testosterone secretion. Prolactin, also secreted by the anterior pituitary, reduces end organ responsiveness to LH and thereby reduces the conversion of testosterone to its active metabolites. Phenothiazines, butyrophenones and, to a lesser extent, some antidepressants suppress LH and stimulate prolactin release by blocking prolactin-inhibiting factor (Langer *et al.*, 1977). Increased levels of prolactin have been reported in association with impotence (Franks *et al.*, 1978). Brown *et al.* (1981) noted lower LH and testosterone levels in a group of schizophrenic patients on chronic thioridazine medication, while control group patients who were on other neuroleptics or who were drug-free showed significantly less suppression. Arato *et al.* (1979) found that sexually active males on fluphenazine decanoate had low testosterone but high LH levels. Less sexually active patients had lower LH values. The possibility that thioridazine may have an adverse effect on CNS mediation of sexual function has been supported by Meltzner & Fang's (1976) observations that a greater elevation in prolactin occurs with thioridazine than with any other neuroleptic. Ghadarian *et al.* (1982), however, related elevated prolactin levels to moderate and severe sexual dysfunction in 54 per cent of the patients receiving a variety of antipsychotic drugs.

Peripheral effects

Although reported far less than ejaculation disorders, the peripheral causes of impotence with neuroleptics may be related to their anticholinergic properties. Kotin *et al.* (1976) in a study of 115 patients on a variety of neuroleptics, reported that 44 per cent of the thioridazine patients had difficulty in achieving erection as compared with 19 per cent for all other neuroleptics, and that 35 per cent of these thioridazine-treated patients also had difficulty in sustaining their erections. These rather high percentages did not support the data of Kline *et al.* (1968), however, and they suggested that further studies were still necessary to resolve the dispute.

Aspermia, ie the absence of an external ejaculate in the presence of an erection, occurs as a side effect with several neuroleptics. Again, this is most common with thioridazine (Grigis, 1968). This phenomenon has also been reported with chlorpromazine, piperacetazine, mesoridazine, butaphenazine, perphenazine and trifluoperazine. Aspermia with thioridazine is not clearly dose-related and may develop with a dose as low as 50 mg per day. It has been estimated that some 30 per cent of male patients treated with thioridazine may develop aspermia (Blair & Simpson, 1966). The mechanism of drug-induced aspermia has been related to alpha-adrenergic blocking activity (Schwarz, 1982). Why thioridazine should produce this effect, is however, unclear since although its alpha-adrenergic effects are similar to those of other neuroleptics, patients with aspermia do not exhibit other peripheral alpha-adrenergic effects.

Alpha-adrenergic agonists have been used in the treatment of retrograde ejaculation and, interestingly, imipramine has been successfully used in aspermia secondary to diabetic neuropathy (Brooks *et al.*, 1980). Conversely, drugs such as thioridazine have been used in the treatment of premature ejaculation (Fraschini, 1966; Lingjaerde, 1969). Similarly, pimozide, a butyrophenone, has been used in the treatment of premature ejaculation and impotence, although its beneficial effects on impotence are as yet unclear (Mattelear, 1974).

Conclusions

Given that neuroleptic drugs have a variety of detrimental effects on sexual functioning, it could be expected that their introduction would have even further decreased the low reproductive rates of schizophrenics. In studying a pre-neuroleptic cohort of patients relative to those in a post-neuroleptic cohort, Erlenmeyer-Kimling *et al.* (1969), however, found reproductive rates to be comparable. Slater *et al.* (1971) also found rates for the latter group to be similar to those obtained in the pre-neuroleptic era by Essen-Moller (1935). The introduction of neuroleptic drugs, therefore, seemed to be associated with little change in the reproductive rates of schizophrenics. It should be remembered, however, that together with the introduction of neuroleptics, there was a dramatic change in the sociotherapeutic treatment of patients which led to alterations in their life-style as well as to changes in the attitude of society in general.

It must also be recognized that the antipsychotic effect of neuroleptics may facilitate sexual functioning by alleviating anxiety and thought disorganization, thereby permitting patients to engage in greater and more effective social interrelationships (Nestros *et al.,* 1981). Neuroleptics may also have increased the reproductive rates of schizophrenics by altering the ratio among the various subtypes of schizophrenia. Morrison (1974) found that in the post-neuroleptic era, the incidence of hebephrenia and catatonia, known to have lower reproductive rates than other subtypes, had markedly decreased.

Clearly, there are a multiplicity of factors involved in the relationship of neuroleptic treatment and sexual functioning in the male schizophrenic. Since dopamine plays an excitatory role in sexual behavior, one might expect schizophrenic patients to be hypersexual. Since neuroleptics block dopamine receptors, one would expect these drugs to suppress sexual behavior. The research findings, however, are not so clear-cut. The level of sexual dysfunction seen in male schizophrenics appears to vary with age, duration and subtype of illness. Neuroleptics may interact with neurotransmitters to exacerbate sexual dysfunction or may, through their antipsychotic properties, aid in the re-establishment of a rewarding level of functioning. The relationship between neuroleptic treatment and male sexual functioning is a complex one calling for a multidisciplinary approach into the psychological, sociological, biochemical and pharmacological factors involved.

References

Akhtar, S., Croker, E., Dickey, N., Helfrich, J. & Rheuban, W.J. (1977): Overt sexual behavior among psychiatric inpatients. *Dis. Nerv. Syst.* **38,** 359-361.

Angrist, B. & Gershon, S. (1976): Clinical effects of amphetamine and L-dopa on sexuality and aggression. *Compr. Psych.* **17,** 715-722.

Arato, M., Erdos, A. & Polgar, M. (1979): Endocrinological changes in patients with sexual dysfunction under long-term neuroleptic treatment. *Pharmakopsychiat.* **12,** 426-431.

Ban, T.A. (1972): *Schizophrenia: a psychopharmacological approach.* Springfield: Thomas.

Blair, J.H. & Simpson, G.M. (1966): Effect of antipsychotic drugs on reproductive functions. *Dis. Nerv. Syst.* **27,** 645-647.

Brambilla, F. & Penati, G. (1970): Hormones and behavior. In *Influences of hormones on the nervous system.* ed Ford, D.H. Karger: Basel. Pp 482-494.

Brooks, M.E., Berezin, M. & Braf, J. (1980): Treatment of retrograde ejaculation with imipramine. *Urology* **15,** 353-355.

Brown, W.A., Laughren, T.P. & Williams, B. (1981): Differential effects of neuroleptic agents on the pituitary-gonadal axis in men. *Archs Gen. Psychiat.* **38,** 1270-1272.

Carlsson, A. (1978): Antipsychotic drugs, neurotransmitters, and schizophrenia. *Am. J. Psychiat.* **135,** 164-173.

Creese, I., Burt, D.R. & Snyder, S.H. (1976): Dopamine receptor binding predicts clinical and pharmacological potencies of anti-schizophrenic drugs. *Science* **192,** 481-483.

Erlenmeyer-Kimling, L., Nicol, S., Rainer, J.D. & Deming, W.E. (1969): Changes in fertility rates of schizophrenic patients in New York State. *Am. J. Psychiat.* **125,** 916-927.

Essen-Moller, E. (1935): Untersuchungen Über die Fruchbarkeit gewisser Gruppen von Geisteskranken. *Acta Psychiat. Neurol. Scand.,* Suppl. 8.

Franks, S., Jacobs, H.S., Martin, N. & Navarro, J.D.N. (1978): Hyperprolactinemia and impotence. *Clin. Endocrinol.* **8,** 277-287.

Fraschini, A. (1966): Contributions to the therapy of ejaculation praecox and some forms of impotentia. *Minerva Med.* **5,** 3823-3824.

Freud, S. (1911): Psychoanalytic notes upon an autobiographical account of a case of paranoia (dementia paranoides). In *Collected papers,* Vol. 3 (first published 1925). London: The Hogarth Press Ltd. & the Institute of Psycho-Analysis. Pp 387-470.

Gessa, G.L. & Tagliamonte, A. (1975): Role of brain serotonin and dopamine in male sexual behavior. In *Sexual behavior: pharmacology and biochemistry,* eds Sandler, M. & Gessa, G.L. New York: Raven Press. Pp 117-128.

Ghadrian, A.M., Chouinard, G. & Annable, L. (1982): Sexual dysfunction and plasma prolactin levels in neuroleptic-treated schizophrenic outpatients. *J. Nerv. Ment. Dis.* **170,** 463-647.
Grigis, S.M. (1968): Aspermia, a survey of forty-nine cases. *Fert. Steril.* **19,** 580-588.
Harrow, M., Grinker, R.R., Sr., Holzmann, P.S. & Kayton, L. (1977): Anhedonia and schizophrenia. *Am. J. Psychiat.* **134,** 794-797.
Jaspers, K. (1962): *General psychopathology.* Translated by Hoenig, J. & Hamilton, M.W. Chicago: University of Chicago Press.
Larczmar, A.G. (1980): *Drugs, transmitters and hormones, and mating behavior.* In *Modern problems of pharmacopsychiatry: drug treatment of sexual dysfunction,* Vol. 15, eds Ban, T.A. & Freyhan, F. Basel: Karger. Pp 1-76.
Kline, N.S., Blair, J., Cooper, T.B., Esser, A.H., Hackett, E. & Vestergaard, P. (1968): A controlled seven year study of endocrine and other indices in drug treated schizophrenics. *Acta Psychiat. Scand.,* Suppl 44, 206.
Kotin, J., Wilbert, D.C., Verburg, D. & Soldinger, S.M. (1976): Thioridazine and sexual dysfunction. *Am. J. Psychiat.* **133,** 82-85.
Krafft-Ebbing, R. von (1965): *Psychopathia sexualis,* 12th ed. Eng. Translation. New York: Stein and Day.
Langer, G., Sachar, E.J., Gruen, P.H. & Halpern, F.S. (1977): Human prolactin response to neuroleptic drugs correlated with antischizophrenic potency. *Nature* **266,** 639-640.
Lingjaerde. O. (1969): Use of thioridazine during ejaculation praecox. *T. Norsk Laegeforen* **89,** 1433.
Lukianowicz, N. (1963): Sexual drive and its gratification in schizophrenia. *Int. J. Soc. Psychiat.* **9,** 250-258.
Matsumoto, K., Berlet, H., Bull, C. & Himwich, H. (1966): Excretion of 17-hydroxycorticosteroids and 17- ketosteroids in relation to schizophrenic symptoms. *J. Psychiat. Res.* **4,** 1-12.
Mattelaer, I. (1974): Pimozide in the treatment of male impotence. A pilot trial. *Acta Urol. Belg.* **42,** 478-483.
Meltzer, H.Y. & Fang, V.A. (1976): The effect of neuroleptics on serum prolactin in schizophrenic patients. *Archs Gen. Psychiat.* **33,** 279-286.
Morrison, J.R. (1974): Changes in subtype diagnosis of schizophrenia: 1920-1966. *Am. J. Psychiat.* **131,** 674-677.
Nestoros, J.N., Lehmann, H.E. & Ban, T.A. (1980): Neuroleptic drugs and sexual function in schizophrenia. *Mod. Problems Pharmacopsychiat.* **15,** 111-130.
Nestoros, J.N., Lehmann, H.E. & Ban, T.A. (1981): Sexual behavior of the male schizophrenic: The impact of illness and medications. *Archs Sexual Behav.* **10,** 421-442.
Petrie, W.M. (1980): The sexual effects of antipsychotic, antidepressant and psychomotor stimulant drugs. *Mod. Problems Pharmacopsychiat.* **15,** 77-90.
Pfeiffer, C.C., Iliev, V. & Goldstein, L. (1973): Blood histamine basophil counts and trace elements in the schizophrenias. In *Orthomolecular psychiatry: treatment of schizophrenia,* eds Hawkins, D. & Pauling, L. San Francisco: W. H. Freeman.
Pinderhughes, C.A., Grace, E.B. & Reyna, L.J. (1972): Psychiatric disorders and sexual functioning. *Am. J. Psychiat.* **128,** 1276-1283.
Rado, S. (1962): Schizotypal organization: A preliminary report on a clinical study of schizophrenia. In *Psychoanalysis of behavior.* New York: Grune and Stratton. Pp 1-10.
Rozan, G.H., Tuchin, T. & Kurland, M.L. (1971): Some implications of sexual activity for mental illness. *Ment. Hyg.* **55,** 318-323.
Schwarz, G. (1982): Case report of inhibition of ejaculation and retrograde ejaculation as side effects of amoxapine. *Am. J. Psychiat.* **139,** 233-234.
Slater, E., Hare, E.H. & Price, J.S. (1971): Marriage and family of psychiatric patients compared with national data. *Soc. Biol.* **18,** (Suppl.), 60-73.
Stein, L. & Wise, C.D. (1971): Possible etiology of schizophrenia: Progressive damage to the noradrenergic reward system by 6-hydroxydopamine. *Science* **171,** 1032-1036.
Tourney, G. & Hatfield, L.M. (1973): Androgen metabolism in schizophrenics, homosexual and normal controls. *Biol. Psychiat.* **6,** 23-36.

9

The sexual effects of antipsychotic, antidepressant and psychomotor stimulant drugs

W. M. Petrie

Tennessee Neuropsychiatric Institute Nashville, Tennessee 37217, USA.

Introduction

While antipsychotic and antidepressant drugs produce marked effects on sexual behavior, a clear understanding of these effects is hindered by the lack of controlled, comprehensive studies and the limitations of the anecdotal reports which largely make up this literature. That symptoms of sexual dysfuntion usually accompany the illness for which these drugs are prescribed (Beck, 1967; Molcan 1968) further confounds the issue.

Assessment

Sexual side-effects are not specifically investigated in the majority of psychotropic drug trials and little additional data have been gathered through post-marketing drug surveillance. Because non-structured interviews and voluntary reporting of sexual effects by patients are likely to be inadequate (Shenn, 1982), the focus has shifted towawrds a structured approach in the assessment of sexual side-effects. Two recent scales (Rozan *et al.*, 1971; Beaumont, 1973) provide a more complete measurement of premorbid functioning, of changes in sexual function during drug treament, and of changes in sexual function related to other symptom changes (eg improved libido following improvement of depression). Even with detailed questioning, however, it may still be difficult to differentiate clearly the relative roles of premorbid sexual adjustment, psychiatric illness, and pharmacological intervention in any particular sexual dysfuntion (Beaumont, 1977).

The majority of the data focus on male sexual function and generally assume that male sexuality is more vulnerable to drug effects than female sexual function. Virtually no reliable data exist which describe the effects of these drugs on female sexuality. Extrapolating the effects, by analogy from the male to the female will remain an inadequate approach, but one likely to be adopted until additional data are available. Although new research is badly needed in all areas relating to the sexual effects of psychotropic drugs, the greatest need is certainly in the area of drug effects on *female* sexual behavior.

Central mechanisms of sexual function

Sexual motivation and behavior is a complex of interrelationships between central mechanisms which are probably mediated in part by central monoamines, and the sexual organs that are controlled by peripheral autonomic input. Antidepressants, antipsychotics and stimulants produce both central and peripheral effects.

At the central level, both cortical and subcortical influences are important in sexual function. A growing and increasingly complex animal literature has linked the central effects of dopamine, norepinephrine and serotonin to sexual activity (Karczmar, 1980). Dopamine has clear facilitory effects on animal mating behavior (Gessa & Tagliamonte, 1974*a*). Data from humans also suggest that L-Dopa affects sexual function (Goodwin *et al.*, 1971; Hyyppa *et al.*, 1975). It is known that rats engage in compulsive mounting behavior following treatment with parachlorophenylalanine (PCPA), a serotonin synthesis inhibitor; the addition of an MAO inhibitor enhances this effect, but administering 5-hydroxytryptophan (5-HTP) abolishes it (Gessa & Tagliamonte, 1974*b*). These data suggest an increase in sexual activity associated with increased dopamine activity and decreased serotonin activity. Conversely, there is suppression of sexual activity with increased serotonin and decreased dopamine levels. More complete reviews are available elsewhere (Everett, 1974; Karczmar, 1980). Studies have also supported roles for both central dopamine and norepinephrine in the regulation of the pituitary-gonadal system (Frohman & Stachura, 1975).

The mechanisms for the control of testosterone secretion are complex. Luteinizing hormone (LH), arising from the anterior pituitary and under the influence of hypothalamic gonadotropin releasing hormones, is the major direct stimulus. Prolactin, also secreted by the anterior pituitary, reduces end organ responsiveness to LH and, thus, reduces conversion of testosterone to its active metabolites. Antipsychotics, and to a lesser degree some antidepressants, increase prolaction secretion by blocking prolactin inhibiting factor (Langer *et al.*, 1977). In the female, LH controls the steps of follicular growth and ovulation. Follicle stimulating hormone (FSH) acts in synergism with LH throughout the menstural cycle. While such central effects are highly complex, it should at least alert clinicians to the point that among their multiple effects, psychotropic drugs can influence sexual behavior through several possible central mechanisms.

Peripheral mechanisms of sexual function

The autonomic innervation in sexual function can be simplified to an arousal phase (erection in the male, genital vasocongestion in the female) mediated largely by parasympathetic fibres from S_2, S_3, and S_4 spinal segments and an orgastic phase directed largely by sympathetic fibre (Hotchkiss, 1970; Weiss, 1972). Purely psychogenic erections, however, are mediated through T_{12} - L_1 spinal segments and damage to these ganglia may impair erection. Male erection and female vasocongestion are vascular phenomena which result from blood flow being shunted away from the genital structures. Ejaculation occurs with the contraction of the seminal vesicles and ejaculating ducts and simultaneous closure of the internal sphincter of the urethra. Visceral aspects of the ejaculatory reflex are controlled by sympathetic fibre. Emission is an adrenergic function (L_2, L_3), while ejaculation involves the tonic-colonic contraction of the bulbocavernosus and ischiocavernosus muscles which are under partial parasympathetic control. Female orgasm is less well understood, although it has been concluded that lubrication and swelling occur through parasympathetic innervation of the circumvaginal plexus. The female vascular response is more undifferentiated than the equivalent in the male, and is, therefore, assumed to be less vulnerable to drug effects than erection (Kaplan, 1974). Female orgasm consists of contractions of the perineal bulbar and pubococcygeal musculature. Whereas emission in the male is sensitive to anticholinergic agents, the female response without emission is less sensitive to drug effects.

Antipsychotics

Antipsychotic agents produce a broad spectrum of sexual effects, almost all inhibitory in nature. Case reports and more systematic studies in patients taking antipsychotics have documented decreased libido, erectile impotence and ejaculation disorders (Haider, 1966; Kline *et al.*, 1968; Greenberg, 1971). In addition, antipsychotics may impair spermatogenesis (Simpson *et al.*, 1964; Karczmar, 1980).

The assessment of sexual dysfunction in patients receiving antipsychotics generally involves schizophrenic populations. However, because the sexual lives of schizophrenics have been investigated in only a limited number of studies (Lucianowicz, 1963; Nesteros *et al.*, 1980), conclusions about drug effects in this population are limited because of the confounding effects of the illness itself.

Although many patients were concurrently receiving antipsychotics, Rozan *et al.* (1971), for example, describe a decrease in the level of reported sexual activity associated with the onset of schizophrenia. Nesteros *et al.* (1980) report on a group of chronic schizophrenic patients, who had received considerable antipsychotic treatment. These patients were described as having globally impaired sexuality which further deteriorated throughout the course of their illness.

Antipsychotics clearly have inhibitory effects on the pituitary-gonoadal axis in rats (De Weid, 1967). Both the phenothiazines and the butyrophenones suppress LH and FSH and stimulate prolactin release (Givant & Sulman, 1976). Central dopamine blockade may also provide a biochemical rationale for the impaired libido observed in patients treated with antipsychotics.

Although loss of sexual interest has been reported with almost all antipsychotics, this side-effect cannot be ascribed to central mechanisms (Bartholemew, 1968; Greenberg, 1978). Arato *et al.* (1979) identified only a non-specific trend towards increased prolactin in sexually dysfunctional schizophrenics, but increased levels of prolactin have been reported in association with impotence (Franks *et al.*, 1978). Brown *et al.* (1981) identified lowered LH and testosterone levels in a group of schizophrenic patients taking thioridazine chronically: control patients taking other neuroleptics, or who were drug-free showed significantly less LH and testosterone supression. Lowered testosterone levels in patients taking thioridazine has also been noted by other authors (Kales *et al.*, 1975; Laughren *et al.*, 1978. Moreover, whereas the patients of Brown *et al.* showed low LH values with thioridazine, Arato *et al.* reported low testosterone levels with high LH values in sexually active males taking fluphenazine decaonate. Patients who were less sexually active had lower LH values. The possibility that thioridazine may have a particularly adverse effect on CNS mediation of sexual function (Brown *et al.*, 1981)is supported by Meltzer & Fang's (1976) observations that a greater elevation in prolactin level occurs with thioridazine than with other antipsychotics.

In another recent study involving male schizophrenic outpatients being treated with a variety of antipsychotics, a correlation was demonstrated between elevated plasma prolactin levels and sexual dysfunction. Fifty-four percent of the patients reported sexual difficulty of a moderate to severe degree (Ghadirian *et al.*, 1982).

Peripheral effects of antipsychotics

Although impotence is reported far less than ejaculation disorders (Small & Small, 1976), Antipsychotic-induced impotence is possibly related to the drugs' peripheral anticholinergic properties. Nevertheless, impotence certainly occurs. Kotin *et al.* (1976) report that of 115 patients taking thioridazine and other antipsychotics, 44 per cent of thioridazine-treated patients reported difficulty achieving erection (compared with 19 per cent for all other antipsychotics) and 35 per cent of this same group reported difficulty sustaining an erection. Physician reports to regulatory agencies or industry do not agree with these high figures (Kline *et al.*, 1968), and further evaluation is certainly needed. Priapism has been infrequently reported with chlorpromazine (Meiraz & Fishelovitch, 1967) and mesoridazine (Gotlieb & Lustberg, 1977). Kotin *et al.* (1976) report a decrease in sexual arousal and decreased satisfaction with orgasm in a 57-year-old woman.

Another report (Ghadirian *et al.*, 1982) indicates that 30 per cent of female schizophrenia patients had difficulty with sexual function following antipsychotic drug use. The most common complaint was a change in the quality of orgasm. Eighty per cent of male patients report a decreased ability to achieve orgasm and a decline in the quality of orgasm. The most frequently used drugs in this study were fluphenazine, chlorpromazine, trifluoperazine and chlorprothixene.

Aspermia, the absence of external ejaculate in the presence of erection, ejaculation and orgasm, occurs as a side-effect of several drugs (Grigis, 1978) and has been most commonly reported with thioridazine. Sperm may or may not enter the urinary bladder and be later eliminated in urine. While it is now a widely recognized effect of thioridazine (Singh, 1961; Blair & Simpson, 1966; Schwarz, 1982), it may also occur with chlorpromazine (Greenberg, 1971), piperacetazine (Jeffries, 1974), mesoridazine (Shader, 1972), butapherazine, perphenazine and trifluoperazine (Simpson & Blair, 1964; Blair & Simpson, 1966). Phenoxybenzamine, reserpine, pargyline, guanethidine and methyldopa have also been related to aspermia (Shader & Elkins, 1980).

Aspermia with thioridazine is not clearly dose related since it may develop with doses as low as 50 mg/day and as high as 600 mg (Shade & Elkins, 1980). Some authors estimate that up to 30 per cent of male patients treated with thioridazine will develop aspermia (Blair & Simpson, 1966).

The mechanism of antipsychotic-induced aspermia has been related to an alpha-adrenergic blocking action (Schwarz, 1982) which interferes with the actions of the vas deferens, seminal visicles, ejaculatory ducts and the bladder neck. Thus, alpha-blockage may impair the propulsion of ejaculate through the ejaculatory ducts (Edwards, 1976) and may reduce the contractions of the detrusor muscle of the bladder, thus retarding the anterograde movement of ejaculate through the membranous urethra. At the same time, the contractions of the external urethral sphincter and bulbospongiosus, unaffected by alpha-blockade, may force the ejaculate back through the relaxed detrusor into the urinary bladder (Shader, 1980). The most predictable non-pharmacological cause of aspermia involves surgery of the prostate or bladder, when the incidence may be as high as two-thirds of patients (Marberger, 1974). Aspermia may also occur after colonic surgery with damage to the hypogastric plexus (Peterson, 1973) and in the peripheral neuropathy of diabetes (Ellenberg & Weber, 1966).

Why thioridazine should produce this effect so prominently is unclear. Its alpha-adrenergic effects are shared by other antipsychotic drugs and patients with aspermia are not notable for other peripheral alpha-adrenergic effects. In many cases, thioridazine has also been associated with complete ejaculatory failure (Singh, 1966). Kotin *et al.* (1976) report that about 60 per cent of their sample of male outpatients on thioridazine therapy had ejaculatory disorders compared to 25 per cent of those taking other antipsychotics. Pain on ejaculation has been reported with both trifluoperazine and haloperidol (Berger, 1979).

Alpha-adrenergic agonists have been used to treat retrograde ejaculation and, interestingly, imipramine has been successfully used in aspermia secondary to diabetic neuropathy (Brooks *et al.*, 1980). Conversely, drugs such as thioridazine, with their impairment of ejaculation, have been used to treat premature ejaculation (Fraschini,

1966; Molcan, 1968; Lingjaerde, 1969). Similarly, pimozide, a butyrophenone, has been used for the treatment of premature ejaculation and impotence, although the nature of its beneficial effects on impotence is still unclear (Mattelaer, 1974).

Effects of antidepressants on sexual function

Sexual behavior in depression

Clinicians have always been aware of the changes in sexual function in affective illness — an increase in sexual behavior in mania and a decrease in libido in depression (Small & Small, 1976; Lief, 1977). Beck (1967) describes loss of interest in sex in two-thirds of a depressed sample compared to 27 per cent in a non-depressed control group. Such a decline in sexual interest, experienced by both males and females, was associated with other 'melancholic' symptoms such as loss of appetite, depressed mood and loss of interest in others. Other surveys have described reduced or absent libido in up to 80 per cent of depressed patients (Lief, 1977). A decline in the frequency of intercourse, impotence in males and reduced orgastic capacity in females has also been reported (Lief, 1977).

Arguing that many sexual complaints are under-reported, Beaumont (1977) devised a structured interview to assess sexual function in depressed patients. Sixty-eight per cent of depressed males (13 of 19 patients) and 57 per cent (20 of 35) of depressed women reported that their illness had adversely affected sexual function.

With antidepressant therapy, the frequency of intercourse increases (Beaumont, 1977). Even in neurotic depressive patients who present for treatment because of sexual complaints, significant improvement in sexual function follows antidepressant therapy with drugs such as doxepin (Renshaw, 1975).

Acetylcholine (parasympathetic stimulation), which is important in mediating digestion, defecation and urination, also facilitates sexual behavior. Sympathetic activity, on the other hand, is important in 'fight-flight' responses. Thus, anticholinergic drugs will generally inhibit sexual responsiveness and produce impotence via parasympathetic pathways in the sacral segment (S_2, S_3, S_4) (Mills, 1975; Snyder & Yamamura, 1979). Almost all anticholinergic agents and ganglion blockers are capable of producing impotence. Therefore, because of the prominent anticholinergic effects of most antidepressants, depressed sexual dysfunction is not unexpected.

Impotence

Impotence has been a frequent complication of antidepressant therapy. At least four different reports have cited imipramine's ability to produce impotence (Ruskin, 1959; Greenberg, 1965; Simpson *et al.*, 1965; Couper-Smartt, 1973). In Simpson *et al.*'s study (1965), doses as low as 10 mg/day were able to produce impotence, and discontinuation of imipramine resulted in the return to normal of erectile function. Impotence has also been noted with protriptyline (Shader & Elkins, 1980), amitriptyline (Couper-Smartt, 1973) and clomipramine (Beaumont, 1977; Yassa, 1982). Ananth *et al.* (1979) report that impotence with clomipramine occurred during the first two weeks of therapy, but disappeared thereafter. The incidence of these effects is difficult to estimate; a five per cent rate of impotence has been reported with imipramine (Greenberg, 1965) and a 20 per cent rate with clomipramine (Beaumont, 1977). Use of the United States Food and Drug Administration (USFDA, 1977) post-marketing report system, however, resulted in only 14 cases being identified, with desipramine and imipramine occurring most frequently. We might have expected there to be frequent reports on amitriptyline which, at one point, was the most widely used tricyclic antidepressant and which is certainly the most anticholinergic of all tricyclics (Snyder & Yamamura, 1979). However, this has not been the case. It seems reasonable to assume that the newer antidepressants, with minimal or no anticholinergic effects (eg mianserin, trazadone), may produce fewer episodes of impotence.

Of the monoamine oxidase inhibitors, phenelzine (Wyatt *et al.*, 1979) and tranylcypromine (Shader, 1970) have been associated with impotence, although both these agents are far less anticholinergic than tricyclic compounds (Snyder & Yamamura, 1979). At least one study has reported impotence with lithium therapy, with return of potency during a double-blind placebo period (Vinarova *et al.*, 1972).

Ejaculation disorders

Ejaculation disorders have been noted to occur with almost all antidepressant drugs and are likely to be a function of the blockade of alpha-adrenergic activity. The adrenergic activity of antidepressants varies with both the drug used and dose given and potentiation of peripheral adrenergic blockade occurs as the dose is increased (Osborne & Sigg, 1960). For example, mild increases in blood pressure may be noted at low doses, while lowering of pressure is more frequent with higher doses. Similar biphasic responses have been noted in the urinary bladder of animals (Osborne & Sigg, 1960). Clinically, adrenergic blockade is much more common with tricyclics, tetracyclics and MAOI's. Of the tricyclics, secondary amines exert a more marked anti-adrenergic effect than do the tertiary amines (Hafeley *et al.*, 1964).

As noted previously, ejaculation may be influenced by both sympathetic and paramsympathetic dysfunction and antidepressants possess both these properties (Snyder & Yamamura, 1973; U'Prichard *et al.*, 1978). Total inhibition and painful or delayed ejaculation have been reported with imipramine (Simpson *et al.*, 1965; Couper-Smartt, 1973; Glass, 1981), amitriptyline (Couper-Smartt, 1973; Nininger, 1978) and clomipramine (Couper-Smartt, 1973; Eaton, 1973; Quirk & Einarson, 1982). Beaumont (1977) noted that ejaculation symptoms with clomipramine occurred particularly at higher doses. The new antidepressant amoxapine has produced both painful ejaculation (Quirk & Einarson, 1982) and retrograde ejaculation (Schwarz, 1982), unusual with antidepressants. Amoxapine's demethylated derivative, loxapine (Cherman *et al.*, 1979), may account for this effect which is more commonly seen with antipsychotics.

Monoamine oxidase inhibitors also produce adrenergic blockade and have been associated with reports of inhibition or retardation of ejaculation (Bennett, 1961; Simpson *et al.*, 1965; Eaton, 1973; Barton, 1979; Glass, 1981). Rapp (1979) reported 2 cases of a dose-related retardation of ejaculation with phenelzine at 75 mg, with return to normal function when the dose was reduced to 60 mg. Such an effect is similar to that observed with both phenoxybenzamine and thioridazine.

Orgasm in women has also been slowed or blocked by antidepressants. Beaumont (1973) has reported this effect with clomipramine, and similar effects have been described with imipramine (Couper-Smartt, 1973) and amoxapine (Shenn, 1982).

The use of antidepressants to treat sexual dysfunction capitalizes on these antiadrenergic effects. Clomipramine has been used in two studies; and although in one study significant differences were not observed (Goodman, 1980), individual adjustment of the dose generally produces positive results (Eaton, 1973; Goodman, 1980). Although we have observed ejaculation disorders with viloxazine, it still remains to be seen whether the newer non-tricyclic antidepressants will be free from these side-effects.

Other effects

Blair *et al.* (1962) reported an increase in sperm count and motility with the MAOI, phenelzine. Sperm counts doubled in two of their three patients. In animal studies, however, massive doses of MAOI's have not produced any morphological changes in the testes and this effect has been hypothesized to occur in the hypothalamus and anterior pituitary with resultant increases in gonadotropin output. Similar effects have not been observed with the tricyclic antidepressants. In an attempt to utilize these effects in patients with low sperm counts, therapeutic effects have been recorded and have been most clearly evident in patients with moderate oligosperma, while those with a lower sperm count showed less response.

Psychomotor stimulants

Stimulant agents are used to a limited extent in medicine, for minimal brain dysfunction, narcolepsy and, by some, in the short-term treatment of obesity. The majority of the information on stimulants and their effects in sexual behaviour derive from anecdotal reports and from the literature on stimulant abuse. It is clear that abusers and non-abusers differ both in terms of psychiatric symptoms (Ellinwood, 1967) and sexual behavior (Bell & Trethowan, 1961). Sociopathic, schizophrenic and other unstable personalities are drawn toward stimulant abuse (Ellinwood, 1967) and normal premorbid sexual adjustment is likely to be rare in such individuals (Bell & Trethowan, 1961; Angrist & Gershon, 1976). Those effects which have been noted suggest the need for further investigation and enable us to offer preliminary hypotheses.

Pharmacologically, amphetamine stimulates post-synaptic norepinephrine and dopamine receptors indirectly through release into the synapse of newly synthesized neurotransmitters (Weissman *et al.*, 1965). Re-uptake blockade potentiates this effect, leading to increased post-synaptic activity (Scheel-Kruger, 1972).

Indirect evidence from animal experiments indicates that dopamine may stimulate sexual behavior in males (Gessa & Tagliamonte, 1974*b*). L-Dopa and apomorphine have both been associated with increased rates of copulation (Butcher *et al.*, 1969). Amphetamine also increases copulation in male rats (Leavitt, 1969; Ahlenius *et al.*, 1971) but apparently inhibits copulation in female rats (Mayer-Gross *et al.*, 1965).

Shortly after nasal inhalants containing amphetamine came into general use in the 1930's, increased libido in amphetamine users was noted (Waud, 1938). Subsequently, other observations of increased sexual stimulation and imagery in amphetamine users appeared (Bett, 1946; Carr, 1954). With more intense use of amphetamines, researchers noted that the increase in sexuality took the form of increased sexual energy and pressure to engage in sex, often with a driven quality (Connell, 1958). Angrist & Gershon (1976) state that 20 per cent of their sample of male patients reported increased libido with amphetamine. In surveys of stimulant abusers, Bell & Trethowan (1961) reported than 5 out of 14 individuals reported a clearly increased sex drive, while Schorring (1977) report that 85 per cent of addicts (34 of 40) noted strong sexual stimulation with this drug. In a Californian sample, 83 per cent reported that their sex drive was augmented by intravenous amphetamine. They described the injection as a flash, similar to orgasm, which was frequently associated with spontaneous arousal or erection (Gay & Sheppard, 1974).

Violence and perversion

One of the behavioral properties of stimulants is that they move their users towards action, unlike psychotomimetic agents such as LSD, or psilocybin (Ellinwood & Petrie,

1979). Thus, the stimulant abuser is likely to act out his feelings. Aggression and sexual behavior have been noted even under controlled experimental conditions (Angrist & Gershon, 1973). Perversions and compulsive sexual behavior have been seen to emerge after amphetamine administration. Transvestism and homosexuality have appeared in individuals apparently without these traits prior to drug exposure (Connell, 1958; Beamish & Kiloh, 1977). Polymorphous perverse sexual activity, sado-masochistic behavior, compulsive orogenital activity, pedophiolia, exhibitionism and genital mutilation have also been observed (Bell & Trethowan, 1961; Ellinwood, 1967; Ellinwood & Rockwell, 1975). Reports have showed amphetamine as facilitating promiscuity and group sexual behavior (Gay & Sheppard, 1973; Ellinwood & Rockwell, 1975), although the setting may also be an important facilitating factor. Women particularly note an increase in sexual excitement and pleasure in sexuality (Bell & Trethowan, 1961).

Cocaine has recently been widely used and cited for its sexual effects. Even Freud described this (Freud, 1884). Cocaine differs from amphetamine in that is possesses a local anesthetic action and there is less striking evidence for tolerance following chronic use. However, as with amphetamine, spontaneous erection and priapism have been noted after acute administration (Gay & Sheppard, 1973). Cocaine also produces sexual excitement (Clark, 1940; Mayer-Gross *et al.*, 1955); in circles of abuse, it is prized for its sexual effects and preferred to all other drugs of abuse because of these effects (Gay, 1981). Reporting on a Californian survey of sexual effects, young people rated cocaine as increasing sexual desire, enhancing sexual enjoyment, affecting orgasm and facilitating sexual activity more than any other drug (Gay, 1981). Grinspoon & Bakalar (1978) report that cocaine enhances sexuality, particularly in female users.

In practice, cocaine is topically applied to the genitalia, thus producing a tingling sensation and partial anesthetization of the area. Extended intercourse may then ensue with local trauma not infrequently being reported.

Sexual dysfunction with stimulation

Despite increases in sexual energy or activity, delay or complete inhibition of orgasm has also been reported in both male and female amphetamine users (Bell & Trethowan, 1961; Gay & Sheppard, 1973). This common observation is noted with both amphetamine and cocaine. Impotence and a decrease in sexual interest occur in some stimulant users (Bell & Trethowan, 1961; Angrist & Gershon, 1973), but generally become more prominent after extended use when neurochemical depletion of norepinephrine and dopamine stores may have occurred (Ellinwood & Escalante, 1971).

Summary

Both antipsychotic and antidepressant agents produce a variety of effects on sexual function. These are related to the drugs' therapeutic effects as well as to other central and peripheral effects. The effects of antipsychotics are largely inhibitory in nature, with probable effects on the pituitary-gonadal axis. In addition, their blockade of central dopamine receptors may also account for diminished libido and sexual response. Aspermia and impotence also occur as peripheral parasympatholytic and sympatholytic effects. Although antidepressant agents are effective against sexual dysfunction resulting from depression, they produce both erectile and ejaculatory dysfunction in a significant number of cases. Monoamine oxidase inhibitors cause ejaculation disorders but have been reported to increase sperm count in a small number of cases.

Psychomotor stimulants, especially amphetamine and cocaine, have been reported to be associated with increases in sexual energy, sexual drive and sexual behavior in humans. However, perverted sexual behaviors have also appeared under the influence of these stimulants. Most reports are either anecdotal or come from surveys of drug abusing populations and the findings cannot, therefore, necessarily be generalized to wider populations.

References

Ahlenius, S., Eriksson, H., Larsson, K., Modigh, K. & Södersten, P. (1971): Mating behavior in the male rat treated with p-chlorophenylalanine methyl ester alone and in combination with pargyline. *Psychopharmacol.* **20,** 383-388.

Ananth, J., Pecknold, J.C., van den Steen, N. & Engelsman, F. (1979): Double-blind comparative study of clomipramine in obsessive neurosis. *Curr. Ther. Res.* **25,** 703-709.

Angrist, B. & Gershon, S. (1976): Clinical effects of amphetamine and L-dopa on sexuality and aggression. *Compreh. Psychiat.* **17,** 715-722.

Arato, M., Erdos, A. & Polgar, M. (1979): Endocrinological changes in patients with sexual dysfunction under long-term neuroleptic treatment. *Pharmakopsychiat.* **12,** 426-431.

Bartholomew, A.A. (1968): A long-acting phenothiazine as a possible agent to control deviant sexual behavior. *Am. J. Psychiat.* **124,** 917-923.

Barton, J.L. (1979): Orgasmic inhibition by phenelzine. (Letter.) *Am. J. Psychiat.* **136,** 1616-1617.

Beaumont, G. (1973): Sexual side-effects of clomipramine (anafranil). *J. Int. Med. Res.* **1,** 469-472.

Beaumont, G. (1977): Sexual side-effects of clomipramine (Anafranil). *J. Int. Med. Res.* **5** (suppl), 37-44.

Beamish, P. & Kiloh, L.G. (1977): Psychoses due to amphetamine consumption. *J. Ment. Sci.* **5** (suppl), 37-44.

Beck, A.T. (1967): *Depression, causes and treatment.* Philadelphia: University of Pennsylvania Press. Pp 35.

Bell, D.S. & Trethowan, W.H. (1961): Amphetamine addiction and disturbed sexuality. *Archs Gen. Psychiat.* **4,** 74-78.

Bennett, D. (1961): Letter to the editor on use of MAOI's for premature ejaculation. *Lancet* **3,** 109.

Berger, S.H. (1979): Trifluoperazine and haloperidol: sources of ejaculatory pain. *Am. J. Psychiat.* **136,** 350.

Bett, W.R. (1946): Benzedrine sulfate in clinical medicine: a survey for the literature. *Postgrad Med. J.* **22,** 205-222.

Blair, J.H. & Simpson, G.M. (1966): Effect of antipsyuchotic drugs on reproductive functions. *Dis. Nerv. Syst.* **27,** 645-647.

Blair, J.H., Simpson, G.M. & Kline, N.S. (1962): Monoamine oxidase inhibitors and sperm production. *J. Am. Med. Ass.* **181,** 192.

Brooks, M.E., Berezin, M. & Braf, Z. (1980): Treatment of retrograde ejaculation with imipramine. *Urology* **15,** 353-355.

Brown, W.A., Laughren, T.P. & Williams, B. (1981): Differential effects of neuroleptic agents on the pituitary-gonadal axis in men. *Archs Gen. Psychiat.* **38,** 1270-1272.

Butcher, L.L., Butcher, S.G. & Larsson, K. (1969): Effects of apomorphine, (+)-amphetamine and nialamide on tetrabenazine-induced suppression of sexual behavior in the male rat. *Eur. J. Pharmacol.* **7,** 283-288.

Carr, R.B. (1954): Acute psychotic reaction after inhaling methylamphetamine. *Br. Med. J.* **1,** 1476-1483.

Chermat, R., Simon, P. & Boissier, J.R. (1979): Amoxapine in experimental psychopharmacology: a neurolpetic or an antidepressant? *Arzneimittel-Forsch.* **29,** 814-820.

Clark, A.J. (1940): *Applied pharmacology.* London: Churchill.

Connell, P.H. (1958): *Amphetamine psychosis.* Maudsley Monograph No. 5. London: Chapman and Hall.

Couper-Smartt, J.D. (1973): A technique for surveying side-effects of tricyclic drugs with reference to reported sexual effects. *J. Int. Med. Res.* **1,** 473-476.

Davis, J., Clyman, M.J., Decker, A., Bronstein, S. & Roland, M. (1966): Effect of phenylzine on semen in infertility: a preliminary report. *Fertil. Steril.* **17,** 221-225.
De Weid, D. (1967): Chlorpromazine and endocrine function. *Pharmacol. Rev.* **19,** 251-258.
Eaton, H. (1973): Clomipramine (anafranil) in the treatment of premature ejaculation. *J. Int. Med. Res.* **1,** 432-434.
Edwards, L. (1976): The pharmacology of the bladder and its sphincter. In *Scientific foundations of urology,* Vol. II, eds Williams, D.I. & Chishalin, G.D. Yearbook, Pp 75-76.
Ellenberg, M. & Weber, H. (1966): Retrograde ejaculation in diabetic neuropathy. *Ann. Intern. Med.* **65,** 1237-1239.
Ellinwood, E.H., Jr. (1967): Amphetamine psychosis. I. Description of the individuals and process. *J. Nerv. Ment. Dis.* **144,** 273-283.
Ellinwood, E.H., Jr. & Esclante, O.D. (1970): Behavior and histopathological findings during chronic methedrine intoxication. *Biol. Psychiat.* **2,** 27-39.
Ellinwood, E.J. & Petrie, W.M. (1979): Drug-induced psychosis. In *Psychiatric factors in drug abuse,* eds Pickens, R.W. & Heston, L.L. New York: Grune & Stratton. Pp 301-332.
Ellinwood, E.H. & Rockwell, W. (1975): Effect of drug use on sexual behavior. *Med. Asp. Hum. Sex.* **9,** 10-32.
Everett, R.M. (1975): Role of biogenic animals in the modulation of agressive and sexual behavior in animals and man. In *Sexual behavior — pharmacology and biochemistry,* eds Sandler, M. & Gessa, G.L. New York: Raven Press. Pp 81-84.
Franks, S., Jacobs, H.S., Martin, N. & Nabarro, J.D.N. (1978): Hyperprolactinemia and impotence. *Clin. Endocrinol.* **8,** 277-287.
Fraschini, A. (1966): Contributions to the therapy of ejaculation praecox and some forms of impotentia. *Minerva Med.* **57,** 3823-3824.
Freud, S. (1884): Uber coca. Centralblatt fur die geammte. *Therapie* **2,** 289-314.
Frohman, L.A. & Stachura, M.F. (1975): Neuropharmacologic control of neuroendocrine function in man. *Metabolism* **24,** 211-234.
Gay, G.R. (1981): You've come a long way, baby! Coke time for the new American lady of the eighties. *J. Psychoactive Drugs* **13,** 297-318.
Gay, G.R. & Sheppard, C.W. (1973): 'Sex-crazed dope fiends' myth or reality. *Drug Forum* **2,** 125-139.
Gessa, G.L. & Tagliamonte, A. (1974*a*): Possible role of brain serotonin and dopamine in controlling male sexual behavior. In Serotonin — new vistas, eds Costa, E. Gessa, G.L. & Sandler, M. New York: Raven Press. Pp 217-228.
Gessa, G.L. & Tagliamonte, A. (1974*b*): Roles of brain monoamines in male sexual behavior. *Life Sci.* **14,** 425-426.
Ghadirian, A.M., Chouinard, G. & Annable, L. (1982): Sexual dysfunction and plasma prolactin levels in neuroleptic-treated schizophrenic outpatients. *J. Nerv. Ment. Dis.* **170,** 463-467.
Glass, R.M. (1981): Ejaculatory impairment from both phenelzine and imipramine, with tinnitus from phenelzine. *J. Clin. Psychopharmacol.* **1,** 152-154.
Grigis, S.M. (1968): Aspermia, a survey of forty-nine cases. *Fert. Sterl.* **19,** 580-588.
Givant, Y. & Sulman, F.G. (1976): Endocrine effects of psychotherapeutic drugs. In *Psychotherapeutic Drugs,* ed Usdin, E. New York: Dekker. Pp 387-435.
Goodman, R.E. (1980): An assessment of clomipramine (Anafranil) in the treatment of premature ejaculation. *J. Int. Med. Res.* **8,** (Suppl), 53-59.
Goodwin, F.K., Murphy, D.L., Brodie, H. & Bunney, W.E. (1971): Levdopa. Alternations in behavior. *Clin. Pharmaco. Ther.* **12,** 383-396.
Gottlieb, J.I. & Lustberg, T. (1977): Phenothiazine-induced priapism. A case report. *Am. J. Psychiat.* **134,** 1445-1446.
Greenberg, H.R. (1965): Erectile impotence during the course of tofranil therapy. *Am. J. Psychiat.* **121,** 1021.
Greenberg, H.R. (1971): Inhibition of ejaculation by chlorpromazine. *J. Nerv. Ment. Dis.* **152,** 364-366.
Grinspoon, L. & Bakalar, J.B. (1976): *Cocaine: a drug and its social evolution.* New York: Basic Books.
Hafely, W., Hurlimann, A. & Thoenen, H. (1964): Scheinbar paradoxe Beeinflussung von

peripheren Noradrenal in Wirkungen durch einige Thymoleptica. *Helv. Physiol. Pharmacol. Acta* **22,** 15-33.
Haider, I. (1966): Thioridazine and sexual dysfunctions. *Int. J. Neuropsychiat.* **2,** 255-257.
Hotchkiss, R.S. (1970): Physiology of the male genital system as related to reproduction. In *Urology* Vol. I, eds Campbell, M.F. & Harrison, J.H. Philadelphia) Saunders. Pp 161-196.
Hyyppa, M.T., Falck, S.C. & Rinne, U.K. (1975): Is L-dopa an aphrodisiac in patients with Parkinson's disease? In *Sexual Behavior, Pharmacology and Biochemistry,* eds Sandler, M. & Gessa, G.L. New York: Raven Press. Pp 315-327.
Jeffries, J.J. (1974): Piperacetazine-induced failure to ejaculate. *Can. Psychiat. Ass. J.* **193,** 322-323.
Kaplan, H.S. (1974): *The new sex therapy: active treatment of sexual dysfunction,* New York: Brunner Mazel.
Kales, A . Kales, J.D., Soldatos, C.R. *et al.* (1975): Effects of thioridazine (Mellaril) on anterior pituitary secretion: changes in testosterone and prolactin. *Sleep Res.* **4,** 278.
Karczmar, A.G. (1980): *Drugs, transmitters and hormones, and mating behavior,* In Modern problems of pharmacopsychiatry: drug treatment of sexual dysfunction, eds Ban, T.A. & Freyham, F.A. Vol. 15, Basel: Karger. Pp 1-76.
Kline, N.S., Blair, J., Cooper, T.B., Esser, A.H., Hackett, E. & Vestergaard, P. (1968): A controlled seven year study of endocrine and other indices in drug treated chronic schizophrenics. *Acta Psychiat. Scand.* **44** (Suppl), 206.
Kotin, J., Wilbert, D.C., Verburg, D. & Soldinger, S.M. (1977): Thioridazine and sexual dysfunction. *Am. J. Psychiat.* **133,** 82-85.
Langer, G., Sachar, E.J., Gruen, D.H. & Halpern, F.S. (1977): Human prolactin response to neuroleptic drugs correlated with antischizophrenic potency. *Nature* **266,** 639-640.
Laughren, T.P., Brown, W.A. & Petrucci, J.A. (1978): Effects of thioridazine on serum testosterone. *Am. J. Psychiat.* **135,** 982-984.
Leavitt, F.I. (1969): Drug-induced modifications in sexual behavior and open field locomation of male rats. *Physiol. Behav.* **4,** 677-683.
Lief, H.I. (1977): Sexual survey No. 5: current thinking on sex and depression. *Med. Asp. Human. Sex.* **11,** 22-23.
Lingjaerde, O. (1969): Use of thioridazine during ejaculation praecox. *T. Norsk Laegeforen* **89,** 1433.
Lucianowicz, N. (1963): Sexual drive and its gratification in schizophrenia. *Int. J. Soc. Psychiat.* **9,** 250-258.
Marberger, H. (1974): The mechanisms of ejaculation, Physiology and genetics of reproduction, Part B, eds Coutinho, E.M. & Fuchs, F. New York: Plenum Press. Pp 99-110.
Mattelaer, I. (1974): Pimozide in the treatment of male impotence. A pilot trial. *Acta Urol. Belg.* **42,** 478-483.
Mayer-Gross, W., Slater, E. & Roth, M. (1955): *Clinical psychiatry,* 3rd edition. London: Casswell.
Meltzer, H.Y. & Fang, V.A. (1976): The effect of neuroleptics on serum prolactin in schizophrenic patients. *Archs Gen. Psychiat.* **33,** 279-286.
Meiraz, D. & Fishelovitch, J. (1967): Priapism and largactil medication. *Israel J. Med. Sci.* **5,** 1254-1255.
Mills, L.C. (1975): Drug-induced impotence. *Am. Fam. Phy.* **12,** 104-106.
Molcan, J. (1968): On the treatment of male sexual dysfunction and mesoridazine. *Acta Nerv. Super.* **10,** 261-262.
Nestoros, J.N., Lehmann, H.E. & Ban, T.A. (1980): Neuroleptic drugs and sexual function in schizophrenia. In *Modern problems of psychopharmacology,* eds Ban, T.A. & Freyhan, F.A. Vol. 15. Basel: Karger. Pp 111-130.
Nininger, J.E. (1978): Inhibition of ejaculation by amitriptyline. *Am. J. Psychiat.* **35,** 750-751.
Osborne, M. & Sigg, E.B. (1960): Effect of imipramine on the peripheral autonomic nervous system. *Archs Int. Pharmacodyn. Ther.* **129,** 272-289.
Peterson, I. (1973): EMG study of behavior of spincter and related muscles during orgasm and ejaculation. In *New developments in electromyography and clinical neurophysiology,* Vol. 2. Desmedt, J.E. Basel: Karger. P 439.
Quirk, J.C. & Einarson, T.R. (1982): Sexual dysfunction and clomipramine. *Can. J. Psychiat.* **27,** 228-231.

Rapp, M.S. (1979): Two cases of ejaculatory impairment related to phenelzine. *Am. J. Psychiat.* **136,** 1200-1201.
Renshaw, D.C. (1975): Doxepin treatment of sexual dysfunction associated with depression. In *Sinequan (doxepin HCl): a monograph of recent clinical studies,* ed Mendels, J. Amsterdam: Excerpta Medica. Pp 23-31.
Rozan, G.H., Tuchin, T. & Kurland, M.L. (1971): Some implications of sexual activity for mental illness. *Ment. Hyg.* **55,** 318-323.
Ruskin, D.B. & Goldner, R.D. (1959): Treatment of depressions in private practice with imipramine. *Dis. Nerv. Sys.* **20,** 391-399.
Scheel-Kruger, J. (1972): Behavioral and biochemical comparison of amphetamine derivates, cocaine, benztropine and tricyclic antidepressant drugs. *Eur. J. Pharmacol.* **18,** 63-73.
Schorring, E., (1977): Changes in individuals and social behavior induced by amphetamine and related compounds in monkeys and man. In *Cocaine and other stimulants,* eds Ellinwood, E. & Kilbey, M.M. New York: Plenum Publishing, Pp 481-522.
Schwarz, G. (1982): Case report of inhibition of ejaculation and retrograde ejaculation as side effects of amoxapine. *Am. J. Psychiat.* **139,** 233-234.
Shader, R.I. (1964): Sexual dysfunction associated with thioridazine hydrochloride. *J. Am. Med. Ass.* **188,** 1007-1009.
Shader, R.I. (1970): Ejaculation disorders. In *Psychotropic drug side effects,* eds Shader, R.I. and Dimascio, A. New York: Williams and Wilkins. Pp 73-74.
Shader, R.I. (1972): Sexual dysfunction associated with mesoridazine besylate. *Psychopharmacologia* **27,** 293-294.
Shader, R.I. & Elkins, R. (1980): The effects oif antianxiety and antipsychotic drugs on sexual behavior. *Mod. Probl. Pharmacopsychiat.* **15,** 91-110.
Shenn, W.W. (1982): Female orgasmic inhibition by amoxapine. (Letter.) *Am. J. Psychiat.* **139,** 1220-1221.
Simpson, G.M., Blair, J.H. & Amuso, D. (1965): Effects of antidepressants on genitourinary function. *Dis. Nerv. Syst.* **26,** 787-789.
Simpson, G.M., Blair, J.H. & Cranswick, E.H. (1964): Cutaneous effects of a new butyrophenone drug. *Clin. Pharmacol. Ther.* **5,** 310-321.
Singh, H. (1961): A case of inhibition of ejaculation as a side effect of Mellaril. *Am. J. Psychiat.* **117,** 1041-1042.
Small, I.F. & Small, J.G. (1976): Sexual behavior and mental illness. In *Comprehensive textbook of psychiatry,* 2nd edition, eds Freedman, A.M. Kaplan, H.I. & Sadlock, B.J. Baltimore: Williams and Wilkins.
Snyder, S.H. & Yamamura, H.I. (1977): Antidepressants and the muscarinic acetylcholine receptor. *Archs Gen. Psychiat.* **34,** 236-239.
Tuchmann-Duplessis, H. & Mercier-Parot, L. (1962): Influence de la niamide sur la sphere sexuelle et la fertilite de rat. *Chemotherapia* **4,** 304.
United States Food and Drug Administration (USFDA) (1977): *Computer assisted search: stimulant and antidepressant side effects.* Rockville: USFDA.
U'Prichard, D.C., Greenberg, D.A., Sheehan, P.P. & Snyder, S.H. (1978): Tricyclic antidepressants: therapeutic properties and affinity for alpha-noradrengeric receptor binding sites in the brain. *Science* **199,** 197-198.
Vinarova, E., Uhlir, O., Stika, L. *et al.* (1972): Side effects of lithium administration. *Act. Nerv. Super.* (Praha) **14,** 105-107.
Warner-Lambert Research Institute (1965): Unpublished data (Morris Plains).
Waud, S.P. (1938): The effects of toxic doses of benzylmethyl carbinamine (Benzedrine) in man. *J. Am. Med. Ass.* **110,** 206.
Weiss, H.D. (1972): The physiology of human penile erection. *Ann. Intern. Med.* **76,** 793-797.
Weissman, A., Koe, B.K. & Tenen, S.S. (1965): Antiamphetamine effects following inhibition of tyrosine hydroxylase. *J. Pharmac. Exp. Ther.* **151,** 339-345.
Wyatt, R.J., Fram, D.H., Buchbinder, R. *et al.* (1971): Treatment of intractable narcolepsy with a monoamine oxidase inhibitor. *N. Engl. J. Med.* **285,** 987-991.
Yassa, R. (1982): Sexual disorders in the course of clomipramine treatment: a report of three cases. *Can. J. Psychiat.* **27,** 148-149.

10

Sexual dysfunction in male patients: biological indices and classification

O. BENKERT and F. HOLSBOER

Department of Psychiatry, University of Mainz, 6500 Mainz, FEDERAL REPUBLIC OF GERMANY

Introduction

Various efforts have been made in recent years to classify sexual dysfunction (synonym: sexual impotence) in a more precise manner. Advances in highly sensitive bioanalytic determination methods, which allow assessment of low concentrations of hormones in various body fluids, has contributed to this development. In addition to this biochemical progress, refinements in psychophysiological techniques, such as nocturnal penile tumescence (NPT), are increasingly important in characterising sexual dysfunction (SD). A group of patients suffering from SD exists in whom no apparent acute or chronic psychogenic factor appears to precipitate the disorder. In a large percentage of these patients, no organic (eg endocrine, neurological or tissue) disease of etiological importance can be identified. Evidence is accumulating to show that, within this group, certain physical conditions (according to the DSM III Classification [Diagnostic and statistical manual of mental disorders, 1980]) are present, eg lowered testosterone or reduced NPT, which contribute to the development of the disorder. The magnitudes of these disturbances are not, however, sufficient to explain the disorder exclusively on those grounds.

At one time, there was general consensus that about 90 per cent of SD was psychogenic in origin (Strauss, 1950; Cooper *et al.*, 1970). Current opinion, however, relates no more than 70 per cent of sexual dysfunction to psychogenic factors (Shrom *et al.*, 1979; Spark *et al.*, 1980). The advent of more sophisticated laboratory methodologies has encouraged and allowed investigators to specifically identify a subgroup of patients with SD in whom some minor laboratory disturbances are indeed present. These individuals are characterized by laboratory data at the extreme ends of normal ranges rather than by a full symptom pattern of clinical (eg endocrine, vascular, neurological) disease.

To classify these patients simply as having SD of psychogenic origin is, therefore, no longer acceptable. In this research area we may face a similar development as seen in cardiovascular disease, where new techniques have reduced the patient sample that used to be classified as having functional heart disorders.

This article reviews material which may be relevant for a more adequate classification of SD than the basic psychogenic/organic dichotomy. Emphasis is placed on endocrine data because, at present, hormonal disturbances are apparently the most promising indices through which a subclinical disorder that contributes to precipitating SD can be identified. On the basis of these laboratory indices, subtypes of SD are identified which can be incorporated into a multi-axial system of classification.

Endocrine investigations

In the following sections we refer to some of our own investigations. Unless otherwise mentioned, the criteria for study admission were:
a) difficulty in achieving or maintaining erection during intercourse;
b) persistent dysfunction for at least one year with unknown etiology;
c) a prior history of normal penile erection;
d) age under 60 and having a regular female sexual partner;
e) at least one attempt at coitus per week; and,
f) normal findings in an andrological investigation.

All men who participated in the studies had normal neurological and medical status. There were also no signs of abnormality in the EEG, in the skull X-ray or in the routinely collected laboratory data. No patient presented with a history of psychosis or had had an acute conflict with his sex partner at the time of the study or just before it. No drug medication had been used for at least three months prior to the investigation.

Testosterone

Testosterone in sexual dysfunction (SD). Most studies agree that normal testosterone plasma-concentrations are found in those patients with SD in whom no medical disease (eg liver disease, cryptorchism, varicocele, cardiac incompensation) is evident (Racey *et al.*, 1973; Lawrence & Sawyer, 1974; Ansari, 1975; Comhaire & Vermeulen, 1975; Davies *et al.*, 1977; Legros *et al.*, 1978; Pirke *et al.*, 1979). Other investigators, however, have observed decreased testosterone levels in males suffering from SD (Legros *et al.*, 1973*a*; Forti *et al.*, 1974; Raboch *et al.*, 1975; Villani *et al.*, 1978). In a sample of 32 males (aged 45-75 y), we detected only seven individuals (21.8 per cent) with pathologically low total plasma testosterone levels (≤300 ng/ml) (Benkert, 1977; Benkert & Witt, 1980). When the total sample was subdivided into two age groups (under 60 and 60 years and over) (see Fig. 1), no differences in mean plasma testosterone concentration

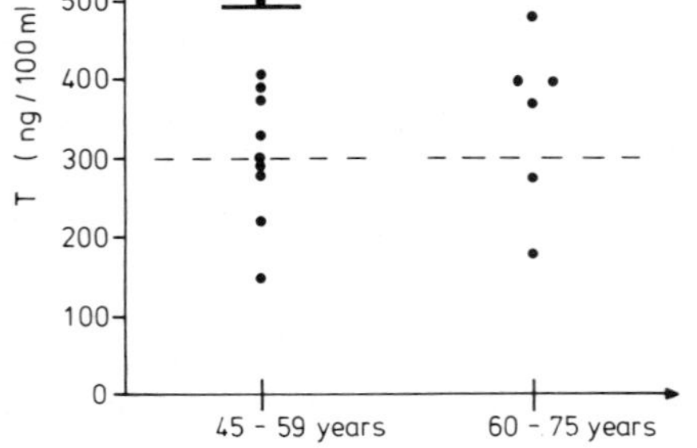

Fig. 1. *Means (solid lines) and inidividual testosterone (T) plasma concentrations (ng/100 ml) of 18 patients aged 45-59 and 14 males aged from 60-75 yrs.* Both groups suffered from sexual dysfunction (SD). The broken line indicates the lower end of the normal plasma testosterone range (300 ng/100 ml). No significant differences of plasma T-levels were apparent between the two age-groups. Seven individuals showed T-values beyond the normal limit (Benkert & Witt, 1980).

were observable between the two groups. Spark *et al.* (1980) determined serum testosterone levels in 105 patients with SD and detected an abnormality of the hypothalamic-pituitary-gonadal system in 37 (35 per cent). Twenty patients showed signs of hypogonadotrophic-hypogonadism (low LH, low testosterone); seven, of hypergonadotrophic-hypogonadism (high LH, low testosterone); eight, of hyperprolactinemia with or without hypogonadism; and two, showed symptomless hyperthyroidism. These authors claim that adequate somatic treatment successfully restored sexual function in most of their patients. In a further attempt to evaluate the association between impotence and the status of relevant hormones, we studied 117 male patients consecutively admitted to the department of psychiatry. Forty-two subjects were excluded for medical reasons (n=27) or refused to participate (n=15). The morning total testosterone levels in those who complained of impaired sexual function (n=31) were significantly lower ($P < 0.001$) than those of a control sample (n=25) within the same age range (see Fig. 2). After clearing the sample of subjects taking psychotrophic drugs, the same differences in total testosterone were still seen in patients with or without SD (see Fig. 3).

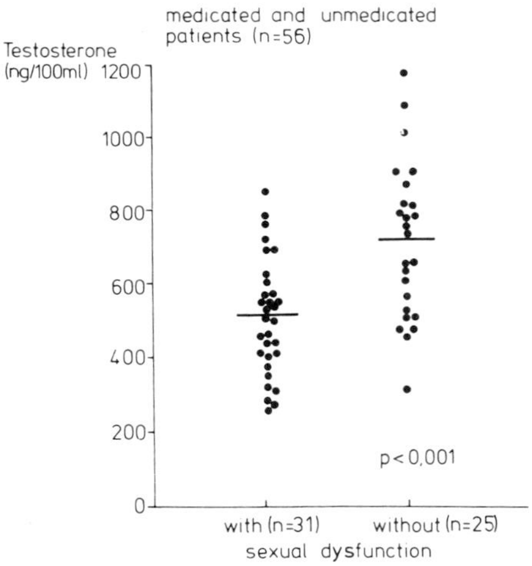

Fig. 2. *Individual testosterone plasma concentrations (ng/100 ml) of 31 patients with and of 25 age controlled comparison patients without SD.* The difference of the mean testosterone plasma levels was statistically significant (*t*-test, $P < 0.001$).

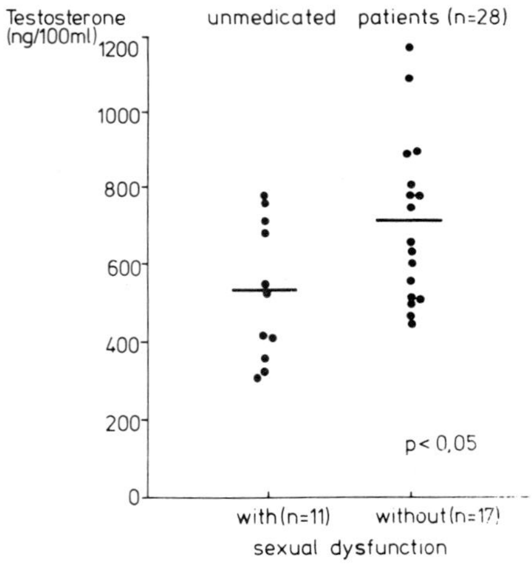

Fig. 3. *Individual testosterone plasma concentrations of 28 unmedicated psychiatric patients with (n = 11) and without (n = 17) SD.* The difference of the mean values was statistically significant (*t*-test, $P < 0.05$). Between groups there were no age differences. The patients documented in this figure represents a subpopulation which is also incorporated in Fig. 2.

These data, together with related reports in the literature, suggest that, in some patients at least, sexual dysfunction is associated with low testosterone plasma concentrations. However, whether these patients with abnormally low testosterone concentrations are potential responders to testosterone substitution therapy still remains to be established. Moreover, the relationship between these total testosterone-concentrations, the free testosterone fraction and the testosterone-estrogen-binding globulin (TEBG, syn: sex hormone binding globulin=SHBG) in this group of patients also remains to be established. In addition, no data on reproducibility, influence of weight-loss and motor-activity in males with SD are to hand.

Testosterone and age. It is well documented that SD is present more frequently in old age (Kinsey *et al.*, 1948; Newman & Nichols, 1960; Masters & Johnson, 1966; Pfeiffer *et al.*, 1968; Martin, 1977). Furthermore, there is agreement that the concentration of plasma testosterone begins to decrease at about 60 years of age (Vermeulen *et al.*, 1972; Nieschlag *et al.*, 1973; Pirke & Doerr, 1973; Steinbeck & Neumann, 1974; Baier *et al.*, 1974). However, whether there is a continuous decline in testosterone secretion that begins at between 40 to 50 years of age (Nieschlag *et al.*, 1973; Baker *et al.*, 1976), or whether a distinct decline occurs at the age of about 60 (Vermeulen *et al.*, 1972; Pirke & Dörr, 1973; Haug *et al.*, 1974) has yet to be clarified. Greenblatt *et al.* (1976) compared men aged 51 to 84 who complained of clinical symptoms which were attributed to a so-called male climacteric syndrome with symptomless males between 30 and 50 years, and recorded higher serum testosterone in the latter group. Other investigators (Harman & Tsitouras, 1980; Sparrow *et al.*, 1980) were not able to confirm these results and failed to observe a decrease in either the total or in the free serum testosterone fraction with increasing age.

Another research area has addressed the role of testosterone-estrogen-binding globulin. Some data indicate that increased binding of testosterone in senescence is due to the rise in TEBG concentration in old age (Pirke & Dörr, 1973). It has been demonstrated that the percentage of free plasma testosterone in younger subjects (22–61 y) is higher (2.24 per cent) than in an older (aged 67–93) comparison group (1.65 per cent) (Pirke & Dörr, 1975). The decrease in *total* testosterone between young and old males is less significant. In a recent study, data on total testosterone, free testosterone, its precursor and androstendione and TEBG concentrations were collected in a group aged from 20 to 88 years (Purifoy *et al.*, 1981). These investigators demonstrated a marked decrease in free testosterone, associated with a linear rise in TEBG (syn: SHBG) across all ages. The total testosterone decrease was comparatively less pronounced, whereas androstendione decreased from age 20 to age 50, and increased again thereafter.

The reasons for this lack of consistency among the different research centers are manifold, and include variability in bioanalytical methods, sampling times, subject characteristics, concomitant weight changes (Stanik *et al.*, 1981), drug intake and the status of other endocrine glands which may affect gonadal activity (ie adrenals, thyroid). Salivary testosterone correlates well with free serum testosterone (Wand *et al.*, 1981), the biologically active fraction of testosterone, and might be a promising parameter for future investigation. Recent developments indicate that at least one estrogen-binding protein exists distinct from TEBG which binds both estrogen and testosterone (O'Brien *et al.*, 1982). Knowledge of these concentrations and the steroid affinities of these transport proteins in relation to age are, therefore, of importance. This will aid our understanding of the physiological meaning of changing androgen and estrogen ratios in male senescence, an age range in which the likelihood of SD is increased.

Testosterone and hypo- or hypergonadal status. In *hypogonadal* men (serum testosterone concentration below 150 ng/100 ml) with sexual dysfunction, Davidson *et al.* (1979) and Spark *et al.* (1980) claim that testosterone substitution improves sexual performance. These authors report that frequencies of erections, including nocturnal erections and coitus responded in a dose-related manner to treatment with a testosterone preparation. Salmimies *et al.* (1982) studied the effect of testosterone injections in males with abnormally low serum testosterone concentrations (≤200 ng/ml). Their data indicate that all patients with levels below this testosterone threshold responded favourably to substitution therapy. These reports, however, contradict an earlier report by Kinsey *et al.* (1953) who could not recognize a specific role for androgens in human sexual behavior. A review by Bancroft (1978) also concluded that no clear evidence existed for a direct association between gonadal hormones and sexual performance.

In patients who demonstrate offensive sexual behaviors, antiandrogen treatment reduces testosterone levels and favourable therapeutic effects are well documented. In these individuals a reduction in initial normal testosterone levels results in diminished sexual drive and fantasies and normalized deviant sexual behavior (Money *et al.*, 1976; Berlin & Meinecke, 1981).

A relationship between sexual activity and the *hypergonadal* state has not as yet been demonstrated.

Testosterone and sexual responsiveness to stimuli. Lange *et al.* (1980) report that the correlation between penile diameter and serum testosterone concentration changes in response to erotic stimuli. These workers showed that the latency to achieving maximum penile tumescence was negatively correlated to testosterone levels. From these objective measures, it was hypothesized that long latency to erection in combination with low testosterone concentration may predispose to the development of SD. However, no clear association between sexual stimulation responsiveness and testosterone plasma levels are available. Sexual activity either by coitus (Fox *et al.*, 1972) or by masturbation (Purvis *et al.*, 1976) increases testosterone levels. The specificity of these hormonal changes to sexual activity is questionable. Other motor activities, for example, bicycle ergometer exercise, also result in testosterone surges (Brisson *et al.*, 1977; Jezova & Vigas, 1981). All in all, however, there is no conclusive evidence that correlates testosterone concentration with sexual behavior and interest variables.

Testosterone, nocturnal penile tumescence and sleep patterns. The literature consistently supports the theory that nocturnal penile tumescence is closely associated with rapid eye movement sleep (REM) (Fisher *et al.*, 1965; Karacan *et al.*, 1966). The relationships between testosterone and sleep structure are conflicting. Although Schiavi *et al.* (1977) found increased nocturnal secretory patterns of testosterone, they could not correlate this with REM or non-REM sleep patterns. Other investigators have also failed to demonstrate a relationship between testosterone secretion and REM-stage sleep (Alford *et al.*, 1973; Judd *et al.*, 1974). Recently, Roffwarg *et al.* (1982) documented an interaction between the testosterone secretion pattern and sleep stage variables. However, no clear relationships exist between testosterone and sleep paramaters like REM and non-REM as do for sleep and NPT. Assessment of NPT, however, appears to be a promising aid in diagnostic categorisation of SD (Fisher *et al.*, 1979).

Testosterone and therapeutic efficacy in male patients with SD. Androgen therapy is a common method of treatment in SD even when no signs of gonadal insufficiency are present (Benkert, 1980*a*). Until recently, the studies which attempted to resolve this issue had methodological flaws (for a review, see Bancroft, 1978).

Applying a rigidly controlled double-blind protocol, we evaluated the clinical benefits of treating patients with testosterone undecanoate (TU). This study involved 29 patients aged between 45 and 75 with SD (Benkert *et al.*, 1979). All patients received placebo for two weeks. Then, TU was administered at a daily dose of 120 mg to 13 patients selected at random, while the other patients continued receiving the placebo. After a treatment period of eight weeks, all patients again received placebo treatment for a further two weeks. Sexual performance was reported to be improved in five patients on active TU-treatment, while eight patients responded favourably to the placebo. Accordingly, pharmacotherapy with gonadal steroids is generally not superior to placebo in men with SD. Further research, however, is needed to establish biological indices which would help to identify those patients in whom restoration of sexual function is most likely to occur with testosterone.

Gonadotrophins (LH-FSH)

The gonads are regulated through feedback mechanisms by pituitary luteinizing hormone (LH) and follicle-stimulating hormone (FSH). Since the interrelationships between gonadal function and sexual behavior are reasonably well documented, investigators have tried to establish whether SD is reflected, in part, by circulating levels of gonadotrophins. To date, however, the majority of findings have not revealed disturbances in basal gonadotrophin levels (Legros *et al.*, 1973*a*, 1978; Benkert *et al.* 1976; Davies *et al.*, 1977; Delitala *et al.*, 1977; Pirke *et al.*, 1979).

Luteinizing hormone-releasing hormone (LHRH) and LH/FSH response. Stimulation of LH and FSH with the related releasing hormone LHRH has induced normal LH/FSH responses in patients with SD (Legros *et al.*, 1978). Stimulation with high doses (500 μg) also resulted in normal gonadotrophin response (Davies *et al.*, 1977).

In our own experiments, we examined 32 males (aged 45–75) with sexual dysfunction and seven healthy controls. Twenty-five minutes after LHRH infusion (100 μg), LH increased significantly in older patients (those aged 61–75 y) in comparison to the younger group (aged 45–60 y). Increases in both gonadotrophins (LH and FSH) after 25 μg of LHRH were significantly higher only in the older group. Thus, abnormal LH-responses to LHRH in some of the older patients with SD are not easily explained. Increased LH levels with age, despite the maintenance of normal testosterone concentrations in plasma, is consistent with an age-related decrease of Leydig-cell synthesizing capacity. Thus, an abnormally high LH response to a test dose of LHRH is possibly an indication of a subclinical condition which may contribute to the development of SD.

It should be recognized, however, that LHRH, gonadotrophins, gonadal steroids and other modulating substances active on this axis interact delicately to regulate each other. For this reason, an exaggerated response of LH following an LHRH challenge may be secondary to an altered secretory capacity of the gonads.

Therapeutic effects of LHRH. To evaluate the therapeutic effectiveness of LHRH, a placebo controlled study was conducted (Benkert *et al.*, 1979). Eighteen patients received four daily administrations from a nasal-spray containing placebo. After two weeks, half the study group received LHRH in four daily doses of 250 mg. After a further four weeks, the active drug group was switched back to placebo for two further weeks. In the original placebo group, inactive treatment was maintained for the same period of time. Although no significant therapeutic effect was observable at the end of the trial, a significant improvement was observed six weeks after cessation of LHRH administration. On the other hand, patients receiving placebo did not show this time-lagged therapeutic action.

Interpretation of these findings is difficult. The present discussion of this and related phenomena focuses on the receptor-regulation model. It is conceivable that continuous administration of synthetic LHRH (HOE-766) down-regulates related receptors. Thus, the therapeutic effect observed after treatment cessation may be due to some kind of rebound-phenomenon.

Prolactin

Thorner & Besser (1977) often observed sexual impotence as the first clinical sign in male patients with hyperprolactinemia due to pituitary adenomas. Increased serum prolactin levels were found in a diagnostically heterogeneous sample complaining of SD (Villani *et al.*, 1978). Among 136 men with SD, Schwartz *et al.* (1982) recently identified 11 hyperprolactinemic individuals. They reported that restoration of sexual performance was achieved when circulating prolactin levels were normalized either by drug treatment (dopamine agonist) or by microsurgery (removal of the pituitary adenoma). The mechanism by which hyperprolactinemia induces SD is poorly understood. Several investigators observed hyperprolactinemia concurrent with low (Goodman *et al.*, 1980) and normal or low-normal circulating testosterone levels (Franks *et al.*, 1978; Nagulesparen *et al.*, 1978). Excessive activity of the pituitary lactotroph can decrease the sensitivity of pituitary gonadotrophin to LHRH (Vasques *et al.*, 1980). To what degree hypergonadotrophic hypogonadism contributes to SD in hyperprolactinemia is unclear, and it remains to be established whether prolactin exerts a physiologically meaningful action at the level of the gonads or at the target organ receptor site. In our study of 75 psychiatric patients consecutively admitted, those complaining of SD did not show signs of hyperprolactinaemia in comparison to psychiatric patients without SD. One source of variance across studies may be the heterogeneity of the populations investigated. In departments of internal medicine, for instance, the likelihood of an obvious organic disorder (eg hyperprolactinemia) may be higher than among patients in a department of psychiatry.

Other hormones

Estrogen treatment for medical reasons precipitates SD in the male. Under physiological conditions, however, no conclusive evidence is at hand, which suggests that elevated estrogen levels play a key role in the development of SD (Benkert & Witt, 1980). In addition, the thyroid axis has been shown to function normally in 12 men with SD (Benkert, 1977). Moreover, the pituitary response of thyroid stimulating hormone (TSH) to the related releasing hormone (TRH) is indicative of euthyroid function in these patients (Benkert, 1977). Whether the well established blunted responses of TSH to TRH in older men contributes to the increased likelihood of developing SD in senescence is highly questionable (Loosen & Prange, 1982). In hyperthyroid men, testicular responses to exogenous gonadotrophins were blunted. These findings were concordant with increased total testosterone plasma levels and clinically apparent sexual dysfunction, which was restored to normal after successful treatment of hyperthyroidism (Kidd *et al.*, 1979). Increased testosterone levels in combination with hyperthyroidism and SD reflect increased testosterone-estrogen binding globulin in these patients and not increased production rates of the gonads (Chopra & Tulchinsky, 1974). To evaluate the possible therapeutic effect of TRH in SD, a double-blind placebo controlled study was conducted (Benkert *et al.*, 1976) and it was shown that daily administration of TRH was not superior to placebo in twelve males suffering from SD.

Classification

The indicators of laboratory abnormalities outlined above in patients with SD lend support to the hypothesis of a subclinical disorder which provides a contributory mechanism in the pathogenesis of SD. Therefore, slightly aberrant laboratory data (biochemical, psychopharmacological, EEG/NPT) should be incorporated into a system classifying sexual dysfunction. To adequately consider the various contributing factors, we propose the introduction of several additional distinct subtypes of SD: subtype Ia (sexual dysfunction, organic disorder); subtype Ib (sexual dysfunction, physical condition), and subtype III (sexual dysfunction, pharmacological condition). The phrases 'organic disorder' and 'physical condition' were adapted to the definitions given in the manual of the DSM III system. Subtypes IIa and IIb address sexual dysfunction related to psychiatric disorders or to psychosocial stresses. Since there is still a large proportion of patients in whom no clear association between SD and possible etiological factors can be established, a further subtype IV (sexual dysfunction, cryptogenic disorder) needs to be added. From a multi-axial system classifying SD, the following scheme was developed (Benkert *et al.*, 1985):

Subtypes of Sexual Dysfunction based on a Multi-axial Classification

Subtype Ia *Sexual dysfunction (organic disorder)*
Sexual dysfunction with concurrent presence of a defined organic disorder (eg endocrine disease, diabetes, varicocele tissue disease) being pathogenetically relevant to the development of SD.

Subtype Ib *Sexual dysfunction (physical condition)*
Sexual dysfunction with concurrent presence of a laboratory abnormality (eg lowered testosterone plasma concentration or a level at the low end of normal, aberrant nocturnal penile tumescence) — applicable only if sub type Ia is excluded.

Subtype IIa *Sexual dysfunction (psychiatric disorder)*
Sexual dysfunction with concurrent presence of a defined psychiatric disorder (including personality disorders).

Subtype IIb *Sexual dysfunction (psychosocial condition)*
Sexual dysfunction in association with psychosocial stresses (eg partner conflict. Applicable only if subtype IIa is excluded.

Subtype III *Sexual dysfunction (pharmacological condition)*
Sexual dysfunction due to concurrent medical drug treatment (eg hor mones, antihypertensives, neuroleptics, lithium) or drug abuse (eg opiates, analgesics, alcohol, benzodiazepines.

Subtype IV *Sexual dysfunction (cryptogenic disorder)*
Sexual dysfunction not being classifiable into one of the above subtypes.

Note: Subtype I (a *or* b) may be present together with subtype II (a *or* b) and subtype III.

Conclusions

Biochemical and electrophysical experiments have consistently demonstrated the frequent coexistence of minor laboratory abnormalities and sexual dysfunction. The future availability of more refined methods to discover subtle neurophysiological or biochemical disturbances will continue to reduce the proportion of cases of SD classified with diagnosis based only on the history.

As outlined above, our present knowledge of the etiological importance of subtle laboratory aberrations is too incomplete to state whether or not they are responsible for precipitating SD. It is, however, fair to say that their inclusion in a classification system is a meaningful approach towards a more adequate diagnosis of SD:

1. The omission of laboratory indices in those cases where their magnitude does not allow the diagnosis of an organic disorder would consequently lead to low diagnostic reliability. Depending on theoretical and therapeutic bearings, the same patient would receive different diagnoses across study centers.
2. Irrespective of its etiological role, the presence of a subtle laboratory disturbance (eg low testosterone, hyperprolactinemia, NPT-disturbance) might serve as a clue for adequate somatic treatment. This information would be lost were the traditional organic/psychogenic dichotomy to be maintained.
3. This approach does not allow a psychogenic etiology of SD on grounds of absent biological findings. It is necessary to define in a positive way psychosocial or psychiatric reasons for SD.
4. The scheme proposed above avoids the pitfalls seen with some recent developments which classify sexual dysfunction according to specific empirical criteria (DSM III, Schover *et al.,* 1982). These problem-orientated categories suffer from broadness (DSM III) or from the difficulty of obtaining precise data (Schover *et al.,* 1982). Attribution to one of the axes (desire, arousal, orgasm, coital pain, dissatisfaction with frequency) is subject to various preoccupations resulting in low reliability.

In terms of our present understanding of the etiology and treatment of sexual dysfunction attempts to dichotomize exclusively psychogenic and exclusively organic factors are inadequate. Data emerging from different laboratories consistently demonstrate that SD is frequently associated with organic factors whose etiological importance is as yet unclear. A similar situation may appear in affective disorders where, to varying degrees, some derangement(s) of the endocrine axes are observable. We do not know whether these hormonal changes are simply ancillary aids in constructing symptom patterns which include biological abnormalities; it may well be that these abnormalities contribute to the course of the illness. Data exist which lend support to the fact that the return to normalcy of endocrine abnormalities (eg adrenal dysfunction) is necessary for a beneficial outcome in affective psychoses (Holsboer *et al.,* 1982). Moreover, hormones by themself have a strong impact as modulators of neurotransmission in those areas of the brain thought of as relevant for human behavior (see Rubin *et al.,* 1982; Holsboer, 1982). Since it is acceptable that sexual function is the fragile outcome of a cascade of known and (mostly) unknown biological factors whose synchronous functioning is delicately regulated, any omission of available objective data is not advisable. The proposed inclusion of the subtypes of sexual dysfunction: organic disorder (Ia), physical condition (Ib), psychiatric disorder (IIa), psychosocial condition (IIb), pharmacological condition (III) and cryptogenic disorder (IV) satisfies the obvious requirements for an adequate diagnosis based on a multi-axial system.

References

Alford, F.P., Baler, H.W.G., Burger, H.G., de Kretser, D.M., Hudson, B., Johns, M.W., Masterton, J.P., Patel, Y.C. & Rennie, G.C. (1973): Temporal patterns of integrated plasma hormone levels during sleep and wakefulness. II. Follicle stimulating hormone, luteinizing hormone, testosterone and estradiol. *J. Clin. Endocrinol. Metab.* **37,** 848-854.

American Psychological Association (1980): *Diagnostic and statistical manual of mental disorders.* Washington, DC: American Psychological Association. Pp 261-281.

Ansari, J.M.A. (1975): A study of 65 impotent males. *J. Psychiat.* **127,** 337-341.

Baier, H., Biro, G. & Weinges, K.F. (1974): Serum levels of FSH, LH and testosterone in human males. *Hormone Metabol. Res.* **6,** 514-516.
Baker, H.W.G., Burger, H.G., de Kretser, D.M., Hudson, B., O'Connor, S., Wang, C., Mirovics, A., Court, J., Dunlop, M. & Rennie, G.C. (1976): Changes in the pituitary-testicular system with age. *Clin. Endocrinol.* **5,** 349-372.
Bancroft, J. (1978): The relationship between hormones and sexual behavior in humans. In *Biological determinants of sexual behavior,* ed J.B. Hutchison. Chichester, New York, Brisbane, Toronto: Wiley & Sons. Pp 493-519.
Benkert, O. (1977): *Sexuelle Impotenz. Neuroendokrinologische und pharmakotherapeutische Untersuchungen.* Berlin, Heidelberg, New York: Springer-Verlag.
Benkert, O. (1980): Pharmacotherapy of sexual impotence in the male. *Mod. Probl. Pharmacopsych.* **15,** 158-173.
Benkert, O., Maier, W. & Holsboer, F. (1985): Multiaxial classification of male sexual dysfunction. *Br. J. Psychiat.* (In press.)
Benkert, O., Horn, K., Pickardt, C.R. & Schmid, D. (1976): Sexual impotence: studies of the hypothalamic-pituitary-thyroid axis and the effect of oral thyrotropin-releasing factor. *Archs Sex. Behav.* **5,** 275-281.
Benkert, O. & Witt, W. (1980): Age-related alteration of the hypothalamic-pituitary-gonadal axis in sexually impotent males. *Archs Psychiat. Belg.* **80,** 465-475.
Benkert, O., Witt, W., Adam, W. & Leitz, A. (1979): Effect of testosterone undecanoate on sexual potency, and hypothalamic-pituitary-gonadal-axis of impotent males. *Archs Sex. Behav.* **6,** 471-479.
Berlin, F.S. & Meinecke, C.F. (1981): Treatment of sex offenders with antiandrogenic medication: conceptualization, review of treatment modalities, and preliminary findings. *Am. J. Psychiat.* **138,** 601-607.
Brisson, G.R., Volle, M.A., Desharnais, M., Dion, M. & Tanaka, M. (1977): Pituitary-gonadal axis in exercising men. *Med. Sc. Sp.* **9,** 47.
Chopra, I.J. & Tulchinsky, D. (1974): Status of estrogen-androgen balance in hyperthyroid men with Graves' disease. *J. Clin. Endocrinol. Metab.* **38,** 269-277.
Comhaire, F. & Vermeulen, A. (1975): Plasma testosterone in patients with varicocele and sexual inadequacy. *J. Clin. Endocrinol.* **40,** 824-829.
Cooper, A.J., Ismail, A.A.A. & Smith, C.G. (1970): Androgen function in "psychogenic" and "constitutional" types of impotence. *Brit. Med. J.* **3,** 17-20.
Davidson, J.M., Camargo, C.A. & Smith, E.R. (1979): Effects of androgen on sexual behavior in hypogonadal men. *J. Clin. Endocrinol. Metab.* **48,** 955-958.
Davies, T.F., Comez-Pan, A., Watson, M.J., Mountjoy, C.Q., Hanker, J.P., Besser, G.M. & Hall, R. (1977): Reduced gonadotropin response to releasing hormone after chronic administration to impotent men. *Clin. Endocrinol.* **6,** 213-218.
Delitala, G., Masala, A., Alagna, S. & Lotti, G. (1977): Luteinizing hormone, follicle stimulating hormone and testosterone in normal and impotent men following LHRH and HCG stimulation. *Clin. Endocrinol.* **6,** 11-15.
Fisher, C., Gross, J. & Zuch, J. (1965): A cycle of penile erection synchronous with dreaming (REM) sleep. *Archs Gen. Psychiat.* **12,** 29-45.
Fisher, C., Schiavi, R.C., Edwards, A., Davis, D.M., Reitman, M. & Fine, J. (1979): Evaluation of nocturnal penile tumescence in the differential diagnosis of sexual impotence. *Archs Gen. Psychiat.* **36,** 431-437.
Forti, G., Pozzagli, M., Calabresi, E., Fiorelli, G. & Serio, M. (1974): Radioimmunoassay of plasma testosterone. *J. Clin. Endocrinol.* **3,** 5-17.
Fox, C.A., Ismail, A.A.A., Love, D.N., Kirkham, D.E. & Loraine, J.A. (1972): Studies of the relationship between plasma testosterone levels and human sexual activity. *J. Endocrinol.* **52,** 51-58.
Franks, S., Jacobs, H.S., Martin, N. & Nabarro, J.D.N. (1978): Hyperprolactinaemia and impotence. *Clin. Endocrinol.* **8,** 277.
Greenblatt, R.B., Oettiner, M. & Bohler, C.S.-S. (1976): Estrogen-androgen levels in aging men and women: therapeutic considerations. *J. Amer. Geriat. Soc.* **24,** 173-178.
Goodman, R.H., Molitch, M.E., Post, K.D. & Jackson, I.M.D. (1980): Prolactin secreting

adenomas in the male. In *The pituitary adenoma*, eds Goodman, R.H., Molitch, M.E., Post, K.E. & Jackson, I.M.D. New York: Plenum Medical Book Press. Pp 91-108.

Harman, M. & Tsitouras, P.D. (1980): Reproductive hormones in aging men. I. Measurement of sex steroids, basal luteinizing hormone, and leydig cell response to human chorionic gonadotrophin. *J. Clin. Endocrinol. Metab.* **51,** 35-40.

Haug, E., Aakvaag, A., Sand, T. & Torjesen, P.A. (1974): The gonadotrophin response to synthetic gonadotrophin-releasing hormone in males in relation to age, dose and basal serum levels of testosterone, oestradiol-17ß and gonadotrophins. *Acta Endocrinol.* (Copenahgen) **77,** 625-635.

Holsboer, F. (1982): Hormones. In *Psychopharmacology 1, Part 2: Clinical psychopharmacology*, eds Hippius, H. & Winokur, G. Amsterdam, Oxford, Princeton: Excerpta Medica. Pp 144-161.

Holsboer, F., Liebl, R. & Hofschuster, E. (1982): Repeated dexamethasone suppression test during depressive illness. *J. Affect. Dis.* **4,** 93-101.

Ježŏvá, D. & Vigaš, M. (1981): Testosterone response to exercise during blockade and stimulation of adrenergic receptors in man. *Hormone Res.* **15,** 141-147.

Judd, H.L., Parker, D.C., Rakoff, J.S., Hopper, B.R. & Yen, S.S.C. (1974): Elucidation of mechanism(s) on the nocturnal rise of testosterone in men. *J. Clin. Endocrinol. Metab.* **38,** 134-141.

Karacan, I., Goodenough, D.R., Shapiro, A. & Starker, S. (1966): Erection cycle during sleep in relation to dream anxiety. *Archs Gen. Psychiat.* **15,** 183-189.

Kidd, G.S., Glass, A.R. & Vigerski, R.A. (1979): The hypothalamic-pituitary-testicular axis in thyreotoxicosis. *J. Clin. Endocrinol. Metab.* **48,** 798-802.

Kinsey, A.C., Pomeroy, W.B. & Martin, C.E. (1948): *Sexual behavior in the human male.* Philadelphia: Saunders.

Kinsey, A.C., Pomeroy, W.B., Martin, C.E. & Gebhard, P.H. (1953): *Sexual behavior in the human female.* Philadelphia: Saunders.

Lange, J.D., Brown, W.A., Wincze, J.P. & Zwick, W. (1980): Serum testosterone concentration and penile tumescence changes in men. *Hormones Behav.* **14,** 267-270.

Lawrence, D.M. & Sawyer, G.I.M. (1974): Plasma testosterone and testosterone binding affinities in men with impotence, oligospermia, azoospermia, and hypogonadism. *Brit. Med. J.* **1,** 349-351.

Legros, J.J., Franchimont, P., Palem-Vliers, M. & Servais, J. (1973): FSH, LH and testosterone blood level in patients with psychogenic impotence. *Endocrine. Exp.* **7,** 59-64.

Legros, J.J., Mormont, C. & Servais, J. (1978): A psychoneuroendocrinological study of erectile "psychogenic impotence": a comparison between normal patients and patients with abnormal reaction to glucose tolerance test. In *Clinical psychoneuroendocrinology in reproduction*, eds Ziehella, L. & Pancheri, P. New York: Academic Press. Pp 301-319.

Loosen, P.T. & Prange, A.J. (1982): Serum thyrotropin response to thyrotropin-releasing hormone in psychiatric patients: a review. *Am. J. Psychiat.* **139,** 405-416.

Martin, C.E. (1977): Sexual activity in the aging male. In *Handbook of sexology*, eds Money, J. & Musaph, H. Amsterdam: Excerpta Medica. Pp 813-824.

Masters, W.H. & Johnson, V.E. (1966): *Human sexual response.* Boston: Little, Brown.

Money, J., Wiedeking, C. & Walker, P. (1976): Combined antiandrogenic and counseling program for treatment of 46 XY and 47 XYY sex offenders. In *Hormones, behaviors, and psychopathology*, ed Sachar, E.J. New York: Raven Press.

Nagulesparen, M., Ang, V. & Jenkins, J.S. (1978): Bromocriptine treatment of males with pituitary tumours, hyperprolactinaemia, and hypogonadism. *Clin. Endocrinol.* **9,** 73.

Newman, G. & Nichols, C.R. (1960): Sexual activities and attitudes in older persons. *J. Am. Med. Ass.* **173,** 33-35.

Nieschlag, E., Kley, H.K., Wiegelmann, W., Solbach, H.G. & Krüskemper, H.L. (1973): Lebensalter und endokrine Funktion der Testes des erwachsenen Mannes. *Dtsch. Med. Wschr.* **98,** 1281-1284.

O'Brien, T.J., Hiogashi, M., Kanasugi, H., Gibbons, W.E. & Morrow, C.P. (1982): A plasma/serum estrogen-binding protein distinct from testosterone-estradiol-binding globulin. *J. Clin. Endocrinol. Metab.* **54,** 793-797.

Pfeiffer, E., Verwoerdt, A. & Wang, H.S. (1968): Sexual behavior in aged men and women. *Archs Gen. Psychiat.* **19,** 753-758.

Pirke, K.M. & Dörr, P. (1973): Age related changes and interrelationships between plasma testosterone, oestradiol and testosterone binding globulin in normal adult males. *Acta Endocrinol.* (Copenahgen) **74,** 792-800.
Pirke, K.M. & Dörr, P. (1975): Age related changes in free plasma testosterone, dihydrotestosterone and oestradiol. *Acta Endocrinol.* (Copenahgen) **80,** 171-178.
Pirke, K.M., Kockutt, G., Aldenhoff, J., Besinger, U. & Feil, W. (1979): Pituitary gonadal system function in patients with erectile impotence and premature ejaculation. *Archs Sex. Behav.* **8,** 41-48.
Purifoy, F.E., Koopmans, L.H. & Mayes, D.M. (1981): Age differences in serum androgen levels in normal adult males. *Human Biol.* **53,** 499-511.
Purvis, K., Landgren, B.-M., Cekan, Z. & Diczfalusy, E. (1976): Endocrine effects of masturbation in men. *J. Endocrinol.* **70,** 439-444.
Raboch, J., Mellan, J. & Starka, L. (1975): Plasma testosterone in male patients with sexual dysfunction. *Archs Sex. Behav.* **4,** 541-545.
Racey, P.A., Ansari, M.A., Rowe, P.H. & Glover, T.D. (1973): Testosterone in impotent men. *J. Endocrinol.* **59,** 23.
Roffwarg, H.P., Sachar, E.J., Halpern, F. & Hellman, L. (1982): Plasma testosterone and sleep: relationship to sleep stage variables. *Psychosomat. Med.* **44,** 73-84.
Rubin, R.T., Reinisch, J.M. & Haskett, R.F. (1981): Postnatal gonadal steroid effects on human behavior. *Science* **211,** 1318-1324.
Salmimies, O., Kockott, G., Pirke, K.M., Vogt, H.J. & Schill, W.B. (1982): Effects of testosterone replacement on sexual behavior in hypogonadal men. *Archs Sex. Behav.* **11,** 345-353.
Schiavi, R.C., Davis, D.M., Fogel, M., White, D., Edwards, A., Igel, G., Szechter, R. & Fisher, C. (1977): Luteinizing hormone and testosterone during nocturnal sleep: relation to penile tumescent cycles. *Archs Sex. Behav.* **6,** 97-104.
Schover, L.R., Friedman, J.M., Weiler, S.J., Heiman, J.R. & Lopiccolo, J. (1982): Multiaxial problem-oriented system for sexual dysfunctions. An alternative to DSM III. *Archs Gen. Psychiat.* **39,** 614-619.
Schwartz, M.F., Bauman, J.E. & Masters, W.H. (1982): Hyperprolactinaemia and sexual disorders in men. *Biol. Psychiat.* **17,** 861-876.
Shrom, S.H., Lief, H.I. & Wein, A.J. (1979): Clinical profile of experience with 130 consecutive cases of impotent men. *Urology* **13,** 511-515.
Spark, R.F., White, R.A. & Connolly, P.B. (1980): Impotence is not always psychogenic. Newer insights into hypothalamic-pituitary-gonadal dysfunction. *J. Amer. Med. Ass.* **243,** 750-755.
Sparrow, D., Bosse, R. & Rowe, J.W. (1980): The influence of age, alcohol consumption, and body build on gonadal function in man. *J. Clin. Endocrinol. Metab.* **51,** 508-512.
Stanik, S., Dornfeld, L.P., Maxwell, M.H., Viosca, S.P. & Korenman, S.G. (1981): The effect of weight loss on reproductive hormones in obese men. *J. Clin. Endocrinol. Metab.* **53,** 828-832.
Steinbeck, H. & Neumann, F. (1974): Androgene und Alter. *Acta Geront.* **4,** 531-539.
Strauss, E.B. (1950): Impotence from a psychiatric standpoint. *Brit. Med. J.* **1,** 697-699.
Thorner, M.O. & Besser, G.M. (1977): Hyperprolactinaemia and gonadal function: results of bromocriptine treatment. In *Prolactin and human reproduction,* eds Crosignani, P.G. & Robyn, C. London: Academic Press. Pp 285-301.
Vasquez, J.M., Ellegood, J.C., Nazian, S.J. & Mahesh, V.B. (1980): Effect of hyperprolactinaemia on pituitary sensitivity to luteinizing-hormone-releasing hormone following manipulation of sex steroids. *Fertil. Steril.* **33,** 543.
Vermeulen, A., Rubens, E. & Verdonck, L. (1972): Testosterone secretion and metabolism in male senescence. *J. Clin. Endocrinol.* **4,** 730-735.
Villani, C., Aragona, C., Pozzi, V., Tamburello, A. & Feliciotti, M. (1978): Plasma prolactin (PRL), FSH, LH and testosterone (T) in 71 male patients with sexual disturbances. In *Clinical psychoneuroendocrinology in reproduction,* Vol. 21. eds Carenza, L., Pancheri, P. & Zichella, L. London, New York, San Francisco: Academic Press. Pp 457-464.
Wang, C., Plymate, S., Nieschlag, E. & Paulsen, C.A. (1981): Salivary testosterone in men: further evidence of a direct correlation with free serum testosterone. *J. Clin. Endocrinol. Metab.* **53,** 1021-1024.

11

Apomorphine and other dopamine modifiers of human sexual and nociceptive tonus*

E. DEL BENE, M. FANCIULLACCI, M. POGGIONI, L. PRINCIPE and F. SICUTERI

Institute of Internal Medicine and Clinical Pharmacology, University of Florence, Florence, ITALY

Introduction

The presumed effect of dopamine (DA) agonists and antagonists on sexuality can be tested by using subjects with enhanced DA reactivity or enhanced or depressed sexual activity. In animals, dopaminomimetics are considered aphrodisiacs, and DA antagonists, sexual inhibitors (Tagliamonte *et al.*, 1974; Da Prada *et al.*, 1977).

Patients with Parkinson's disease, who are known to have supersensitive post-synaptic DA receptors, have been sexually stimulated by L-Dopa treatment, a precursor of DA capable of crossing the blood-brain barrier.

Quite separately, previous observations have indicated that headache sufferers can be considered suitable subjects for the study of sexual activity.

The mechanism of migraine and other associated headaches is still unknown; the classification 'vascular, muscular and mixed headache' is, therefore, completely arbitrary and acceptable only as a working hypothesis. Our personal interpretation assumes that idiopathic headaches are the clinical expression of a dysfunction of the nervous apparatus which subserves the nociception. This dysfunction is not organic in nature; in these pain diseases attention has been given to the turnover of neurotransmitters as well as to their action on pre- and post-synaptic receptors. Some evidence of impairment in neurotransmission has been observed for the antinociceptive system, particularly for its transmitters (endogenous opioids, serotonin (5-HT) and DA) and related receptors (Sicuteri, 1974, 1977, 1979, 1982).

In this chapter, in accordance with our theory, the spontaneous pain syndromes are classified as 'nocipathies'. In using this term we wish to stress the assumption that, in the headache area, we are referring to 'pathological' pain (ie pain due to an impairment of the nociceptive-antinociceptive system) and not to 'physiological' pain which depends on the occasional activation of a physiologically functioning nociceptive system. However, the conventional category of circulatory or muscular (vascular, tensional) headaches involves 'physiological' pain, since this would be evoked at the periphery by stimuli (dilation of arteries, contraction of scalp muscles) which are not usually painful.

**This paper comes within the programme of the Finalized Groups, 'Chimica Fine e Secondaria e Medicina Preventiva' of the National Research Council (CNR) Rome, Italy.*

More than one sign of excessive reactivity to different mediators, especially to DA (Sicuteri, 1979; Sicuteri *et al.*, 1980*a*), is detectable in nocipathies. This excessive reactivity is probably caused by a deficiency of opioid modulation. It could also be due to a receptoral supersensitivity (pre- and/or post-synaptic) caused by a decreased concentration of the agonist (a supersensitivity similar to that arising from denervation). It could also be due to a post-receptoral hyperreactivity, ie to an increase in the cell's intrinsic energy (like that witnessed in opiate abstinence — Sicuteri *et al.*, 1979; Collier, 1980).

There are two principal manifestations of direct or indirect superreactivity to DA agonists in nocipathies:

The orthostatic reflex. Malfunctioning of this reflex is not rare; it is demonstrated by orthostatic hypotension and the well-known central nervous system syndrome including loss of consciousness (syncopal migraine). It seems credible that these phenomena are due to a supersensitivity of the DA pre-synaptic receptor, located on the sympathergic neuron, which innervates the smooth muscles of the arterioles and plays a fundamental role in orthostasis.

It is known that the neuronal DA receptor modulates the intra-synaptic norepinephrine (NE) release. Patients with syncopal migraine, expressed by seriously impaired orthostasis, exhibit a dramatic intolerance to the DA agonist, bromocriptine; an oral clinical dose of 2.5 mg resulting in their being unable to stand for several hours (orthostasis induces a presyncopal phenomenon or frank syncope within a few seconds or minutes — Fanciullacci *et al.*, 1980; Boccuni *et al.*, 1981). The mechanism of the bromocriptine test undermines the theory that syncopal migraine is primarily due to a spasm of the basilary artery (Bickerstaff, 1961). Domperidone, a peripheral DA antagonist, prevents and reverts the loss of the orthostatic reflex produced by bromocriptine (Sicuteri *et al.*, 1982). Since pre-synaptic receptors of DA and other transmitters are physiologically more sensitive than post-synaptic ones, their supersensitivity produces a response (inhibition of NE release) that is exaggerated in intensity and duration. It is known that the transition from lying down to standing up produces strong stimulation of neuronal NE release, as demonstrated by the constant and long-lasting doubling of NE plasma concentration. In our bromocriptine-treated patients, the concentration of plasma NE remains unchanged during orthostasis, even when a standing position is possible in the absence of syncope (Boccuni *et al.*, 1981).

Nociception. In the most seriously affected headache sufferers, the acute administration of different DA agonists evokes or increases pain. However, *chronic* treatment with a gradually increasing dose frequently induces a type of tachyphylaxis (ie increased tolerance) and frequently ameliorates the clinical picture (Sicuteri, 1977; Sicuteri *et al.*, 1977).

Orally administered L-Dopa (1 g), bromocriptine (2.5 mg) and sublingual apomorphine (100 mcg) are capable of exacerbating pain in headache sufferers for many hours (Sicuteri *et al.*, 1984). These drugs all induce or enhance pain after a latency of 1-2 h which suggests that their effect is indirect. The almost pure dopaminomimetic agent apomorphine, in particular, not only mimics the type and localization of pain but also other concomitant phenomena, both in quality and chronological occurrence. Yawning, somnolence, nausea, shivering, depression, hyperestesia to noise, odours and light and headaches (throbbing, if intense) are the usual phenomena of a migraine attack and these are the manifestations evoked in these patients by apomorphine administration. No other drug can mimic a migraine attack as exactly as apomorphine does. The same doses of L-Dopa, bromocriptine or apomorphine, given to healthy volunteers completely free from any type of headache, do not induce pain. This suggests that headache sufferers have a peculair pain susceptibility.

Sexual reactivity to dopamine modifiers in nocipathics

Supersensitivity of the mating centres which control sexual behaviour could represent another aspect of the hyperreactivity of the structures in the central nervous system of nocipathics. Sexual arousal is, in fact, a possible clinical manifestation of a migraine attack. This sexual arousal is experienced at the end of the headache crisis, and is often accompanied by erotic fantasies (Del Bene *et al.*, 1982). We have ourselves studied the effects of some dopaminomimetic drugs on the sexual activity of migraine sufferers.

In one experiment, 28 male volunteer outpatients (mean age 32.4) were studied for three months. A personal chart was given to each patient; on this chart the subject recorded his sexual behaviour using the following categories: erotic dreams, sexual arousal, penile erection, masturbation and coitus. During the first month, the patients were drug-free; in the second month a placebo was administered; and in the third month patients were treated with lisuride (75 mcg/day, orally). The record of sexual behaviour was kept for the entire three-month period.

Patients were classified into two groups, according to the degree of sexual change observed during the placebo or lisuride treatment relative to sexual behaviour in the same individual during the drug-free period. In the first group of patients, sexual activity either showed no change or, if there was an increase, it was limited to less than double the number of episodes (see group 2). In the second group, the number of penile erections or the number of episodes of coitus was at least doubled during placebo or lisuride treatment; erotic fantasies and dreams were also crudely taken into consideration. None of the 28 placebo-treated patients exhibited a two-fold increase in sexual behaviour (six of them slightly increased their sexual tonus). During lisuride treatment, sexual behaviour more than doubled in five of the 28 cases (eight patients showed slight enhancement of sexual tonus). No patient reported a decrease in sexual activity during lisuride or placebo treatment. Lisuride significantly increased sexual tonus over placebo ($P < 0.05$).

In the second experiment, 10 inpatients suffering from migraine (three women, mean aged 37.6 y and seven men, mean age 35.2 y) were studied for 20 days. The patients were treated with a physiological solution (250 ml iv daily) for 10 days; they then received 250 ml of physiological solution and apomorphine for the remaining 10 days (the infusion rate was always 30 drops/min). The first dose of apomorphine was 0.5 mg. This was increased by 0.5 mg every day until a dose of 3.0 mg was reached, and this was maintained for the remaining days of the treatment. Each day, a chart was

Table 1. *The effect of apomorphine on sexual behavior in 10 headache sufferers.* The sexual parameters were recorded hourly each day, and each annotation was arbitrarily considered as '1'.

Mean no. of events per subject in a 10 day period	*Placebo*	*Apomorphine*	*Statistical analysis*
Females (3), mean age 37.6 y			
Sexual ideas and fantasies	5.3	6.6	NS
Erotic dreams	0.7	3.3	$P < 0.05$
Males (7), mean age 35.2 y			
Sexual ideas and fantasies	5.4	15.7	$P < 0.001$
Erections	3.6	11.3	$P < 0.001$
Erotic dreams	0	0	NS

given to the patients to record their sexual behaviour (erotic dreams, sexual thoughts and fantasies and penile erections) on an hourly basis.

Although apomorphine did not significantly modify female sexual thoughts and fantasies, the numbers of erotic dreams were significantly increased ($P < 0.05$). In the seven men tested, apomorphine significantly increased both sexual fantasies and the number of penile erections ($P < 0.001$). However, no erotic dreams were reported by this group of men either during placebo treatment or apomorphine administration (see Table 1).

Discussion

Clinical pharmacology offers several advantages over animal pharmacology. First, there is the possibility of observing the effects of drugs in spontaneous pathological conditions which are usually difficult to reproduce in animals. Secondly, the minimal subjective effects of the drugs, certainly not detectable in animals, can be studied in man. Finally, humans seem to be particularly sensitive to drugs which act upon the central nervous system. The disadvantages are primarily ethical. The use of healthy volunteer subjects to provide a basis of comparison when testing drug effect on delicate functions such as sex, vigilance and pain is fraught with difficulties that are exacerbated when the pharmacological investigation is of long duration. Moreover, Italian law forbids any payment to those who volunteer for such experiments. The present investigation has been affected by these constraints. Although we have been able to compare the effects of drugs capable of modifying sexuality with a placebo in the same subjects, comparison of the drugs' pharmacological effects in healthy and unhealthy subjects has not been possible. In comparison with the placebo, DA agonists such as apomorphine and lisuride, significantly stimulate sexual tone, inducing penile erections, erotic dreams and sexual fantasies in some nocipathics. The question, crucial to this discussion, is whether or not clinical doses of dopaminomimetics cause erotic activity in some subjects because they exhibit a peculiar pathology.

If we compare our results with those of others (Hamburger-Bar & Rigter, 1975; Liuzzi *et al.*, 1978; Gopinatham *et al.*, 1981; Parkes *et al.*, 1981), we support the assumption of a relationship in headache sufferers. However, the fact that other clinical parameters, that did not include sexuality, were considered in these investigations, makes such a comparison have doubtful validity. Patients usually keep their sexual life hidden, only revealing it if expressly asked to do so. Direct and indirect evidence suggests that headache sufferers show an increased reactivity to dopaminomimetics in different structures and apparatus.

Nociception, like orthostatic hypotension, nausea and vomiting, is enhanced by dopaminomimetic agents; sexual function is likewise enhanced. During migraine attacks, sexual excitation (particularly significant given the discomfort of the attack) is not rare and can be detected (only if requested) in both males and females (Del Bene *et al.*, 1982).

The interpretation of the DA supersensitivity is intriguing. In fact, dopaminomimetics act as modulators (in small doses) by binding to the pre-synaptic neuronal autoreceptors, and as excitators by binding to the post-synaptic DA receptors (Carlsson, 1979). Experimental data show that pre-synaptic receptors are more sensitive than post-synaptic ones; this is an almost general biological law. It is, therefore, important to ascertain whether the dopaminomimetics used act upon pre-synaptic, post-synaptic or on both types of DA receptors. Pathological changes in receptoral sensitivity may occur to further complicate the problem of determining the site of action of the DA agonists. DA agonists (or antagonists) are usually administered to patients who have a pathological condition related to some dysfunction of the DA system. For instance, apomorphine is an active drug in the treatment of Parkinson's disease, a condition in which the extrapyramidal DA system is impaired and the DA post-synaptic receptors are supersensitive. Small clinical doses of apomorphine act mainly or exclusively on the DA autoreceptors, causing a depression of DA tonus. The incongruity of apomorphine's therapeutic mechanism in Parkinson's disease is only apparent because the autoreceptors are greatly reduced in number and in function; apomorphine would, therefore, act exclusively as DA substitute therapy at the level of the post-synaptic DA receptors (Corsini *et al.*, 1980*a,b*).

Interpretation of the nociceptive and sexual hyperreactivity to dopaminomimetics observed in headache sufferers is a difficult task. In nociception, DA acts as a partner to the endorphins and 5-HT in increasing the activity of the natural analgesic apparatus (antinociceptive system) (Vanderwende & Spoarlein, 1973; Akil & Liebeskind, 1975; Slater & Blundell, 1978; Sakai *et al.*, 1981). The motor function of the striatum spreads into the antinociceptive area (Krauthamer & Albe-Fessard, 1964). According to our investigations, perlingual, oral and parenteral apomorphine (as well as bromocriptine and lisuride) greatly exacerbate pain in headache sufferers; these drugs are inert on nociception in normal subjects (Sicuteri *et al.*, 1984).

Another fact which has emerged from our investigation is that headache, nausea, yawning, vomiting and somnolence as well as the tendency to orthostatic hypotension induced by dopaminomimetics when they are first administered in naive subjects, gradually decrease during chronic treatment. After a few weeks of therapy, headache sufferers could tolerate, without pain, a dose of apomorphine 10–50 times higher than the dose that was able to provoke or exacerbate the pain and extra-pain phenomena in untreated subjects. Acute administration of apomorphine does not exacerbate tremor and muscular rigidity in patients with Parkinson's disease. In headache sufferers, however, it increases nearly all the spontaneous phenomena (pain, nausea, vomiting, sensory hyperesthesia); it seems credible that this drug acts upon DA autoreceptors reducing the intrasynaptic secretion of the analgesic transmitter, thereby working as an anti-antinociceptive agent. The phenomenon of tolerance and clinical improvement following chronic treatment with increasing doses of apomorphine could, therefore, be correlated with a reduction in the number of and/or the affinity for autoreceptors.

As previously reported, L-Dopa acts similarly to the dopaminomimetics in the treatment of headache. We have observed that several patients, acutely administered very small doses of L-Dopa (4 mg/kg orally), complained of intense exacerbation of chronic headache. On the basis of their pain exacerbation, they succeeded in distinguishing L-Dopa from placebo (Sicuteri, 1977).

Interpretation of the activity of the dopaminergic system in nociception is made more complex by the anatomical, functional and pharmacological correlations between endogenous and exogenous opioids and DA.

The questions raised about nociception can, equally, be directed to the sexual area. In some headache sufferers, small doses of dopaminomimetics are able to provoke sexual excitation, either as penile erection or as erotic fantasies and dreams. After about an hour's latency from the start of venous infusion of apomorphine, males had repeated penile erections of 5–10 minutes duration, with some minutes of non-erection, for a period of 1–2 h. The men also experienced sexual fantasies. During placebo infusion, neither erections nor sexual fantasies occurred. During chronic oral treatment with lisuride, some male migraine sufferers had a significant increase in sexual behaviour. The amounts of apomorphine and lisuride were quite small. As with the nociceptive phenomenon, two main possibilities can be considered. Apomorphine and lisuride could act on DA autoreceptors, causing a reduction of dopamine secretion or, alternatively, these patients' post-synaptic DA receptors could have become supersensitive, so that small doses of DA, acting on post-synaptic receptors, would increase functioning of the DA pathways as has been observed in patients with Parkinson's disease. The effect on the autoreceptors should then be overcome (as happens with large DA doses) and inhibition unmasked by activation.

On the basis of experimental evidence, one can conclude that small amounts of dopaminomimetics act as aphrodisiacs by impinging on DA receptors in mating centres, or more exactly, on DA post-synaptic receptors in a supersensitive condition. The interpretation, which is difficult, assumes acrobatic characteristics when one considers the connection between endorphin and DA systems. All authors agree that DA and the endorphins are concentrated in roughly the same areas of the brain. The striatum, for instance, is the richest central region in DA and endorphins. More than one piece of evidence suggests that the striatum is not just involved in motor function. Evidence of the reciprocal influence between DA and exogenous and endogenous opioids in animals and humans is increasing (Lal, 1978; Van Loon & Kim, 1978). Acute administration of opiate and opioids in animals clearly inhibits multiple DA activities (Gessa & Tagliamonte, 1975; Lal, 1978; de la Baume *et al.,* 1979; McMillen, 1979).

It has been hypothesized that the presumed DA autoreceptor is actually an opiate pre-synaptic receptor (Costa *et al.,* 1978; Moroni *et al.,* 1979). An impairment of the endorphinergic system and its serotoninergic and dopaminergic partners in the antinociceptive area has been postulated in headache (Sicuteri, 1982). A decrease in cerebrospinal fluid and plasma endogenous opioids has been found in headache sufferers (Anselmi *et al.,* 1980).

Profound modifications in the reactivity to DA and 5-HT agonists have also been noted (Fanciullacci, 1979; Sicuteri *et al.,* 1980*a*) in patients suffering from headache.

The results obtained by manipulating headache sufferers with drugs which act on monoamine turnover and receptors seem to suggest that 5-HT and DA agents act in opposite directions, the former depressing, and the latter stimulating sexual activity (Sicuteri *et al.,* 1976). The results in humans are compatible with those obtained in animals (Meyerson, 1968; Meyerson & Lewander, 1970; Salis & Dewsbury, 1971; Zemlan *et al.,* 1973; Gessa & Tagliamonte, 1974).

Endorphins also play a role in sexual behaviour. Opioid agonists reduce and opioid antagonists increase sexual activity in animals (Meyerson & Terenius, 1977; Pellegrini-Quarantotti *et al.,* 1978; McIntosh *et al.,* 1979).

Sexual activity itself in animals acutely stimulates the production of brain opioids and, thus, the antinociceptive system, resulting in analgesia (Komisaruk *et al.,* 1976; Szechtman *et al.,* 1981).

Two significant phenomena are observed during pregnancy. First, sexual desire frequently disappears (particularly in animals), and secondly, relief, partial or total, from pain in headache sufferers is frequently observed with the enhancement of pain threshold. It has been demonstrated that increased concentrations of endorphin are observed in the blood and tissues of pregnant women and animals (Csontos *et al.,* 1979; Sicuteri *et al.,* 1980*b*). Since endorphins inhibit sexuality by modulating DA neuronal secretion, anti-morphine agents can be expected to promote sexual activity in animals and in man. In fact, naloxone induces intense sexual behaviour in sexually indifferent rats but not in sexually normal rats (Gessa & Paglietti, 1979).

Naltrexone provokes erotic excitement in man (Mendelsson *et al.,* 1979); penile erection and sexual fantasies are induced in headache sufferers by the venous infusion of naloxone (unpublished data). Presumably, naltrexone and naloxone attenuate opioid inhibition of the dopaminergic neurons which subserve the mating centres.

The sex stimulating capacity of morphine antagonists supports the hypothesis that apomorphine and lisuride exert their erotic activity by acting on supersensitive DA post-synaptic receptors, rather than on DA autoreceptors. The increase in endorphinergic turnover (perhaps placental in nature) during pregnancy can be correlated with nociceptive and sexual changes (Gintzler, 1980).

In conclusion, both the direct and the indirect evidence supports the following assumptions: small doses of dopaminomimetics can stimulate sexuality in men and women, particularly if they are suffering from diseases in which a multifocal DA hyperreactivity is present; nociception and sexuality exhibit many analogous pharmacological and biochemical characteristics; endorphin-5-HT-DA agonists and antagonists administered to humans with normal or impaired eroticism can provide information on the intimate mechanisms of sexuality.

Summary

Sufferers from migraine and related headaches who are treated with dopaminomimetic agent, such as apomorphine, lisuride and bromocriptine, complain of nausea, somnolence, shivering, headache, orthostatic hypotension (which can manifest itself in presyncopal symptoms) and sexual excitement. The most precocious effects of the dopaminomimetics, administered in small amounts, are penile erection, sexual fantasies and erotic dreams. There are no reports, either in the literature or from the few normal control samples, of sexual excitement resulting from these doses of dopaminomimetics. The sexual hyperreactivity caused by clinical doses of dopaminomimetics in these patients is further evidence of their anomalous reactivity to drugs which stimulate dopamine receptors. It also suggests a connection between the dopaminergic system and sexual arousal.

References

Akil, H. & Liebeskind, J.C. (1975): Monoaminergic mechanism of stimulation-produced analgesia. *Brain Res.* **94,** 279-296.

Anselmi, B., Baldi, E., Casacci, F. & Salmon, S. (1980): Endogenous opioids in cerebrospinal fluid and blood in idiopathic headache sufferers. *Headache* **20,** 294-299.

Bickerstaff, E.R. (1961): Basilar artery migraine. *Lancet* **1,** 15-17.

Boccuni, M., Fanciullacci, M., Michelacci, S. & Sicuteri, F. (1981): Impairment of postural reflex in migraine: the possible role of dopamine receptors. In *Apomorphine and other dopaminomimetics,* Vol. 2. Clinical pharmacology, eds G.U. Corsini & G.L. Gessa. New York: Raven Press. Pp 267-273.

Carlsson, A. (1979): Dopaminergic autoreceptors. In *Chemical tools in catecholamines research,* Vol. 11, eds O. Almigien, A. Carlsson & G. Engel. Amsterdam: Elsevier. Pp 219-225.

Collier, H.O.J. (1980): Cellular site of opiate dependence. *Nature* **283,** 625-629.

Corsini, G.U., Del Zompo, M., Tocco, F., Arca, P. & Gessa, G.L. (1980*a*): Drugs acting on dopamine receptors: the usefulness of a peripheral blocker in Parkinson's disease. *Pharmacol. Res. Commun.* **12,** 699-707.

Corsini, G.U., Piccardi, M.P., Bocchetta, A., Bernardi, F. & Del Zompo, M. (1980*b*): Behavioural effect of apomorphine in man: dopamine receptor implications. In *Apomorphine and other dopaminomimetics,* Vol. 2, Clinical Pharmacology, eds G.U. Corsini & G.L. Gessa. New York: Raven Press. Pp 13-24.

Costa, E., Cheney, D.L., Mao, C.C. & Moroni, F. (1978): Action of antischizophrenic drugs on the metabolism of gamma-aminobutyric acid and acetylcholine in globus pallidus striatum and accumbens. *Fed. Proc.* **37,** 2408.

Csontos, K., Rust, H., Hollt, V., Mahr, W., Kromer, W. & Teschemacher, H.J. (1979): Elevated plasma ß-endorphin levels in pregnant women and their neonates. *Life Sci.* **25,** 835-844.

Da Prada, M., Bonerri, E.P. & Keller, H.H. (1977): Induction of mounting behaviour in female rats by lisuride. *Neurosci. Letters* **6,** 349-353.

De la Baume, S., Patey, G., Marcais, H., Protais,. F., Costantin, J. & Schwarz, J. (1979): Changes

in dopamine receptors in mouse striatum following morphine treatment. *Life Sci.* **24,** 2333-2342.
Del Bene, E., Conti, C., Poggioni, M. & Sicuteri, F. (1982): Sexuality and headache. In *Advances in neurology,* Vol. 33, eds M. Critchley, A.P. Friedman, S. Gorini & F. Sicuteri. New York: Raven Press. Pp 209-214.
Fanciullacci, M. (1979): Iris adrenergic impairment in idiopathic headache. *Headache* **8,** 8-13.
Fanciullacci, M., Michelacci, S., Curradi, C. & Sicuteri, F. (1980): Hyperresponsiveness of migraine patients to the hypotensive action of bromocriptine. *Headache* **20,** 99-102.
Gessa, G.L. & Tagliamonte, A. (1974): Role of brain monoamines in male sexual behaviour. *Life Sci* **14,** 425-436.
Gessa, G.L. & Tagliamonte, A. (1975): Role of brain serotonin and dopamine in male sexual behaviour. In *Sexual behaviour pharmacology and biochemistry,* eds M. Sandler & G.L. Gessa. New York: Raven Press. Pp 117-128.
Gessa, G.L. & Paglietti, E. (1979): Induction of copulatory behaviour in sexually inactive rats by naloxone. *Science* **204,** 203-204.
Gintzler, A.R. (1980): Endorphin-mediated increases in pain threshold during pregnancy. *Science* **210,** 193-195.
Gopinathan, G., Teravainen, H., Dambrosia, J.M., Ward, C.D., Sanes, J.H., Stuart, W.K., Evarts, E.V. & Calne, D.B. (1981): Lisuride in Parkinsonism. *Neurology* **81,** 371-376.
Hamburger-Bar, R. & Rigter, H. (1975): Apomorphine: facilitation of sexual behaviour in female rats. *Eur. J. Pharmacol.* **32,** 357-360.
Komisaruk, B.R., Ciofalo, V. & Latranyi, M.B. (1976): Stimulation of the vaginal cervix is more effective than morphine in suppressing a nociceptive response in rats. *Advances in Pain Res. and Therapy* **1,** 439-443.
Krauthamer, G.M. & Albe-Fessard, D. (1964): Electrophysiologic studies of the basal glanglia and striopallidal inhibition of non-specific afferent activity. *Neuropsychologia* **2,** 73-83.
Lal, H. (1978): Narcotic dependence, narcotic action and dopamine receptors. *Life Sci.* **17,** 483-496.
Liuzzi, A., Chiodini, P.G., Oppizzi, G., Botalla, L., Verde, G., De Stefano, L., Colussi, G., Graf, K.L. & Horowski, R. (:1978): Lisuride hydrogen maleate: evidence for a long lasting dopaminergic activity in human. *J. Clin. Endocrinol. Metab.* **46,** 196-202.
McIntosh, T.K., Vallano, M.L. & Barfield, R.J. (1979): Effects of morphine ß-endorphins and naloxone on catecholamine levels and sexual behaviour in the male rat. *Pharmac. Bioch. and Behaviour* **18,** 435-4411.
McMillen, B.A. (1979): On the mechanism of morphine action on rat striatal dopaminic metabolism. *Bioch. Pharmac.* **29,** 1432-1435.
Mendelson, J., Ellingboe, J., Kenhule, J. & Mello, N. (1979): Effects of naltrexone on mood and neuroendocrine function in normal adult males. *Psychoneuroendocrinol.* **3,** 231-236.
Meyerson, B.J. (1968): Amphetamine and 5-hydroxytryptamine inhibition of copulatory behaviour in the female rat. *Ann. Med. Exp. Fenn.* **46,** 394-398.
Meyerson, B.J. & Lewander, T. (1970): Serotonin synthesis in inhibition of estrous behaviour in female rats. *Life Sci.* **9,** 661-671.
Meyerson, B.J. & Terenius, L. (1977): ß-Endorphins and male sexual behaviour. *Eur. J. Pharmacol.* **72,** 191-192.
Moroni, F., Peralta, E., Cheney, D.L. & Costa, E. (1979): On the regulation of gamma-aminobutyric acid neurons in caudatus, pallidus and nigro: effects of opioids and dopamine agonists. *J. Pharmac. Exp. Ther.* **208,** 190-194.
Parkes, J.D., Schacter, H., Marsden, C.D., Smith, B. & Wilson, A. (1981): Lisuride in Parkinsonism. *Ann. of Neurol.* **9,** 48-52.
Pellegrini-Quarantotti, B., Corda, M.G., Paglietti, E., Biggio, G. & Gessa, G.L. (1978): Inhibition of copulatory behaviour in male rats by D-ALA-Met-Enkephalinamide. *Life Sci.* **29,** 673-678.
Sakai, U., Nishijima, Y., Nicuni, N. & Iwata, N. (1981): Inhibitory mechanism of the hyper-irritability caused by picrotoxin in the rat. *Pain* **11,** 21-35.
Salis, P. & Dewsbury, D.A. (1971): P-Chlorophenylalanine facilitates copulatory behavior in male rats. *Nature* **232,** 400-401.
Sicuteri, F. (1974): Headache biochemistry and pharmacology. *Archs Neurobiol.* **37,** 27-65.

Sicuteri, F. (1977): Dopamine, the second putative protagonist in headache. *Headache* **17,** 129-131.

Sicuteri, F. (1979): Headache as the most common disease of the antinociceptive system: analogies with morphine abstinence. In *Advances in pain research and therapy,* Vol. 3, eds J.J. Bonica, J.D. Liebeskind & D.G. Albe-Fessard, New York: Raven Press. Pp 359-364.

Sicuteri, F. (1982): Natural opioids in migraine. In *Advances in neurology,* Vol. 33, eds M. Critchley, A.P. Friedman, S. Gorini & F. Sicuteri. New York: Raven Press. Pp 65-72.

Sicuteri, F., Anselmi, B. & Del Bianco, P.L. (1980*a*): Dopamine and 5-HT supersensitivity in non-organic central pain and in morphine abstinence; fortuitous or real analogy? In *Neural peptides and neural communications,* eds Costa, E. & Trabucchi, M. New York: Raven Press. Pp 523-533.

Sicuteri, F., Baldi, E., Branconi, F., Cappelli, G. & Salmon, S. (1980*b*): Hyperendorphinemia in pregnancy: its relevance to the disappearance of migraine. In *Psychopharmacology,* eds Brambilla, P., Rocagni, G. & De Wild, D. Elsevier/North Holland Biomedical Press. Pp 339-346.

Sicuteri, F., Boccuni, M., Fanciullacci, M., D'Egidio, P. & Bonciani, M. (1982): A new non-vascular interpretation of syncopal migraine. In *Advances in neurology,* Vol. 33, eds Critchley, M., Friedman, A.P., Gorini, S. & Sicuteri, F. New York: Raven Press. Pp 199-208.

Sicuteri, F., Del Bene, E. & Fonda, C. (1976): Sex, migraine and serotonin interrelationships. In *Clinical pharmacology of serotonin,* eds Sicuteri, F. & Schoubaum, E. *Monogr. Neurol. Sci.* **3,** 94-101.

Sicuteri, F., Del Bianco, P.L. & Anselmi, B. (1979): Morphine abstinence and serotonin supersensitivity in man: analogies with the mechanism of migraine. *Psychopharmacol.* **65,** 205-209.

Sicuteri, F., Fanciullacci, M. & Del Bene, E. (1977): Dopamine system and idiopathic headache. In *Headache: new vistas,* ed Sicuteri, F. Florence: Biomedical Press. Pp 239-250.

Sicuteri, F., Fanciullacci, M., Pietrini, U. & Cangi, F. (1984): Apomorphine-induced headache. In *Recent advances in pain research and therapy,* Vol. 7, eds Benedett, *et al.* New York: Raven Press.

Slater, P. & Blundell, C. (:1978): The effect of 6-hydroxydopamine on the antinociceptive action of morphine. *Eur. J. Pharmacol.* **48,** 237-247.

Szechtman, H., Simantov, R. & Hershkowitz, M. (1981): Sexual behaviour decreases pain sensitivity and stimulates endogenous opioids in male rats. *Eur. J. Pharmacol.* **70,** 279-285.

Tagliamonte, A., Fratta, W., Del Fiacco, M. & Gessa, G.L. (1974): Possible stimulatory role of brain dopamine in the copulatory behaviour of male rats. *Pharm Biochem. and Behaviour* **2,** 257-260.

Vanderwende, C. & Spoarlein, M.T. (1973): Role of dopaminergic receptors in morphine analgesia and tolerance. *Res. Comm. in Chem. Pathol. Pharmacol.* **5,** 35-43.

Van Loon, G.R. & Kim, C. (1978): ß-Endorphin-induced increase in striatal dopamine turnover. *Life Sci.* **23,** 961-970.

Zemlan, F.P., Ward, L.I. & Crowley, W.R. (1973): Activation of lordotic responding in female rats by suppression of serotoninergic activity. *Science* **179,** 1010-1011.

12

Psychopharmacology of sexual disorders of old age

V. A. KRAL

University of Western Ontario, London, Ontario, CANADA

Introduction

Although there cannot be any doubt that the age-linked decline in sexual functioning in man as in other mammals is biologically determined (Master & Johnstone, 1966), the sex problems encountered in psychogeriatric practice are largely due to neurotic anxiety or to psychotic conditions. It is for this reason that psychopharmacology is becoming an important tool in the treatment of the problem in the elderly.

Needless to say, it is always necessary to obtain, in addition to the patient's sexual history, a detailed medical history with particular emphasis on metabolic disorders in the patient and in his family. In addition, before one accepts the diagnosis of a neurotic or psychotic origin for the patient's sexual dysfunction, an accurate medical and neurological examination must be completed in order to rule out organic reasons.

Neurotic anxiety manifests itself in three forms: withdrawal from all sexual activity in spite of persistent sexual desire; phobic anxiety, in men of not being able to achieve or sustain an erection and in women of not being able to achieve orgasm and, thus, disappointing the partner; and, premature ejaculation.

Withdrawal from sexual activity

The complete withdrawal from sexual activity in spite of persistent sexual desire is frequently found in aging and aged people who believe that sex life at an older age is unhealthy or socially unacceptable or both. This belief forms part of Butler's ageism (Butler & Lewis, 1976). It is frequently enforced by the experience which the aging male has, namely that it takes longer to achieve erection and ejaculation and that the latter is perhaps not as copious as before. The patient sees in these normal age-linked phenomena an an indication of incipient disease and withdraws from all sexual activity.

In our experience, in order to alleviate anxiety, particularly when the partner is cooperative and tactful, it is usually sufficient to explain these phenomena as a normal part of the aging process. Small dosages of benzoadiazepines, such as chlordiazepoxide, oxazepam, lorazepam, are helpful in restoring normal sexual function in these patients.

Postmenopausal women who are widowed or divorced or have remained single throughout their lives also frequently show this neurotic tendency to complete withdrawal from sex life. Here too, supportive psychotherapy, with the aid of one of the benzodiazepines is useful if an appropriate relationship is established.

Phobic anxiety

Phobic anxiety of performance is clinically met in two different forms. The first is frequently found in men who have suffered a cardiac infarction or a cerebrovascular accident or only a transient iaschemic attack, who have recovered sufficiently that their physicians advise that sexual intercourse can be attempted. Many of these patients, at first, refuse any such attempt because they are afraid of suffering another heart attack or cerebrovascular accident. This fear is frequently shared and reinforced by the partner.

In time, the tendency to sexual withdrawal is replaced by phobic performance anxiety, that is, by the fear of not being able to produce an erection and, thus, disappointing the partner. At this stage, the partner usually becomes more encouraging, and supportive psychotherapy, again with the help of a benzodiazepine, is successful.

The second type of phobic performance anxiety seen in men is not related to preceding oprganic disease, aging or any hormonal imbalance. It is interesting, and diagnostically important, that patients with this primary phobic performance anxiety have normal sexual interest and desire, have normal morning erections, normal erections and ejaculations and maturbate. However, when faced with the actual situation the patient becomes panicky and is unable to produce an erection. When this neurotic condition lasts for some time, the patient learns to avoid the embarrassing situation completely and this leads to withdrawal from all sexual activity except masturbation.

This condition is psychodynamically determined, frequently dating back to early adolescence. Treatment is psychotherapy in its various forms, and beneficial results are being reported by therapists of various schools. Some use benzodiazepines or small doses of tricyclic antidepressants as adjuvants, but others consider any medication as unnecessary or even antiproductive (Kral, 1982).

Premature ejaculation

Premature ejaculation, in most cases, also dates back to early adolescence. The treatment is the same as in phobic anxiety of performance. In some cases, premature ejaculation indicates improvement from complete withdrawal from sexual activity as the result of phobic performance anxiety. Needless to say, such patients should continue to be treated until normal sex function is achieved. It should be remembered, though, that premature ejaculation improves spontaneously with increasing age because the ejaculation time of sexual response increases with age.

In treating these neurotic conditions it is frequently necessary also to treat the female partner who suffers sexual excitement without gratification. Many try to achieve it through masturbation, but a great number reject such a solution. Cooperation in the male partner's treatment, in joint or separate sessions, and the adjuvant of benzodiazepine use is also helpful.

In the treatment of the conditions so far discussed, psychopharmacology plays only an adjuvant role. This role becomes of greater, and even of decisive, importance in the treatment of sexual problems in aged patients who are mentally ill (Kral, 1980).

Patients with psychiatric disease

In endogenous depressions, sex drive is diminished and, frequently, is even completely absent in both sexes. Younger women may be amenorrheic, men impotent. In one of our case studies, the patient suffered two periods of impotence, each of three to four months duration, before he developed his first episode of a deep endogenous depression which was also accompanied by impotence. These monopolar depressions recurred at two year intervals until the patient was placed on lithium carbonate. He then became depression-free and his sexual function became and remained normal until his late sixties when he died of a rectal carcinoma.

Many psychiatrists have noted that sexual dysfunction as the result of endogenous depression does not improve on hormone treatment. Hormone therapy is practically useless in restoring sexual interest and potency. However, sexual function becomes normal when the depression subsides either spontaneously or through appropriate treatment. In endogenous depressions, tricyclic antidepressants, monoamine oxidase inhibitors or ECT with supportive psychotherapy are the treatments of choice, while in reactive depressions psychotherapy is the main treatment modality.

With tricyclic antidepressant therapy, we need to note that, in some cases, continuation of antidepressant medication as maintenance treatment can keep libido low even when the depression has subsided. This has been observed in several patients taking imipramine and amitriptyline but not in those taking monoamine oxidase inhibitors (Mitchell & Popkin, 1982).

While depressions reduce sex drive, the manic state, if it affects sexual function at all, increases sexual desire in both sexes, sometimes to such an extent that psychiatric intervention by psychopharmacological means becomes necessary. The following examples should be mentioned. A postmenopausal woman with a history of bipolar depressive illness surprised her husband with a gonorrheal infection. He immediately brought her to a psychiatrist and she was treated with chlorpromazine and later with lithium carbonate. The second case involved a man with a typical bipolar history. In previous manic episodes, he had shown overactivity in socially acceptable business activities. Now, at age sixty, he became sexually overactive, starting affairs with several women and bragging about it even to his wife who approached a lawyer for divorce proceedings. Treatment of the manic state and lithium maintenance solved the problem.

Schizophrenia poses difficult and serious sexual problems. The tendency to delusional loss of contact with reality, incoherent or bizarre thinking and inappropriate emotional reactions may lead, singly or in combination, to situations that require psychiatric intervention. It should suffice to recall the case of the (young) schizophrenic who felt he would gain the love of a young girl by shooting the President of the USA. Every psychiatrist has to treat paranoid patients with ideas of jealousy based on delusional interpretations of harmless events and reinforced by hallucinations. Neuroleptics, such as chlorpromazine or some other phenothiazines or haloperidol, are being effectively used in preventing tragic consequences.

An important factor is the fact that many schizophrenics (of various types) can now be discharged from hospital on adequate dosages of antipsychotic neuroleptics. These patients are frequently able to work and look after their personal needs, including their sexual needs both in and outside marriage. It is, however, not too rare to find that a patient who functions quite well on an adequate dose of chlorpromazine, trifluoperazine or haloperidol can suddenly decompensate when pregnancy and childbirth occur. Interestingly enough, it is not always the schizophrenic mother who suddenly decompensates. Not infrequently, it is the elderly schizophrenic father who does so. In two of our cases, these schizophrenic fathers had to be temporarily hospitalized, mainly in order to protect the child. Furthermore, some aged schizophrenic patients use unusual, sometimes rather sadistic, sexual approaches and are unable to understand the partner's reluctance to cooperate. In all such cases, the neuroleptics are of the greatest help.

Chronic dementing processes of various etiologies not infrequently pose serious problems that require psychiatric intervention and psychopharmacological treatment. A word of caution, however, should be made in this respect. It is necessary to differentiate between aged people in full possession of their mental capacities and those who are suffering from one of the dementing processes of the elderly, such as Alzheimer's dementia or multi-infarct dementia. While old men are frequently accused of sexual assualts of female children or inappropriate sexual approaches to women, closer investigation reveals that these accusations have their origin mostly in sexual taboos of agism of nurses, old folks' homes administrators or even law enforcing agents. In our many years of experienmce, not a single allegation of a mentally well preserved elderly man could be proven. On the other hand, some cases of sexual misbehaviour which could be proved were perpetrated by old men suffering from a dementing process. The charges were dropped and the patients referred for psychiatric treatment, including neuropleptic therapy. Attempts at sexual assault by demented patients already hospitalized are easily managed by neuroleptic treatment. Thioridazine, as a regular medication in a moderate dosage of 25-50 mg tid to qid, has a calming effect generally and also upon the sex drive.

Occasionally, fortunately only rarely, a psychiatrist may be called upon to look after a person apprehended just after a sexual crime. This task is independent of the psychiatric expert testimony which, in many cases, is required during the trial in court. In our experience there are two main ways in which an apprehended sex offender may react. The more frequent one is wild aggressive excitement which leads to attacks on others including the apprehending police officers. The other is depressive stupor which may lead to attempts at suicide.

The treatment of the first type of reaction consists of immediate administration of a neuroleptic, while the second type requires supervision and, if necessary, a relatively fast-acting antidepressant. In our experience, the first type was represented by a homosexual sociopath who, in a jealous rage, attempted to kill his boyfriend. When apprehended by the police he became highly excited, started yelling and shouting and attacked the police officer with a knife; 100 mg of chlorpromazine, with a repeat dose of 50 mg after three hours, calmed the patient. He later stood trial.

The second type of case was represented by a woman who as a child had suffered an Economo encephalitis. As is well known, such patients develop, when growing up, a personality disorder of the sociopathic type. This particular patient behaved usually normally except during the premenstruum, when she developed a strong sexual desire. Then she approached various people, both men and women. On one occasion, she approached a girl of nine who tried to fight her; the patient strangled her and the child died. The patient immediately became depressed and stuporous and had to be admitted to hospital.

Summary

A great proportion of sexual problems of the elderly have a psychogenic origin which responds to psychotherapy. Minor tranquilizers or small doses of antidepressants have been found useful as adjuvants. When functional psychosis interferes with sexual functioning of the aged, neuroleptics, antidepressants and lithium carbonate have been found helpful in treating the sexual dysfunction accompanying the psychosis. Sexual disorders found in the course of dementing processes are responsive to psychopharmacological treatment, although the underlying brain process remains unaffected.

References

Butler, R.N. & Lewis, M.N. (1976): *Sex after sixty.* New York: Harper & Row.

Kral, V.A. (1980): Psychopharmacology of sexual disorders in the aged. *Med. Probl. Pharmacopsych.* **15,** 174-181.

Kral, V.A. (1982): Sexual problems in old age. In *Handbook of studies on psychiatry and old age*, eds Kay, D.W.K. & Burrows, G.D. Amsterdam: Elsevier.

Master, W.H. & Johnson, V.E. (1966): Human sexual response. Boston: Little Brown & Co.

Mitchell, J.E. & Popkin, M.K. (1982): Antipsychotic drug therapy and sexual dysfuntion in men. *Am. J. Psychiat.* **139,** 633-637.

13

Prolactin and sexuality

B. Norman BARWIN

Fertility Centre, University of Ottawa, Ottawa General Hospital, CANADA

Introduction

Sexual dysfunction in the male and female may be endocrinological as well as iatrogenic, neurological, psychiatric or metabolic in origin (Kupperman, 1982). Of all these factors, although the least attention has been paid to endocrine factors, these can be the most easily diagnosed and managed, and the results after appropriate therapy can be most rewarding (Vezina & Sutton, 1974; Bartke, 1978; Tollis & Franks, 1979; Kinch, 1980).

At certain stages of a person's life, sexual dysfunction and desire diminishes, especially, for example, at the climacterium and post partum in the female (Freisen, 1978). At certain stages in a man's life, testicular function may diminish, and this is associated with a decrease in testicular hormonal levels (Bartke, 1978). Vasomotor symptoms, similar to but generally not as severe as those seen in the female at menopause, can also result (Freisen, 1978). Despite these points, patients are often told that the problem is psychological and that psychiatric management is indicated without adequate endocrine assessment (Thorner, 1977; Freisen, 1978; Tolis & Franks, 1979).

Excessive release of prolactin (PRL), hyperprolactinemia, may be due to chronic exposure to tranquilisers, opiates, estrogens and adenomas of the pituitary or, on the other hand, may lack an obvious etiology (Tolis & Frank, 1979; Kinch, 1980; Kupperman, 1982). In women, hyperprolactinemia may be associated with amenorrhea, infertility, anovulation, galactorrhea and sexual dysfunction (Kinch, 1980) (Fig. 1).

Several recent reports indicate that raised prolactin levels may interefere with sexual function in men (Bartke, 1978; Kupperman, 1982). Impotence may be the most common presenting symptom although various degrees of hypogonadism have also been described (Vezina & Sutton, 1974; Tolis & Franks, 1979).

Pathophysiology

The mechanism by which excessive prolactin release intereferes with libido in the male and in the female is not undestood (Reichlin, 1979; Kupperman, 1982). The ability of prolactin to act on dopaminergic neurons in several regions of the brain may be one explanation of the impotence. Such an action would lead to the impairment of gonadotropin release and result in diminished testosterone production in the male with consequent infertility and diminished sexual function (MacLeod, 1976; Sherman *et al.*,

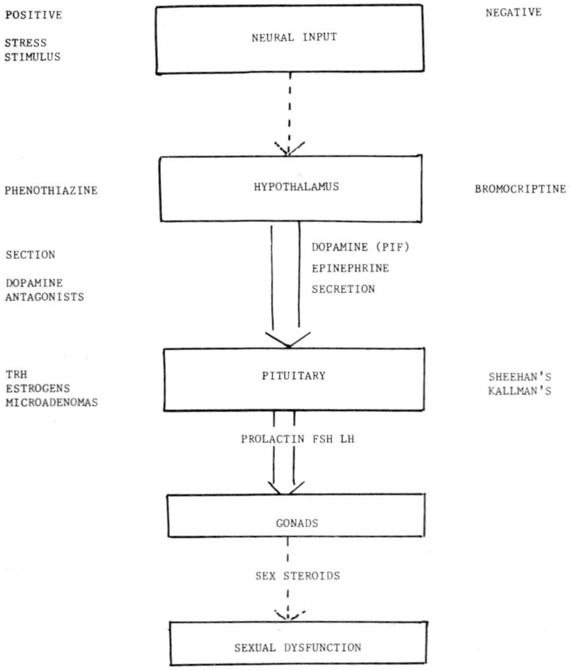

Fig. 1. *Factors controlling prolactin release.*

1978; Labrie *et al.*, in press). In the female, the decreased gonadotropin levels may result in anovulation and reduced estrogen levels with loss of libido (Freisen, 1978; Kupperman, 1982) (Fig. 2).

The fact that gonadotrophin levels are not elevated in the hyperprolactinemic hypogonadal male provides evidence for altered hypothalamic dysfunction (Labrie *et al.*, in press). The adrenal gland activity in hyperprolactinemic males (MacLeod, 1969, 1976; Lamberts & MacLeod, 1978) may also be responsible for the hypergonadism and impotence in this group of patients (Bartke, 1978).

In animal models (rat and mouse), the action of prolactin on the hypothalamic-pituitary testicular/ovarian axis and sexual behaviour indicates that reduced hyperprolactinemia may result in sexual dysfunction. The transplantation of prolactin producing tumors in adult male rats produces testicular atrophy with subsequent suppression of testicular production, raised gonadotropin levels and adrenal enlargement (Calabro & MacLeod, 1978; Caron, 1978).

Pituitary glands transplanted under the renal capsule cause persistent hyperprolactinemia and LH-RH suppression (Bartke, 1978; Calabro & MacLeod, 1978; Kupperman, 1982). Although plasma testosterone and testicular weight are not affected (MacLeod & Fontham, 1970; MacLeod, 1976; Bartke, 1978; Kupperman, 1982), basal gonadotrophin levels are also suppressed with an increase in adrenal weight (MacLeod & Fontham, 1970). Marked reduction of copulatory behaviour has been demonstrated in male rats and mice rendered hyperprolactinemic by multiple pituitary grafts. It is of interest that physiological amounts of prolactin normally stimulate gonadal activity in men (Bartke, 1978) and experimental animals (Bartke, 1978; Kupperman, 1982). Pathological elevation of prolactin, however, may suppress sexual function and delay puberty.

Hyperprolactinemia has also been demonstrated in patients suffering from stress and from infertility of psychosomatic origin (Argostini *et al.*, 1978). The secretion of prolactin is regulated by the secondary tonic inhibition of a hypothalamic hormone known as prolactin inhibiting factor (PIF) (Tolis & Franks, 1979). (Fig. 2). PIF is controlled by dopaminergic neurons in the vertro-medial nucleus and median eminence (MacLeod, 1969; MacLeod & Fontham, 1970).

Loss of libido and sexual function in the male and female may also be secondary to emotional stress (Agostini *et al.,* 1978; Kinch, 1980). The high levels of prolactin in males may also be a function of the constant low levels of testosterone caused by emotional stress (Agostini *et al.,* 1978).

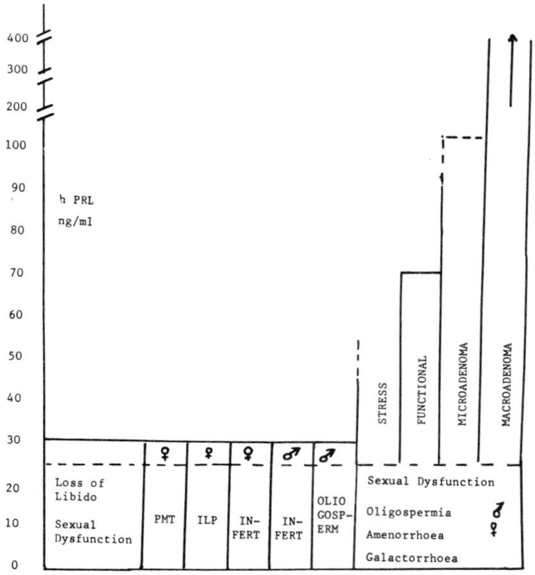

Fig. 2. *Clinical spectrum of hyperprolactinemia.* PMT —premenstrual tension; ILP — inadequate luteal phase; INFERT — infertility; OLIGOSPERM —oligospermia. Modified from Kinch (1980).

Diagnosis

There can be many causes of hyperprolactinemia. These include pituitary adenoma, hypothyroidism, psychotropic drugs and hypothalamic dysfunction (Thorner, 1977; Tolis & Franks, 1979). Organic causes of sexual dysfunction and loss of libido may be associated with generalized illness (chronic renal failure), metabolic disorders (diabetes mellitus), genetic disease preventing the production of gonadal steroids (Turner's syndrome), or because of lack of priming by pituitary luteinizing hormone (LH) through a genetic defect in the elaboration of LH (Kallman's syndrome); other causes may include destruction of the pituitary by an infarct (postpartum Sheehan's syndrome), hemochromotosis, leukemia, craniopharyngioma, non-secreting adenomas are the most frequent and the most easily reversible causes of centrally mediated sexual dysfunction (Kupperman, 1982).

Prolaction levels are higher in females than in males, fluctuating from levels of approximately 12 ng/ml, rising to 14 ng/ml in the evening and doubling during the night (Lamberts & MacLeod, 1978). The normal upper level of prolactin is usually 30 ng/ml. Obtaining an accurate 'normal' prolactin measurement requires taking 3 or 4 samples by an indwelling venous catheter during a 1 h period (Freisen, 1978; Kinch, 1980).

The dignosis of a prolactin secreting adenoma should be suspected on the basis of elevated serum prolactin that demonstrates resistance to stimulatory tests (ie sleep), thyrotrophin releasing hormone (TRH) or chlorpromazine administration (Fig. 3).

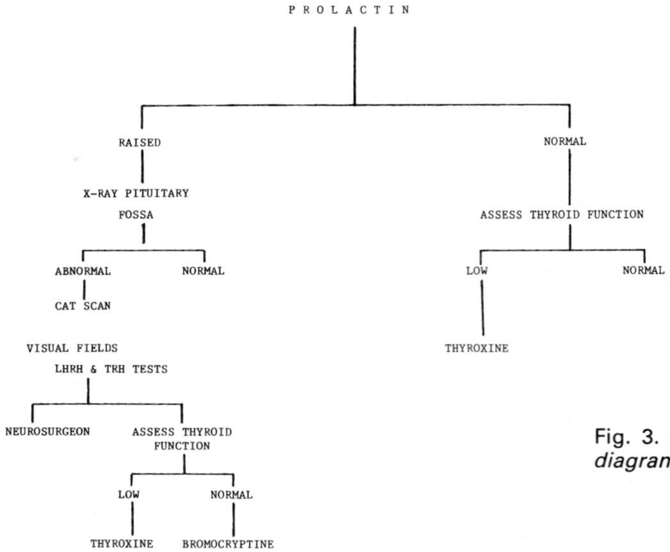

Fig. 3. *Prolactin and sexuality — flow diagram of investigation.*

Small tumors (<10 mm) may be identified by high resolution computed tomography (Thorner, 1977; Cowden, 1979; del Pozo *et al.*, 1979; Tolis & Franks, 1979). In the presence of micro-adenomas, the function of the posterior and anterior parts of the pituitary remains intact except for disturbed gonadoptrophin secretion. Visual fields may help diagnose the presence of a micro-adenoma (Tolis & Franks, 1979). The episodic LH surges which occur every 90–120 minutes during a 24-h cycle may be lost in patients with prolactinomas resulting in reduced Leydig cell function and reduced testosterone levels (but within normal levels). Treatment of raised prolactin levels with bromocriptine will also raise testosterone levels but they still remain within the normal range (Cowden *et al.*, 1979). Normal testosterone levels cannot be used to exclude other endocrine causes for impotence. Small prolactinomas in the male and female will demonstrate prompt release of LH with the administration of LHRH (Cowden *et al.*, 1979; Mehta & Tolis, 1979). This test (with few exceptions) may predict the response of sex steroids secretion to bromocriptine; if no LH is released after LHRH administration, there may be irreversible damage to the pituitary gonadotropes (Reichlin, 1979; Tolis & Frabks, 1979). In such cases, the administration of LH on testosterone/estrogen may result in normal levels of these sex steroids. Libido in a patient with hyperprolactinemia may not improve with the administration of testosterone or estrogen alone (Kupperman, 1982). Elevated prolactin may interfere with androgen metabolism and/ or action upon the sex hormone sensitive structures of the brain ('libido genic area') (Mehta & Tolis, 1979). The demonstration in animals and man of the conversion of testosterone to dihydrotestosterone in hyperprolactinemia is consistent with this hypothesis (Labrie *et al.*, in press).

Hypothyroidism may be seen in patients with hyperprolactinemia (Labrie *et al.*, in press). The increased production of TSH overlaps with the overproduction of other anterior pituitary hormones including prolactin and may result in galactorrhea and decreased sexual function (Kinch, 1980; Kupperman, 1982). Assessment of thyroid function, especially TSH, is essential in cases of raised prolactin levels (Kupperman, 1982). Thyroid supplementation in the case of hypothyroidism will usually result in normal prolactin levels and correct the associated symptoms of hyperprolactinemia.

Treatment

Surgery should be reserved for those patients in whom there is marked enlargement and erosion of the sella turcica as a result of an enlarged or enlarging tumor secreting excessive amounts of prolactin, and where there is encroachment of the visual fields.

If the visual fields are not adversely affected and there is a microadenoma or enlargement of the pituitary gland as demonstrated in the CT scan (Nillius *et al.*, 1978; Sherman *et al.*, 1978; Mehta & Tolis, 1979), bromocriptine is the treatment of choice provided the patient is carefully monitored (CT scan and serum prolactin) every 6–12 months (Parkes, 1977; Nillius *et al.*, 1978; Sherman *et al.*, 1978; Mehta & Tolis, 1979).

Bromocriptine is a semi-synthetic bromate of the ergot alkaloid (2-Bromo-2-ergocriptine) mesilate (Parkes, 1977; del Pozo *et al.*, 1979). Bromocriptine is a dopamine-agonist and in therapeutic dosage produces rapid and prolonged inhibition of prolactin secretion (del Pozo *et al.*, 1979; Kinch, 1980). It has two sites of action (del Pozo *et al.*, 1979). At the level of the central nervous system, the biochemical changes as well as the behavioral effects strongly indicate a dopamine receptor stimulating action, while, at the level of lactroph, there is evidence of dopamine receptors on the cell membrane and bromocriptine, acting as a dopamine receptor agonist thereby stimulated dopaminergic mechanisms (Calabro, 1978; Caron *et al.*, 1978; Cowden *et al.*, 1979; del Pozo *et al.*, 1979). Anterior pituitary function is modified by hypophysiotropic neurosecretion except in the case of dopamine which exerts direct effects on the pituitary that are inhibitory to prolactin and to the release of thyroid-stimulating hormone (TSH) (Labrie *et al.*, in press).

Dopamine is at present the major prolactin inhibitor: dopamine agonists decrease prolactin levels while dopamine agonists enhance them (Caron *et al.*, 1978; del Pozo *et al.*, 1979).

The suggested dosage of bromocriptine is 1.25 mg daily, increasing to 2.5 mg one to three times a day with meals. This may be reduced once normal prolactin levels are achieved in order to allow adequate gonadal function (Kupperman, 1982). Bromocriptine therapy should be reserved only for patients with hyperprolactinemia. Treatment of patients with normal prolactin levels may result in no reversal of their sexual dysfunction due to a psychological origin (Kupperman, 1982). The sexual improvement in patients treated with bromocriptine, because of significant increases in prolactin levels, is clearcut (Kupperman, 1982). When the prolactin levels are brought to normal, an increase in potency and normal sexual activity invariably occurs with a return to a normal sperm count (Agostini *et al.*, 1978; Kupperman, 1982).

If the gonadotropin and testosterone levels remain low despite normal prolactin levels, human chorionic gonatrophin (HCG) 5000 IU IM and 300 mg of testosterone cypionate intramuscularly at two week intervals may be indicated, particularly if sexual dysfunction persists in the male (Kupperman, 1982). HCG stimulates the Leydig cells acting synergistically with the exogenous testosterone in poreventing testicular atrophy (Labrie *et al.*, in press). The endogenous increase in testosterone due to the administration of HCG becomes additive with respect to normal sexual function.

Conclusion

A causal relationship between sexual dysfunction and hyperprolactinemia is strongly suggested (Bartke, 1978; Tolis & Franks, 1979). However, hyperprolactinemia and sexual dysfunction may represent unrelated symptoms of hypothalamic-pituitary disease in adenohypophyseal tumors (Bartke, 1978). Bromocriptine could improve potency by a direct action on central and peripheral dopaminergic neurons involved in the control of the erectile response in men (Thorner, 1977). Conclusive evidence, however, still remains to be demonstrated that the restoration of libido by bromocriptine is due solely to the suppression of prolactin (Bartke, 1978).

A multi-disciplinary approach to the problem of sexual dysfunction is needed in order to clarify the pathophysiological mechanisms and rationale for the various therapeutic approaches.

References

Agostini, R., Patella, Primiero & Castagnino, F. (1978): *The endocrine profile in male sterility due to stress in emotions and reproduction.* eds Carenza, L. & Zichella, L. New York: Academic Press.

Bartke, A. (1978): Hyperprolactinemia and impotence. *Andrology* **1,** 2.

Calabro, M.A. & MacLeod, R.M. (1978): Binding of dopamine to bovine anterior pituitary gland membrane. *Neuroendocrinology* **25,** 32-46.

Caron, M.C., Beaulieu, M., Raymond, V., Gagne, B., Drouin, J., Lefkowitz, R.J. & Labrie, F. (1978): Dopaminergic receptors in the anterior pituitary gland. *J. Biol. Chem.* **253,** 2244-2253.

Cowden, E.A., Thomson, J.A., Doyler, D., Ratcliffe, J.G., MacPherson, P. & Teasdale, G.M. (1979): Tests of prolactin secretion in diagnosis of prolactinomas. *Lancet* **1,** 1155.

Del Pozo, E. & Fluckiger, E. (1979): Pharmacological aspects of the prolactin inhibitor bromocriptine. In *Clinical neuroendocrinology: a pathophysiological approach,* eds Tolis, G., Labrie, F., Martin, J.B. & Naftolin, F. New York: Raven Press. Pp 429.

Friesen, H.G. (1978): Human prolactin. *Ann. R. Coll. Phys. Surg.* Canada **11,** 275-281.

Kinch, R.A. (1980): The use of bromocriptine in obstetrics and gynecology *Fertil. and Steril.* **33,** 43.

Kupperman, H.S. (1982): The role of prolactin in impotence. *Med. Aspects Hum. Sex.* **16,** 9.

Labrie, F., Ferland, L., Dipaolo, T. & Veilleux, R. (In press): Modulation of prolactin secretion by sex steroids and thyroid hormones. In *Central and peripheral regulation of prolactin function,* eds MacLeod, R.M. & Scapagnini, A. New York: Raven Press.

Lamberts, S.W.J. & MacLeod, R.M. (1978): The biphasic regulation of prolactin secretion by dopamine agonist-antagonists. *Endocrinology* **103,** 287-295.

MacLeod, R.M. (1976);: Influence of norepinephrine and catecholamine-depleting agents in the synthesis and release of prolactin and growth hormone. *Endocrinology* **85,** 916-923.

MacLeod, R.M. (1976): Regulation of prolactin secretion. In *Frontiers in neuroendocrinology,* Vol. 4. eds Martini, J.C., & Ganong, W.F. New York: Raven Press.

MacLeod, R.M. & Fontham, F.M. (1970): Influence of ionic environment on the *in vitro* synthesis and release of pituitary hormones. *Endocrinology* **86,** 863-869.

Mehta, A.E. & Tolis, G. (1979): Pharmacology of bromocriptine in health and disease. *Drugs* **17,** 313.

Nillius, S.J., Bergh, T., Lundberg, P.O., Stahle, J. & Wide, L. (1978): Regression of a prolactin-secreting pituitary tumor during long-term treatment with bromocriptine. *Fertil. and Steril.* **30,** 710.

Parkes, D. (1977): Bromocriptine. *Adv. Drug Res.* **12,** 247.

Reichlin, S. (1979): Overview of the anatomical and physiologic basis of anterior pituitary regulation. In *Clinical neuroendocrinology: a pathophysiological approach,* eds Tolis, G., Labrie, F., Martin, J.B. & Naftolin, F. New York: Raven Press. P 1.

Sherman, B.M., Harris, C.E., Schlechte, J., Duello, T., Halmi, N.S., CanGlider, J., Chapler, F.K. & Granner, D.K. (1975): Pathogenesis of prolactin-secreting pituitary adenomas. *Lancet* **2,** 1019.

Thorner, M.O. (1977): Prolactin: clinical physiology and the significance and management of hyperprolactinemia. In *Clinical neuroendocrinology,* eds Martini, J.C. & Besser, G.M. New York: Academic Press. Pp 319-361.

Tolis, G. & Franks, S. (1979): Physiology and pathology of prolactin secretion. In *Clinical neuroendocrinology: a pathophysiological approach,* eds Tolis, G., Labrie, F., Martin, J.B. & Naftolin, F. New York: Raven Press. Pp 291.

Vezina, J.L. & Sutton, T. (1974): Prolactin-secreting pituitary microadenomas. *Am. J. Roentgenol.* **120,** 46.

Author Index

Ahlenius, S., 15
Ban, T. A., 115
Barwin, B. N., 161
Benkert, O., 133
Bowden, N. J., 63
de Jonge, F. H., 63
Del Bene, E., 145
Dikstein, S., 5
Fanciullacci, M., 145
Guy, W., 115
Holsboer, F., 133
Hunter, A. J., 33
Kral, V. A., 155
Larsson, K., 15
Lehmann, H. E., 1
Murphy, M. R., 51
Petrie, W. M., 121
Poggioni, M., 145
Principe, L., 145
Rees, J. M. H., 99
Renshaw, D. C., 79
Schnieden, H., 99
Segal, M., 5
Sicuteri, F., 145
Swanson, H. H., 63
van de Poll, N. E., 63
van Oyen, H. G., 63
Wilson, C. A., 33
Wilson, W. H., 115

Subject index

Affective disorders, drugs for sexual dysfunction in, 3
Aggression, 1, 63
experimental factors in, 63
Aggressive behavior, 70
Agonistic behavior, 1
Alcohol, 79, 80, 99, 107-109
and marital problems, 80
Amenorrhea, 100, 161
Amines, brain, 2
Aminotetralins, 15, 24
effects of, 19
Amitriptyline, 6, 7, 94
Amphetamine, 17, 21, 81, 99, 106-107, 121
Amygdaloid nuclei, 2
Amyl nitrate, 3, 81
Antianxiety drugs, 79, 93-94
non-specific, 99
— see also Anxiolytic drugs
Antidepressants, 3, 79, 94, 117, 121, 155
and ejaculation disorders, 126
and human sexual response, 6
and initial reversal of decreased libido, 6
and sexual behavior, 121-129
and sexual behavior in the rat, 3
classes of, 5
clinical effectiveness of, 5
effectiveness and mechanisms, 5
for sexual problems in the elderly, 3
non-specific 99
Antihistamines, 79, 89
Antihypertensive drugs, 90
and sexual function, 3
Antipsychotic drugs, 3, 93
and sexual behavior, 121-129
and sexual dysfunction, 118
peripheral effects of, 123-124
— see also Neuroleptic drugs
Anxiolytics, 109
— see also under Antianxiety drugs
Aphrodisiacs, 79, 83
Aphrodite, 79
Apomorphine, 2, 17, 21, 151
Aspermia, 100, 118, 121, 124

Barbiturates, 99, 109
Behavior, and central serotenergic systems, 33
agonistic, 64
Benserazide, 16
Benzodiazepines, 109, 155, 156
Brain mechanisms, 51
subcortical, 1
Brain monoamines, 15
Bromocriptine, 2, 20, 57, 79, 151, 161, 164-165
Butoxamine, 7

Catatonia, 119
Catecholamines, 1, 8, 35
Cerebrovascular accident, 156
Chemotherapy, 79
Chlorpromazine, 163
Cimetidine, 90
Clomiphene citrate, 84
Clonidine, 7
Clogyline, 5, 6, 8
Cocaine, 3, 79, 81, 99, 106-107, 121, 128
Cyproterone acetate, 87
Contraceptives, 79

Danazol, 84
Dementia, and pharmacotherapy, 3
Dementing processes, 155, 158
Deprenyl, 5, 8
Depression, 121
and circadian rhythms, 5
and sexual behavior, 125
sleep deprivation therapy in, 5
Diabetes, 163
Diagnostic and Statistical Manual (DSM) III 3
Dihydrotestosterone, 63, 65
Diuretics, 79, 90
Dopamine, 115
antagonists, 161
pathway, 2
receptors, 145
Dopaminergic nerons, 3
Drugs, 51
and sexual functioning, 3
and sexuality, 15
and sexual side-effects, 3, 79, 85, 94
assessment of, 121
illicit, 51
non-prescribed, 79-82
prescribed, 3, 79, 85, 94
pharmacodynamics and sexual side-effects of 86
— see also individual drugs (eg Naloxone, Nomefensine etc) and groups of drugs (eg Benzodiazepines, Diuretics etc)
— see also under Sexual dysfunction

Ejaculation,
delayed, 51, 59
disorders of, 121

premature, 59
use of opiates in, 51
— see also Premature ejaculation
Endorphins, 51, 145
in sexual behavior, 2
Erectile response, problems of, 2
Ergot drugs, 15
effects of, 19
Eros, 2
Estradiol benzoate, 67
Estrogen, 63
Ethanol, 99

Female sexual behavior
— see Sexual behavior, female
Fertility drugs, 79, 83
Freud, 2, 115

Galactorrhea, 161
Gonadotrophins, 133, 161

Hallucinogens, 99, 106
Haloperidol, 17, 25
Hamsters, Syrian golden, 51-53, 58
Headache, 145
Hebephrenia, 119
Helen of Troy, 1, 2
Histamine, 115
Hormones, 51, 79, 161
gonadal, 2, 27
influences on aggression in rats, 63
— see also individual hormones, eg Testosterone
Hyperprolactinemia, 161
and sexual dysfunction, 2
etiology, 163
Hypnotic drugs, 79, 88
Hypotensives, 79
Hypothalamic dysfunction 161
Hypothalamus, 2, 161
Hypothyroidism, 161, 163, 164
Hydralazine, 92
5-Hydroxytryptophan (5-HTP), 17

Imipramine, 5, 6
Impotence, 59, 121, 125-126, 161
and opium, 51
Infarction, 15
Infertility, 51, 161, 162
Insomnia, 79

Kallman's syndrome, 163

L-Dopa, 16, 17, 18, 146, 149
Libido, 51, 59, 161, 163, 164
loss of, 2

Lisuride, 15, 20, 21, 145, 151
Lithium, 3, 79, 93
Love potions, 79
Luteal phase, inadequate, 161
Luteinizing hormone, 57, 117
Luteinizing hormone releasing hormone (LHRH), 58, 133, 138, 161
Lysergic acid diethylamide (LSD), 3, 99, 106, 127

Marijuana, 3, 79, 80, 99, 101-103
Masculine sexual behavior
— see Sexual behavior, male
Maturity-gap, 1
Medications,
non-prescribed, 79
prescribed, 79
— see also Drugs, prescribed & non-prescribed
Metergoline, 25
Methadone, 52, 53, 55
Methaneline, 92
Methaqualone, 89
Methiothepin, 25
Methyldopa, 91
Methylphenidate, 81
Metropolol, 92
Mianserin, 5, 6, 7
Migraine, 2, 145
Mounting behavior, 5

Naloxone, 51
Naltrexone, 51, 53, 55, 150
Neuroleptic drugs, 3, 115, 117, 121, 123, 155, 157
— see also Antipsychotic drugs
Neurotransmitters, 1, 15
Nialamide, 16
Nicotine, 18, 99, 106
Nociception, 146
Nomifensine, 5, 6, 7
Noradrenaline pathway, 2

Old age, 155
Oligospermia, 100, 161
Onanism, 115
Opiate antagonists, 51
in the treatment of sexual dysfunction, 2
Opiates, 3, 51, 99, 103-104
endogenous, 51
effect of copulation on, 55
role in sexual behavior, 51
Oral contraceptives, 87

Parkinson's disease, 150
P-Chlorophenylalanine (PCPA), 2, 5, 17, 33
  and sexual behavior, 7
  and sexual behavior in the rat, 7
  and steroid metabolism, 36
  effect on adrenal, 36
  effects on female sexual behavior, 34
  effects on male sexual behavior, 33
  method of action of, 7
  pharmacological action of, 35
Pergolide, 15, 20
Phenylethylamine (PEA), 3, 5
  receptor 3
Pituitary, 161
  adenoma, 161, 163
Pituitary-gonadal axis, 3
Placebos, 79, 82
Polypeptides, 1
Porgyline, 16
Prednisone, 84
Premature ejaculation, 79, 116, 155, 156
  — see also Ejaculation, premature
Premenstrual tension, 161
Priapism, 124
Progesterone, 40
  and female sexual behavior, 44
Prolactin, 100, 117, 123, 133, 139, 161, 164, 165
  and sexuality, 161-166
  inhibiting factor (PIF), 163
  secretion, 99
Propranolol, 7, 91
Psychomotor stimulants, 121, 127
Psychosis, 155
Psychotherapy, in the elderly, 3
Psychotic disorders, 3
Psychotropic drugs, 93, 99, 161

Rats,
  and aggression, 2
  male, mounting behavior in, 3
  Sprague-Dawley, 18, 66
  S3-Tyron Maze-Dull, 66, 71
  WEzob, 71
  Wistar, 18, 66, 71

Schizophrenia, 115-119, 121, 123, 124, 155, 157
  and sexual behavior, 115-119
  anhedonia in, 116
  gonadotrophin secretion in, 116
Serotonin, 33
  in the control of female sexual behavior, 2
Sex steroids, 161
Sexual behavior, 63, 115, 145
  animal, 51
  compounds for induction of, 6
  female, 33
  in the rat, 65
    methodology for assessment of, 9-12
  in the female rat, 15
  male, 51
    and brain monoamines, 15
  neural mechanisms in, 28
  sex differences in, 63
Sex hormones, 115
  — see individual hormones (eg Estrogen) and Hormones, gonadal
Sexual arousal, 2
Sexual disorders, 3
  diagnosis of in old age, 155-158
Sexual dysfunction, 121, 155, 161
  and drugs of abuse, 99-110
  classification of, 133-141
  endocrine functions in, 161, 164, 165
  endocrine investigations in, 134-139
  etiology of, 161, 163
  role of hormones in the treatment of, 3
Sexual function, 1
  and emotional stress, 163
Sheehan's syndrome, 163
Social behavior, 63
Stein-Leventhal syndrome, 85
Sympathomimetics, 99, 107

Testosterone, 1, 33, 34, 57, 63, 64, 67, 117, 133, 134-138, 161, 164
Testosterone propionate (TP), 67
Thyroid hormone, 87
Tranquillizers, for sexual problems in the elderly, 3
Turner's syndrome, 163

Vitamins, 99